T0182074

Translating National Policy to Improve Environmental Conditions Impacting Public Health Through Community Planning

Beth Ann Fiedler
Editor

Translating National Policy to Improve Environmental Conditions Impacting Public Health Through Community Planning

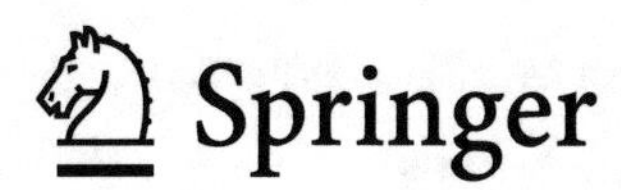

Editor
Beth Ann Fiedler
Independent Research Analyst
Jacksonville, FL, USA

ISBN 978-3-030-09212-2 ISBN 978-3-319-75361-4 (eBook)
https://doi.org/10.1007/978-3-319-75361-4

Softcover re-print of the Hardcover 1st edition 2018

Printed on acid-free paper

This Springer imprint is published by the registered company Springer International Publishing AG part of Springer Nature.
The registered company address is: Gewerbestrasse 11, 6330 Cham, Switzerland

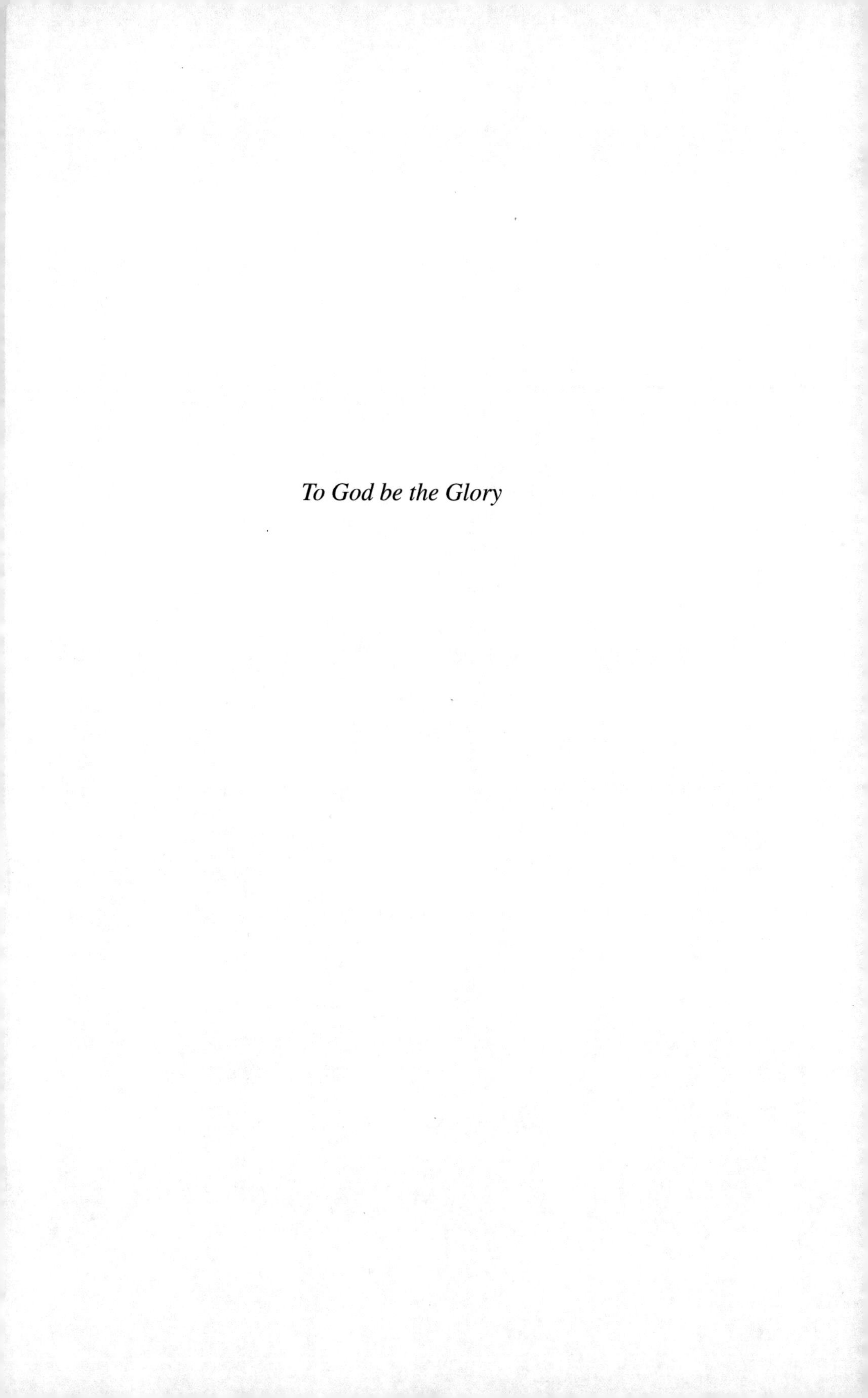

To God be the Glory

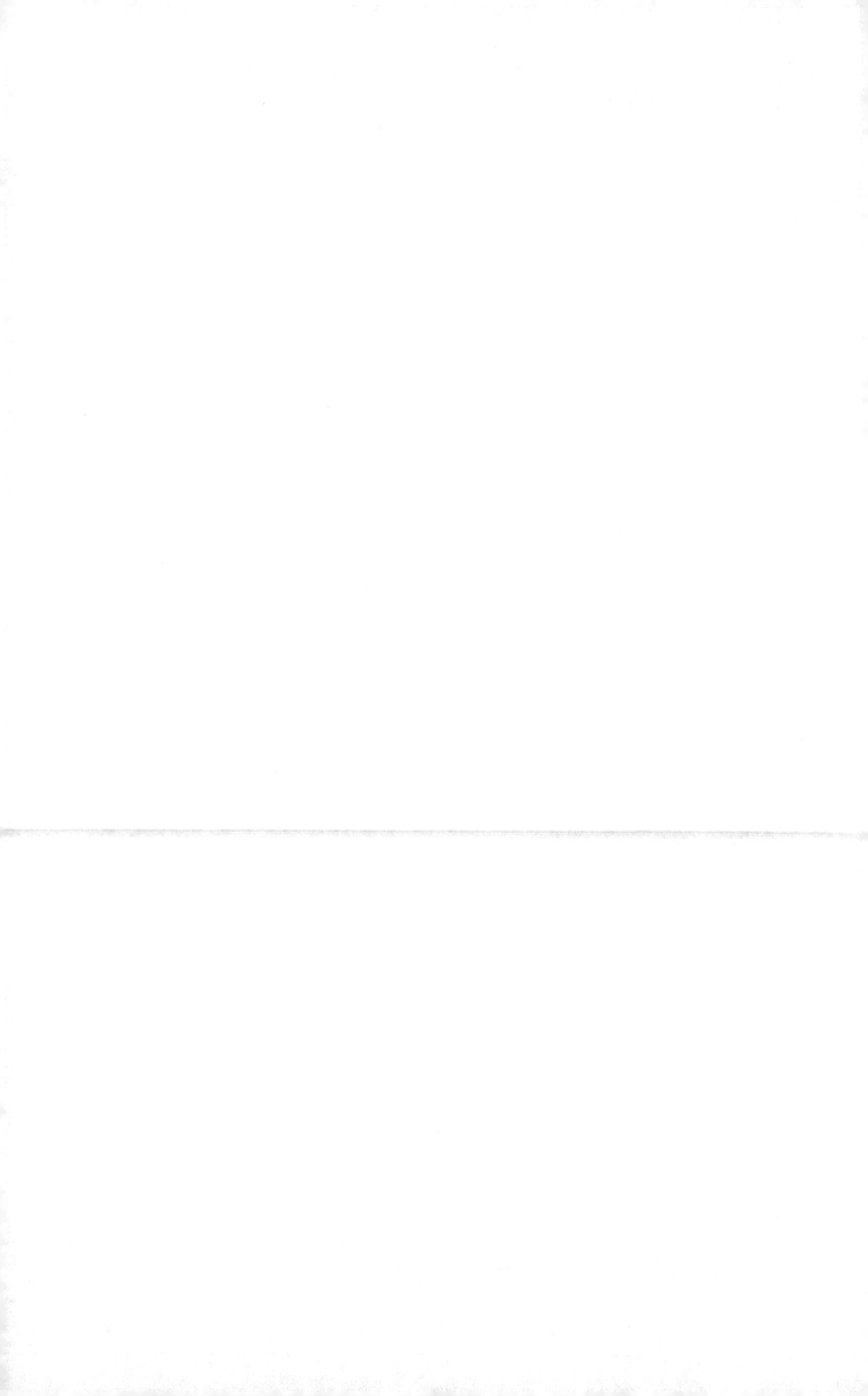

Preface

Translating National Policy to Improve Environmental Conditions Impacting Public Health Through Community Planning came about when I plodded through material documenting scientific confirmation of horrific environmental conditions that presented health hazards to the Earth and its inhabitants. Digging back to preliminary papers in the first year of my doctoral program at the University of Central Florida in Orlando, FL, I came across a rudimentary document I had presented at the Global Network for the Economics of Learning, Innovation, and Competence (GLOBELICS) conference in 2009 held in Dakar, Senegal. The document and the succinct version of the presentation discussed how local community development, via collaboration and the development of social networks, could concurrently meet the needs of community healthcare and economic development. The problem was clear: community planning played a key role in safe development with the least environmental and population impact. Because the paper was housed at the Georgia Institute of Technology in Atlanta, GA, I was enticed by several projects and thesis from graduate researchers that discussed atypical and problematic environmental conditions discovered in the social fabric of community development revealed in their contact with urban development and community planning. Given this information, I knew the addition of understanding policy as a barrier/solution could bring forth a unique book on environmental conditions (e.g., environmental, behavioral, cultural) that impact public health. Linking a foundation of existing policy, a problematic environmental condition impacting population health, and the role of community planning was necessary to formulate credible solutions. Thus, the concept was born.

I generated a preliminary outline in March 2016 enveloping policy with problem and potential solution. The approach differentiated this work from most environmental books that focus on the science of the problem. The concept garnered favor from an alternate publisher but not acceptance because my genre was not in the field of environmental or public health. My prior book focus, as a health generalist with an interest in regulatory policy, has been on hospital and healthcare quality. Collaborating with previous associates was also out of the question on this book. Therefore, months of personal research and recruiting permitted me to submit a second proposal. A first submission in the summer of 2016 to my present publisher added the fruits of my endeavors with potential contributing authors having unique knowledge in addition to my own. This submission to Springer International Publishing, maintaining the general topics and the flexibility of subject matter experts to infuse their interpretation of chapter topics, was accepted. The outcome of which was a Springer invitation to edit the book through contractual obligation in October 2016.

Of course, the proposal and contract were just the beginning of the process. I conducted several systematic literature searches (e.g., EBSCO host, ProQuest ABI, PubMed, and the United States National Library of Medicine at the National Institutes of Health, International Environmental and Public Health Agencies) spanning the chapters of the book to form baseline information. Contributing authors also conducted their own literature searches. The combination of general information and specific literature brought forth many resources informing the chapter and serving to extend the understanding of complex concepts.

I am thankful for the insightful information that the contributing authors who stayed the course provided to add to the overall depth of the book. Our combined efforts have resulted in the emergence of more than a dozen chapters identifying unique and interlinked concepts of international and national policy, economic development, environmental and population health in relation to community development and planning. Indeed, the thread of population health is shown as the foundation of responsible and accountable development in many arenas spanning global geopolitical concerns from aid distribution and policing to fundamental problems with water quality. I have opted to let the reader find the inevitable links between and among each chapter in a path to discovery, instead of categorizing the chapters into sections. I believe that this method further engages the reader into a unique experience. While each chapter offers a certain level of understanding, the combined book endeavors to expand the reader's depth of understanding as tidbits of information from one chapter informs another.

Still, no book is without limitations even with 20 months of dedication. The approach highlights many areas of specific environmental and health conditions merely opening the door to the concept that these elements are intertwined with public administration and community planning. Generating a greater understanding of existing policy, environmental problems and the specific impact on public health, offers an opportunity to enhance critical thinking moving toward problem resolution. I hope this text serves to inspire educators, policymakers, public administrators, planners, and students to inform, improve, and inspire inclusive stakeholder decisions that address public need while balancing resource limits.

Jacksonville, FL, USA Beth Ann Fiedler

Contents

Contributors

Oliva P. Canencia Research Division, College of Science and Mathematics, University of Science and Technology of Southern Philippines, Cagayan de Oro, Misamis Oriental, Philippines

Kirsten Cook Planner, Partnership for Southern Equity, Atlanta, GA, USA

Valeria Costantini Department of Economics, Roma Tre University, Rome, Italy

Beth Ann Fiedler Independent Research Analyst, Jacksonville, FL, USA

Antonio Mele Department of Economics, Roma Tre University, Rome, Italy

Vincent N. Van Ness III Orange County (FL) Sheriff's Office (Retired), Lee, MA, USA

Naz Onel School of Business, Stockton University, Galloway, NJ, USA

Samina Panwhar Oregon Health Authority, Salem, OR, USA

Arthi Rao Center for Quality Growth and Regional Development, College of Design, Georgia Institute of Technology, Atlanta, GA, USA

Catherine L. Ross Center for Quality Growth and Regional Development, College of Design, Georgia Institute of Technology, Atlanta, GA, USA

Angelo Mark P. Walag Department of Science Education, College of Science and Technology Education, University of Science and Technology of Southern Philippines, Cagayan de Oro City, Misamis Oriental, Philippines

Rebecca Webster University of Minnesota Duluth, Duluth, MN, USA

Chapter 1
The Challenge of Implementing Macroeconomic Policy in an Increasingly Microeconomic World

Beth Ann Fiedler and Valeria Costantini

Abstract "How did I get here?" (Byrne and Eno. Once in a lifetime—Talking Heads song (Album). Sire Records, Philadelphia, PA; 1980).

The problem with development and implementation of large-scale policy into small communities is foundational to the basic conflict in an economics-driven society. That is, economic growth normally depletes resources and reduces ecosystem services leading to negative environmental externalities that, in turn, impacts social welfare. But national policy still places economic growth as a leading indicator of societal success, even if success is achieved to the detriment of the global scarcity of resources, contributing to child mortality, obesity, lack of access to clean water, unsafe communities, uncertain citizenship status, and similar concerns. All these negative environmental conditions crucially influence health conditions, whatever undeveloped, emerging, or industrialized country is considered. Reconciling the differences in this multidimensional political, social, economic, behavioral, life science, and public health dilemma is tricky, at best, due to governing models reliant on a foundation of economics, history, and mathematics—a triple bane of every scholar's existence. However, the opportunity to generate progressive and sustainable change absent this foundation would otherwise be missed. Thus, this chapter introduces and then unfolds the economic problem in contrast to human development that is at the root of the challenge of implementing national economic policy and the local impact effecting general human development and quality of life. The chapter addresses the application of new metrics supporting economic, human and sustainable development and closes with the application of these metrics towards reasonable constraints of national equitable distribution and global economic expansion.

B. A. Fiedler (✉)
Independent Research Analyst, Jacksonville, FL, USA

V. Costantini
Department of Economics, Roma Tre University, Rome, Italy
e-mail: valeria.costantini@uniroma3.it

B. A. Fiedler (ed.), *Translating National Policy to Improve Environmental Conditions Impacting Public Health Through Community Planning*,
https://doi.org/10.1007/978-3-319-75361-4_1

1.1 Introduction

Societal problems associated with poverty persist just as the basis of the economic problem has not changed since economist Adam Smith introduced the concept of the distributive and commercial nature of land, labor, and capital into the colonial United States. Though Smith's understanding of opportunity through increasing trade flows came in the form of "agriculture, manufacture, and trade" (Campbell and Skinner 1982, p.172), the key to success remains in output or production capacity. This holds true even as agriculture became secondary to industrialization on the basis that any service or commodity, natural or man-made, can be purchased for a price or exchanged. But Smith was also aware of the need for equal distribution of assets to obtain successful human development for the population who had not inherited wealth (Kim 2009; Sen 2010). Others, such as John Rawls, later developed the imperfect but progressive theoretical premise to infuse justice within the framework of institutions and not exclusively to law administration (Garrett 2005; Rawls 1999) attempting to offset the persistent conditions of wealth distribution inequality.

A specific definition of human development can be found in the Human Development Report by the United Nations Development Programme (UNDP) as "a process of enlarging people's choices, the most critical ones are to lead a long and healthy life, to be educated and to enjoy a decent standard of living" (United Nations Development Programme 2010, p.10). Such approach originates from the contributions by Amartya Sen (1970, 1984) and represents a milestone in the debate on how to go beyond the Gross Domestic Product (GDP) measure by incorporating various concepts raised in earlier development discussions and places them in a comprehensive framework (Costantini and Monni 2008). As a general remark, by combining the capability approach developed by Sen and its operationalization into a synthetic Human Development Index as proposed by the UNDP, the concepts of welfare and utility adopted by the neoclassic utilitarian framework to assess the development level of a nation are completely revised, and the classic utility gains based on achievement of higher income levels are substituted with the satisfaction of a crucial condition that is an even distribution of means and ends. Thus, a higher GDP level is only considered a method to reach a better quality of life in terms of improved functioning and capabilities.

The need to modify Smith's economic approach became apparent in several ways. The notion that land, especially during unconstrained U.S. Western Expansion, was a limitless element that could continue to be exploited to overcome poverty and the overarching objective to achieve social equality halted in the face of dismal reality. Eventually, the cost of achieving social equality became evident in the 1970s as the cumulative impact of environmental decay was the recognizable result of unsustainable economic growth and lessening quality of life evidenced by each successive generation. The U.S. National Environmental Policy Act of 1969 began an aggressive attempt to reduce the negative impact by establishing the foundations of environmental quality in national policy. But with diminishing access to natural resources also came fewer opportunities as large tracts of land had already been swallowed up by developers, resources stripped, and once thriving communities abandoned for greener pastures, both literally and figuratively.

Consequently, reduced and harder to exploit resources increased the cost of extraction and decreased the capacity to move up from depressed environments resulting in a greater economic span between the "haves" and the "have nots." The distribution of that wealth computed from 2012 complete comparative data indicates that "the top 1 percent owns 42 percent of total U.S. wealth, up from 25 percent in the 1970s" (Zucman 2016, p.39) while "the bottom 90 percent collectively owns just 23 percent of total U.S. wealth, about as much as in 1940" (Zucman 2016, p. 42). For most the standard of living is not improving and this weakening in social status, or low socioeconomic status (SES), is linked to limited economic opportunity, social and behavioral conditions spanning diverse regions across the globe (Checkley et al. 2016; Katikireddi 2016; Lilford et al. 2016; Venkataramani et al. 2016) that is concurrent with a decline in public health.

To compensate for declining resources, some theorists have discussed the addition of a fourth factor of production including entrepreneurship (Holcombe 1998), technology (Dewan and Min 1997), and/or a combination of entrepreneurial technology. Still others consider these additions simply to be the mechanism through which labor is employed in the production activities. Certainly, technology has provided a way in which previously inaccessible resources might be reached to extend the "shelf-life" of mineral-rich locations and to provide a mechanism for growth in countries with limited resources. However, this chapter will stick to the foundational elements of production for simplicity.

Thus, the chapter introduces basic economics and production inputs, reviews the historical conflict in the measure of societal success through gross national product (including humanitarian foreign investment) and the impact on public health, discusses some behavioral and environmental factors in public health policy development, and proposes how future international development collaborations can restrain global expansion and the impact of industrialization. Finally, the chapter concludes with recommendations and a high-level summary.

1.2 Basic Economics and Production Inputs

The basic economic components continue to revolve around the capacity to optimize the inputs of land, labor, and capital with the goal of production. This general premise remains consistent despite notable variations caused by factors of post-industrial societies including dynamic political systems (e.g., monarchy, democracy, oligarchy, dictatorships), cultural mores (e.g., religious, provincial, male-dominated, slavery), and environmental landscapes (e.g., soil-rich plains for agriculture, seaside for fishing/tourism, oil-rich) that can adjust independent factors (Annenberg Foundation, Bridging World History 2016). Notable is that the influence of pre-industrial cultural factors, such as slavery and religion, continue to influence national production decisions with policy shifts emphasizing strong beliefs of fairness and lifting oppression. The fact remains, however, that the introduction of policy has also been a source of oppression. Therefore, this section will provide a general description of basic economics and define the three production inputs and in so doing, introduce the problem relating to this dynamic role of oppressor and savior.

We note that prominent factors relating to the economy are continuously monitored but sometimes become lost in the grand scheme of currency reflected in gross national product. They include the seemingly mundane announcement of unemployment statistics often viewed as "someone else's problem" if you are gainfully employed but is a factor that greatly impacts the mental and physical health of individuals, communities, and nations around the world. The global implication of conditions that impact public health spans social and behavioral factors such as criminal, terrorist and geopolitical activities often leading to war. The product of conflict compounds with displaced employees through immigration, cultural clashes, and lack of opportunity. Traditional environmental contaminants—a consequence of industrial development—such as poor air and water quality also contribute to the onset of chronic diseases, reduce the quality of life, and limit opportunity, especially for those unskilled workers.

Thus, the problem boils down to balancing the opportunity for human development and quality of life against the erosion of natural resources because at some point, the cost of short-term economic advantages against long-term environmental decay is unsustainable. Understanding these key elements is important to developing, recognizing, and implementing sustainable solutions that can balance the same overall need to improve the variety of environmental conditions against more effective, efficient, and equitable methods of both achieving and measuring development.

Figure 1.1 illustrates the interaction of the elements of production (e.g., land, labor, and capital), the high-level elements of the economy in the form of the costs of decision-making driving production and exchange of goods and services, and the economic problem: "When faced with unlimited wants, how do you address the problem of limited resources?" Both sides of the economic problem must be balanced against needs and resource depletion such that distribution on the left side of the economic problem takes into consideration the impact on the right side relevant to the distribution of goods. Who benefits from employment by producing goods? Who receives goods? What natural resources are depleted in the process? What part of the population is impacted by environmental destruction leading to poor health? Some items are produced for basic consumption, such as food, while others are made to address a desire (e.g., limited edition vehicles). Both have the potential to generate advantages, such as power for a government providing food for a portion of constituents, or wealth for the entrepreneur or innovator who can provide luxuries for the elite or at least those with disposable income and/or good credit standing.

The seemingly simple decision to build a facility to extract natural gas in Florida seems relatively clear because the facility would generate jobs acting as a mechanism to stimulate the economy. The Florida Everglades location, rich in natural gas that

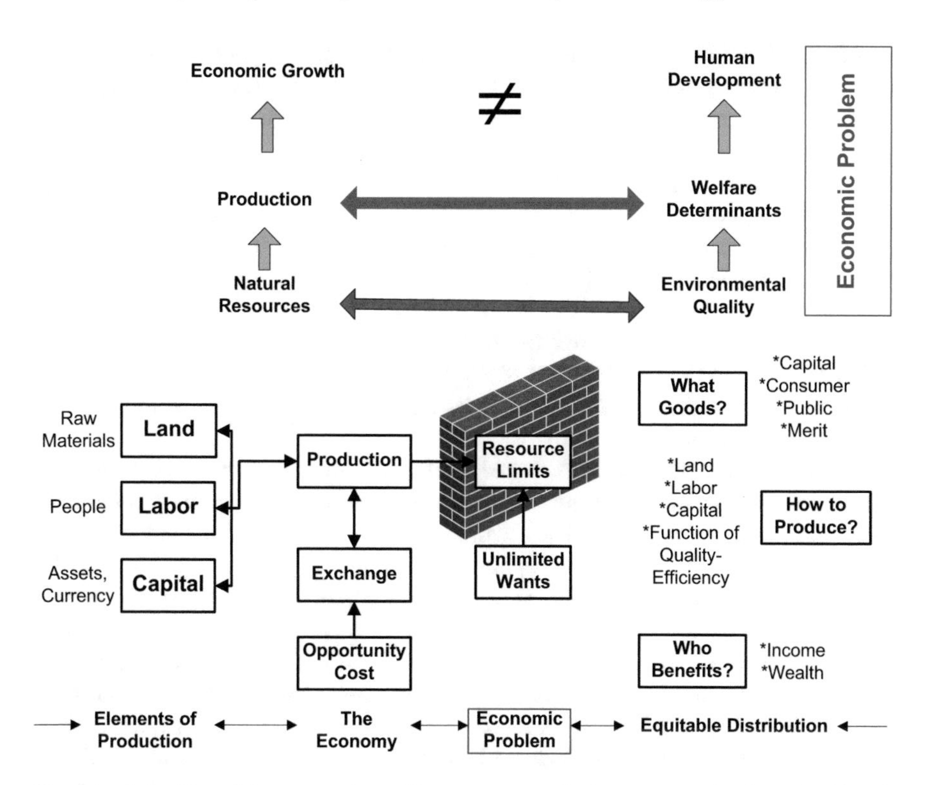

Fig. 1.1 Both sides of the economic problem represent a basic concern—the determination of asset distribution to produce items addressing consumer wants while weighing the cost of asset depletion, limited opportunity, and equitable distribution of products (Fiedler 2009)

can be extracted from limestone, presents a common problem in land use decisions—balancing environmental and population health, especially when the land in question is a vital watershed and a national park (Quest 2015; Russo and Screaton 2016). Simultaneously, a decision to move forward with extraction provides a basis for concern for the perceived, if not actual, long-term effect on land. Short-term gains could successfully elevate the local population income and contribute to national economic growth, but at the expense of destroyed watersheds leading to poor water, increases in vehicle emissions leading to poor air quality, depletion of natural resources and landscapes to accommodate raw materials and infrastructure, and manufacturing waste escaping into the environment as a direct result of production. The local application of national or state economic policy is a complex basis from which to achieve a balance of human development, economic opportunity, and sustainable living conditions resting on the careful manipulation of land, labor, and capital that drive nations.

Land is an asset and a primary factor of production. The term is generally described by The Business Dictionary as a factor of production with limited supply and no cost of production that applies to "all physical elements in the wealth of a nation bestowed by nature (including but not limited to) climate, environment …

(and) minerals." Nations define land in relation to what is on, above, and under the ground "down to the center of the Earth" (http://www.businessdictionary.com). Consequently, even if you could dig your way to China there would be no financial incentive.

Labor is both the physical and literal backbone of society because of the relationship with production that Smith initially refers to as the application of skill, dexterity, and judgment (Campbell and Skinner 1976; Kim 2009; Smith 1776). The concurrent transition from the limitations of the physical aspects of labor to the intellectual and innovative capacity of the work force became evident through improvements in rate of production from technology. This led to the concept of labor as a key to the development of large-scale supply and demand. Supply and demand also brought forth a division of labor often increasing competition for jobs and ultimately, economic opportunity.

Many are politically opposed to the last element of production—capital, because they must acknowledge that the source of economic opportunity must come from some form of existing wealth. The use of capital as a crucial production factor in the mainstream economic literature supposes that wealth is privately held and consequently exchanged on the market as a good fully characterized by perfect competition. In turn, this also implies that perfectly assigned private property rights are in force, and that no externality occurs. All other forms of capital (or more generally endowments, including natural resources) and management (e.g., collective actions) are considered as inefficient. On the contrary, the Nobel laureate Elinor Ostrom would argue that a properly defined property rights regime is strictly connected with the type of resource under consideration, but more importantly with the quality of the formal and informal institutions that are supposed to manage these resources. Especially in poor communities, Ostrom defined some necessary conditions under which common pool resource management is more efficient than private property rights regime (Ostrom 1990). However, others will agree that recognizing capital as some form of existing wealth (i.e., land, cash, buildings) is fundamental to production. The primary difference between the former and the latter is that the latter holds that there must be some form of existing capital.

Capital is the "wealth in the form of money or other assets owned by a person or organization or available for a particular purpose such as starting a company or investing" (Oxford Dictionary at https://www.oxforddictionaries.com/). Innovators, intellectuals, creative artists, and all those not born into wealth may, at some point, rely on investment in some form or another whether funding is direct through novel product development or indirect because you work for someone building their product or service. Access to capital is fundamental to production. Historical references attest to this fact from Italian explorer Christopher Columbus who was funded by Spanish royalty to discover new trade routes, to modern Angel Investors (https://www.entrepreneur.com/article/52742), and Sharks (http://abc.go.com/shows/shark-tank/).

The concept of capital investment is not new, but we recognize that some of the mechanisms to accomplish access are somewhat different from when Columbus approached the throne—an event not to dissimilar to approaching a panel of wealthy entrepreneurs on the American Broadcasting Company television production Shark Tank. Social media is a game changer in the acquisition of funding but while the venue has changed, the players have not. One side has wealth, one side needs the capital to create their product and thus, their own wealth. Whether that exchange occurs is dependent on the ability of the taker to convince the giver to take the risk of investment based on the projected value of the future product.

This section introduced the economic problem of equitable distribution of the input factors of production using endowed national resources of land, labor, and capital. We move to an overview of low SES in relation to public health from this foundation.

1.3 Striving for Innovation: Public Health and Socioeconomic Status

> "For health and health care in the US ... 6 years after the passage of the Affordable Care Act (ACA), nearly 30 million Americans remain uninsured. Americans spend more on health care per person, yet overall life expectancy sits at the bottom of a list of comparable nations. Long the frontrunner in medical innovation, stagnant funding of biomedical research has begun to erode America's edge." (The Lancet 2016, p.388)

The onset of the Trump administration in the USA in 2017 has been viewed negatively by many outside her borders. But for many Americans, restoring foundational governing concepts of life, liberty, and the pursuit of happiness must emphasize a balance between support for local research and development that can simultaneously offer financial and health incentives to the US economy, not just for nations who are benefactors of US foreign investment. More importantly, the growing problem of poverty leading to poor public health (Katikireddi 2016) must be addressed. Therefore, policy development should reflect a variety of stakeholders in relation to health, human, and economic development by designing mechanisms for logical investment in research and novel business opportunities. The basis of this statement is that research leads to innovation that, in turn, increases income opportunity, and thus, economic growth. Income opportunity can help pay for basic needs such as housing, food, and healthcare but must be balanced with sustainable methods that may require a fresh perspective on "money" and out of the box thinking when balancing population needs against alternatives that promote better prospects for those left out of the system.

1.3.1 Money an Unnecessary Evil?

Money makes the world go around. Or does it? The introduction of BitCoin and other virtual currencies has encouraged growth and the exchange of products in unexpected ways. For example, while BitCoin is an acceptable substitute for national currency, there are additional benefits to alternative payment methods. One of these payment options—Blockchain—also offers a platform to resolve the problematic nature of tracking the authenticity of high-ticket products and land ownership (*Napoletano* 2016). Blockchain technology can maintain the provenance of the item, such as diamonds and real estate titles, through shared registration and distribution to relevant parties including owners, insurers, estate attorneys, and law enforcement agencies.

The value of these virtual transactions has been felt on a small scale, primarily between individuals and among organizations. But the recent introduction of a cashless society by India has pushed the implementation scale to the national level with no apparent limits in sight.

Just as India has avoided the US problem of creating digital communication infrastructure over outdated analog infrastructure, they too are investing in ways to skip over two generations of financial technology and thus, laying the foundation for a cashless society (Wadha 2017). This pathway starts with linking digital identification of the population to newly created payment banks that hold but do not lend money. The Aadhaar project, an Indian government sponsored program since 2009, has generated a unique identification number for more than one billion people by linking the number to individual retina and fingerprint scans. The creation of the 12-digit number addresses the problem of unrecorded births that had previously kept these unregistered citizens out of the economy and system of social services. More than that, the Aadhaar number provides a way for banking institutions to transfer money under the Unified Payment Interface (UPI) (Razorpay 2017).

Skeptics may, of course, find these items interesting but limited to small transactions and certainly not applicable to "big" economies. But the inclusion of the forgotten population in India accumulated $10 billion from just over 250,000 accounts that were started in the first 3 years the payment banks were in operation (Wadha 2017).

Both novel ways to exchange goods and services and payment options that incorporate those who have been left out of the economic system can serve to remove some of the evil connotation associated with money. This is especially true since they ultimately offer a platform to improve the quality of life in small ways with large benefits such as the ability to (1) pay for utilities including communication and electricity, (2) build safer environments, and (3) generate an inclusive economy.

1.3.2 Thinking Beyond Boundaries

Innovation, of course, is not limited to research or business development related to healthcare though a growing number of healthcare businesses (Statistics Brain Research Institute 2016) account for employment opportunities. Problem recognition and solution generation in Green Business Development (Green Jobs and Career Network 2017) presents an opportunity with very few constraints on production inputs. The emerging field offers a variety of occupations representing diverse businesses bringing forth the high hope of increasing opportunity in a sustainable fashion. Waste management, natural foods, and cultured meat are areas that show high and continuous growth potential because they solve a problem or need (e.g., increasing population, increasing waste, diminishing food supply, access to fresh food for health), and produce product or services in a manner that sustains the environment.

New York architects from Present Architecture—Andre Guimond, Evan Erlebacher, and Christian Scharzwimmer—unveiled a "Composting Infrastructure Masterplan" in 2013 introducing the concept of a large-scale organic alternative to help eliminate 14 million tons of trash and reduce emissions caused by transporting waste to landfills across state lines while increasing public green space (Present Architecture 2013). Dubbed "The Green Loop," the project brilliantly optimizes existing transportation infrastructure, takes into account the real problem of waste management in a densely populated urban location, and adds 125 acres of public, multi-purpose facilities divided among ten boroughs in the New York metropolitan area (http://presentarchitecture.com/project/green-loop/).

The Green Loop serves to demonstrate alternative ways in which to optimize land use. Another path is the slow but steady emergence of companies who support urban farming that (1) adds thriving green land back into the environment to improve environmental conditions and fresh food resources and (2) provides services and equipment to meet the problem of ways to increase food production for an increasing global population.

For example, Pure Agrobusiness, Inc. (http://www.pureagro.net/) has been asking families, communities, and businesses who are up to the challenge to "Rethink Farming" for the past 20 years. The company kick-starts projects by selling a wide variety of indoor hydroponic technologies and equipment. The west coast company led by Rick Byrd, Chairman and CEO, consolidated with Way to Grow in early 2016 to form the largest US supplier of urban agriculture and hydroponics technologies (Business Wire 2016). Though the business seemingly popped up overnight, Mr. Byrd has steadily built the indoor agriculture enterprise and is positioned to supply equipment for the growing need for urban farming, including medical marijuana. The emerging and controversial market for medical marijuana (ProCon.org 2016) to relieve the effects of chemotherapy in cancer patients (e.g., lack of appetite, nausea, vomiting) and support overall health (e.g., high Omega-3 value in hemp seeds) is another arena in which businesses are making the most of new and growing opportunities for market entry.

Emerging technologies able to produce food from chemical processes rather than through traditional agriculture might help encompassing the global problem of food shortage in a scenario where a rapid population growth is followed by a rapid transition of arable land into urbanized area and a drastic reduction in land productivity. An example might be cultured meat where animal tissue is grown in a controlled environment using cell culture technology rather than obtained by traditional livestock. Industrial livestock production presents the most difficult challenge for the global food system due to production requirements that account for large consumption of natural resources (e.g., pasture lands and water) and is also responsible for a large share of greenhouse gas (GHG) emissions (Sentience Politics 2017). In addition, negative environmental and health impacts from such activity have been increasingly put under the lens of the consumers' attention as freshwater pollution from manure or the increasing resistance to antibiotics due to abuse of them as preventative measure in highly intensive industrial livestock production (Agribusiness Accountability Initiative 2017).

These concepts represent innovation in problem resolution and changing cultural mindsets through small steps that contribute to resolving the overarching problem of low SES and the associated problems that reduce quality of life. Money may or may not be the root of all evil. But the following evidence gathered from across the globe indicates that poverty—the lack of money or some form of capital asset—impacts the human condition that could form the modern definition for evil for many who continue to subsist.

1.3.3 The Global Problem of Low SES

Several recent studies on various global populations bring forth the complex nature of low SES as a determinant of public health based on the social, behavioral, and economic limitations associated with this indicator. The scope of the phenomena of plausible economic growth given environmental conditions (e.g., poor air quality, low socioeconomic status) and consequent decline in public health is demonstrated in the following research conducted in diverse geographic locations.

1.3.3.1 Africa, China, and India: Urbanization and Poor Health Outcomes

The urbanization process, broadly defined as the population shift to large cities, is problematic because dense populations lead to fierce competition for access to scarce resources and satisfaction of basic needs. Specifically, diverse nations such as Africa, China, and India among others across the globe, all face the growing impact of urbanization—minimal employment opportunities and housing shortages in densely populated urban locations, leading to slum development and consequent congestion disamenities (Checkley et al. 2016; Ezeh et al. 2016; Lilford et al. 2016). The United Nations indicates that in 2013 nearly a billion people live in slums divided between undeveloped (863 million) and developed nations (70 million) (United Nations Human Settlements Programme 2014, p.2) and expects that number to continue to escalate.

Slums, according to the United Nations Human Settlements Program, are defined by a combination of conditions that include variables of the environment such as deficient sanitation caused by insufficient infrastructure to preserve and provide access to clean water. This characteristic is causal in 2.5 billion cases of diarrhea in children less than 5 years old alone and kills nearly two million people annually across all ages (United Nations Human Settlements Programme 2015, p.3). A full "80 percent of those [total] cases are in Africa and South Asia" (United Nations Development Programme 2015, p. 3). Other conditions that characterize a slum are the absence of raw materials making development of long-term housing difficult, if not impossible, overcrowding, and the cumulative impact from physical and emotional hazards in the environment.

(Ezeh et al. 2016, p.1):

> Slums are unhealthy places with especially high risks of infection and injury … because health is affected by factors arising from the shared physical and social environment, which have effects beyond those of poverty alone.

The problem of unchecked urban sprawl and the increasing percentage of the population living in slum conditions within urban populations can promote other negative health conditions represented by the onset of pneumonia, asthma, tuberculosis, and other respiratory health problems (Checkley et al. 2016). About 30 million or half of the population that live in slums within India's highly urban population suffers from at least one respiratory ailment in which the cost of medical care and treatment further diminishes their limited earnings by about 10% (Checkley et al. 2016, p.853; Chowdhury 2011). The problem is exasperated because those who dwell in slums are often not granted national rights (e.g., security of tenure), because they do not have any official claims to the land where they have built their makeshift housing (Ezeh et al. 2016, p.5; Subbaraman et al. 2012).

In another scenario, the displacement of Chinese rural farming communities has been persistent for several decades but not very well communicated to the rest of the world. However, the completion of the Three Gorges Dam on the Yangtze River (Vitka 2006) was well publicized and illustrative of the rural farmer population transfer of over one million people adding to the dislocation of millions of Chinese due to various dam projects across the nation (Campbell-Hyde 2012). While forced relocation into urban manufacturing locations is slightly different from the independent movement of a population, the results are still consistent—massive environmental disruption has led to an increase in dangerous social and environmental effects stemming from increased competition for a limited number of jobs and displaced laborers have less opportunity to find work because their skills are often not transferrable. The problem is further exasperated because social networks—a mechanism to find employment—are limited, if available at all.

1.3.3.2 United States

Researchers using a limited sector of the population between the ages of 25 and 35 from self-reported data accumulated from 2009–2012 in the United States Behavioral Risk Factor Surveillance Surveys detect another dimension to the association between economic opportunity and health. "Inequality of economic opportunity, defined as disparities in the prospects for upward social mobility, has come to the forefront of public discourse in the USA and Europe" (Venkataramani et al. 2016, p.1). They explain that options to improve SES conditions are in effect, dependent on location, the assets at that location, and physical access to those assets at a specific point in time (Venkataramani et al. 2016; Chetty et al. 2014). Their perspective is consistent with the fact that environmental conditions are dynamic in that the same piece of land can morph from agriculture development, factory site, depleted or brown land, renewed community development, natural gas resource, and so on. Thus, even in the land of opportunity, opportunity has environmental limitations and the impact of that limitation can be felt in population health status.

The Venkataramani et al. (2016) study reviewed individual attributes such as age, race, income, and marital status that play a role in achieving equal access to economic opportunity. The researchers also indicated that behavior and the consequences of their habits (e.g., smoking, obesity, sexual activity) and the level of physical activity and reported sick days had statistically significant influence on limiting economic opportunity and consequently, the increasing expectation of poor mental and physical health outcomes (Venkataramani et al. 2016).

Overall, the studies herein illustrate the global problem of lack of economic opportunity leading to poor health. Further, the results demonstrate the universal need for sustainable economic development that continues to shatter the global misconception that Americans, and other nations considered historically wealthy, are somehow invulnerable to the consequences of poverty. Wealth inequality and income opportunity impacting public health is a problem shared across the globe.

In this section, we discussed the global problem of low SES and health decline. Next, we move from simple economic definitions and problem awareness to the more complex nature of economics and the changing role of the environment in economic growth towards a sustainable human development and economic model.

1.4 The Changing Role of the Environment: Modeling Sustainable Human and Economic Development

Economics can be explained in simple terms but that is not to imply conceptual simplicity. This is especially true because the dynamic imbalance and the inherent inequality in the economic problem continuously generate a need for a new view of land, labor, and capital. Land becomes a prominent focus in this section because environmentalists have long battled the advancement of civilization in relation to economic growth. The primary reason for this position is that human growth was associated with an increase in industrialization that translated into the recognizable loss of irreplaceable natural resources for short-term gains. Therefore, this section introduces the concept of sustainable human development, illuminates the flaws of increasing acquisition and the reality that income adjustments do not necessarily equate to improved social status or quality of life but may, in fact, decrease quality of life often reflected in health status. Thus, the section provides a foundation for the conflict in human development and the measure of societal growth through common measures of expenditures on health and gross national product (Statista 2017a; Statista 2017b).

Assessment of human well-being independent of economic growth measurements (e.g., personal income, progressive technologies, modernization) was ushered into existence by Amartya Sen who fathered the advance of sustainable human development in terms that did not limit capacity for existing generations "without compromising the capabilities of future generations" (Anand and Sen 2000; Costantini and Monni 2008, p.868; Sen 2000). The basic paradigm shifts from a "vision of environment as a limit to economic growth" (Costantini and Monni 2008, p.868; Meadows et al. 1972) to examining the contribution of the environment in context with the potential the environment may have towards improving the quality of life. These mechanisms simultaneously address ways to reduce poverty, achieve higher standards of living, and increase human development needs by integrating them into a model of sustainable human development.

Modeling builds examples that test the limit of inputs and projects outputs that offer a new way to view observable data. But models are dependent on consistent performance metrics. The United Nations General Assembly recently incorporated elements of Sustainable Development Goals (SDGs) when they adopted the 2030 Agenda for Sustainable Development in the Fall of 2015 (World Bank 2017). Their actions move from Millennium Development Goals to *World Development Indicators* contained in the World Development Database (World Bank 2016) viewed considering SDGs and their overarching twofold agenda to (1) eradicate extreme poverty and (2) bring into equilibrium the distribution of wealth within and between nations.

Understanding the nature of the new performance metrics may be best illustrated by those authors that operationalize the concept of sustainable human development into a measurable metrics. For instance, Costantini and Monni (2008) expand the context of human development over pure economic considerations using World Bank variables that reflect an opportunity to discern (in)efficient use of natural resources at the country level. They also illustrate how institutions could be a crucial support for economic and human development leading to the desired integration of sustainable development proposed by Sen. This is relevant to the scope of this chapter on the premise that good institutions drive good policy. By combining the Recourse Curse Hypothesis (RCH) which measures the effects of naturally endowed resources on economic growth with the Environmental Kuznets Curve (EKC) approach—a measurement of the effects of economic growth on environmental quality indicating the impact of pollution on population health, it is possible to assess the turning point where sustainable human development can be ensured by good institutions.

(Costantini and Monni 2008, p.870):

> The linkages between the resource curse and the role of institutions may be divided into two strands: where the quality of institutions is damaged by resource abundance and constitutes the intermediate causal link between resources and economic performance, and where resources interact with the quality of institutions so that resource abundance is a blessing when institutions are good and a curse when institutions are bad.

The RCH measures the relationships between level of natural resources against economic growth in three main categories: first, ↑ natural resource and ↓economic

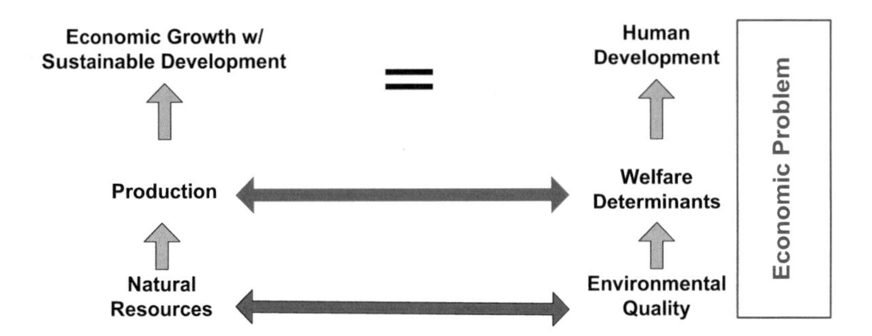

Fig. 1.2 The integration of sustainable development offers a method to balance the twofold goal of economic growth and human development

growth (resource curse); second, ↓ natural resources and ↑ economic growth (e.g., Japan, Hong Kong, Ireland) (resource blessing); and third, ↑relatively high dependence on primary resources, ↑ relatively good growth rate (e.g., Botswana, Norway). Countries like Russia, Nigeria, and Venezuela with an abundance of resources damaged by institutions (curse) could morph into blessed institutions if resource decisions were enhanced at the institutional level. But first, other items with RCH impact had to be taken into consideration such as restrictive trade policies, macroeconomic instability, low human capital accumulation rate, human capital growth through education, and the quality of institutional development and their ability to manage resources.

The relevance of such alternative model is evident in alternate metrics and assessments for the goal of institutional improvements. The model illustrates that (1) strictly economic indicators do not have to be the only measures of advancements in society, (2) these measures provide indicators of institutional disarray that should impact policy decisions in regard to foreign investment and/or foreign aid, and (3) Anand and Sen's Sustainable Human Development promoting the capabilities of people in the present without compromising the capabilities of future generations can be measured, benchmarked, and applied to global economic development to achieve a higher standard of living while maintaining natural capital. Thus, human development can reach a balanced relationship with economic growth with the premise of sustainable development (Fig. 1.2).

The origin of the EKC considers that pure economic growth could only occur at the expense of environmental exploitation but substitutes factors of human development (e.g., health, education) as a measure of the demand perspective to address public opinion. Public opinion represents the desire to reduce environmental decay and introduce structural changes in the economic growth patterns with less industry and higher technology that would equate to a lower global impact of harmful emissions. Here, the inter-relationship of economic growth coupled with the ability to advance technology helps to reduce pollution.

Costantini and Monni's (2008, p.875) integration of the RCH and a modified EKC or (M)EKC was practical because both models introduce factors of human development and can be considered in the determination of causal relationships in the current battle between human development and economic development with sustainable objectives.

This approach has several important outputs. They (1) establish the ability to measure well-being during various stages of development, (2) provide a tool to assess cost of offering social services in developed nations, and (3) propose a policy framework with built-in decision-making metrics for developed countries to determine the level and type of charitable support to developing nations, if any. The first two outcomes reflect internal national measures against other nations. The third reflects an opportunity to discern (in)efficient use of natural resources at the country level to make informed external decisions about humanitarian support, decisions to build infrastructure for sustainable development, and providing mechanisms that increase human development through access to education and daily needs. Thus, foreign investment decisions contributing to GDP can be profitable and sustainable given policy decisions based jointly on economic, human, and sustainable development goals. Domestic economic and population health decision-making using this foundation can also benefit. Therefore, the concept of development as freedom (Sen 1999) come to life as a measure of societal improvement. One in which natural resources, together with national and global institutions, are means to reach equilibrium between the constructs of social justice and human development in concert with the ecosystem.

1.5 Application and Discussion

Many questions emerge from the conflicting nature of economic growth and human development in which primary inputs to production—land, labor, and capital—impose limits impacting opportunity and well-being. The authors suggest one avenue is posed in the question, "When considering the perspective of human development, does the context of the "Economic Problem" change? Another, in cases of extreme poverty, "What good is maintaining the environment if no one can expect to survive to enjoy it?" Also, "How does one account for countries with limited resources but that demonstrate high rates of economic growth that could not be attributed to technology output?" Finally, "Can Anand and Sen's dream of sustainable human development coexist with economic development?"

First, when considering whether the perspective of human development changes in the context of the economic problem, the simple answer is, "Yes." Explaining how the change occurs is not as easy. Suffice it to say that there is a notable shift from the production or product to exchange to the well-being of the person involved in the transaction. The difficulty in expressing that shift lies in the problem of expressing the contribution of the elements of production in relation to the exchange instead of in relation to wants and needs that drive supply and demand through production input selection and utilization. The problem is reflected in the second question involving the balance between unhealthy conditions of poverty and environmental damage resulting from rapid industrial growth that also impacts quality of life. Short-term economic solutions that save a population from hunger often have long-term health implications. But how do you tell the parents of a child who is hungry now that they will not build a factory to provide an income source to meet basic needs because at some distant point in the future the environment surrounding the factory will show evidence of air and water pollution?

The third question of inexplicable economic growth for countries with limited resources suggests a signal in the RCH that there is a misallocation of revenues from resource exploitation demonstrated by such countries as Malaysia and Thailand (Costantini and Monni 2008, p.870). Misallocation of revenues is one of the five dimensions of the three primary RCH measures of economic growth in relation to the level of natural resources mentioned earlier. Other dimensions include the Dutch Disease Effect (when a resource boom diverts money from those activities that promote long-term growth), rent-seeking behavior (concentration of rents in the hands of a few private owners that takes away from human resources and small enterprise), the relationship between the quality of institutions and the capacity to manage resources, and the role of human capital—structural investments in human resources. Evidence of these activities should be a strong indicator to reduce or eliminate trade and charitable donations to these nations, or at least to select strict rules for respecting fundamental human rights.

Finally, "Can Anand and Sen's dream of sustainable human development coexist with economic development?" The investment by the UN in Sustainable Development Goals and the selection of World Bank Development Indicators able to measure the achievements of SDGs seem to suggest that this is plausible but difficult to implement in practice.

First, there is an ethical foundation to attempt to achieve equitable distribution on both sides of the economic problem. Second, there is a realistic expectation that a system that heavily favors social justice can lead to lack of incentive to improve conditions and thus, have far-reaching negative repercussions. The influx of nonprofits and federal funding within the country and in global humanitarian efforts reflects the first instance. The second instance can best be reflected in what may be considered folklore but illustrates a good point. Consider the story of the instructor who agreed to combine everyone's grade to demonstrate the repercussions from striving for too much social equity (You Tube 2014). While low-scoring students initially received higher grades because of students who study and normally receive better grades, the advantage was short-lived. After a short period of time, the students who were diligently studying became complacent because their incentive to study was removed. Their logic could be summed in the statement, "Why study for an 'A' and receive a 'B' because someone else did not work as hard?" Eventually, the lack of individual incentive to achieve had the result of innovators losing interest in studying and followers no longer able to take advantage of those who strived to achieve on their own merits. Everyone received a failing grade by the end of the semester.

The drivers of economics and capitalism may be an imperfect system compared to the initial high hopes of socialism illustrated in the prior story. But the elements exist to improve social status when there is a greater understanding of the economic problem—balancing the needs of the people weighed against diminishing resources. Innovation in policy implementation offering opportunity for human development, abating the division of the wealth inequality or at least addressing the needs of the extremely impoverished, and acting against national fraud or harm against certain peoples provides the opportunity to resolve some of this imbalance by identifying need, recognizing problems, and generating sustainable solutions.

We should now better understand how we got here. Let's imagine where we can go from here.

1.6 Summary

In this chapter, we discussed historical input components of production, touched upon individual behavioral and social determinants, and considered the impact of both social status and environmental pollutants as an outcome of industrialization. We describe how institutional policy can be improved by using indicators reflecting national performance developed by the World Bank that take into consideration a wider scope of factors beyond those limited to economic development. Prominent elements include (1) an introduction to the economic problem in contrast to human development, (2) a foundational basis on the notion of large-scale government policy enveloping the intertwined and complex concepts of economic development, human development, environmental impact, and public health that is the essence of sustainable development, and (3) to address the question of reasonable limits of global economic expansion by understanding ways to induce collective action for civic engagement and provide information to guide policy makers in order to improve government accountability, transparency and reduce internal corruption.

Glossary

Capital A form of currency or asset (e.g., money, land, machinery, technology) that indicates a strong financial status that can be used to support new business development as an investment for profit; a key input in production

Commerce The introduction of logistics (e.g., railroad, truck, aircraft, ship) to transfer finished goods or services to another location for payment

Economics A social science utilizing theories of management and economic systems emphasizing the exchange of natural resources to produce and transfer goods and services to consumers; study of the creation and distribution of wealth to communities with limited natural resources

Economic Growth Increasing opportunities in terms of new technologies, information, communication, and competitiveness

Economic Problem The difficulty in balancing population needs that consume natural resources against the reality of limited resources

Equitable Distribution Ability to balance divergent needs of a population in a manner that accounts for wealth inequality through the interpretation of a variety of inputs including who benefits from labor income, product output, access to land, etc.

Entrepreneur A person or group of people who assumes the investment risk of a new business to try to achieve the benefits of productions, and/or the decision-maker of a new business that organizes the daily operations for profit

Environmental Kuznets Curve (EKC) The effects of economic growth on environmental quality

Gross Domestic Product An accepted annual measure of the cumulative economic activity of a nation representing the total monetary value of production, including finished goods and services, adjusting for imports

Gross National Product (GNP) The sum of gross domestic product and the net income from foreign investment

Human Development Consists of two dimensions that, in turn, permit access to opportunities to progress in other areas of life—(1) directly enhancing human abilities (e.g., quality of life, education, longevity) and (2) generation of conditions to support the first dimension (e.g., civic engagement, environmental sustainability, safe environments, human rights)

Industrialization When a society moves from an agricultural economy to one that relies on the manufacture of goods

Opportunity Cost Views the cost of decision-making in comparison to the next best alternative that was not selected; highlights the value of various options by comparison

Resource Curse Hypothesis (RCH) Measures the effects of naturally endowed resources on economic growth

Socioeconomic Status (SES) A common classification of high, middle, or low SES in the social sciences representing personal or group social status based on a variety of attributes such as level of education, income, and job that is commonly linked to expected levels of health and representative of unequal resource distribution

Sustainable Development The same level of well-being achieved for the present generation that will be maintained at the same level for the benefit of future generations

References

42 U.S.C. National Environmental Policy Act of 1969 (Public Law 91–190) [As Amended Through Dec. 31, 2000].

Agribusiness Accountability Initiative. Environmental and health problems in livestock production: pollution in the food system. Leveling the field– issue brief #2; 2017. http://www.ase.tufts.edu/gdae/Pubs/rp/AAI_Issue_Brief_2_1.pdf. Accessed 22 May 2017

Annenberg Foundation, Bridging World History. Unit 14, land and labor relationships; 2016. http://www.learner.org/courses/worldhistory/unit_overview_14.html. Accessed 12 Feb 2017.

Anand S, Sen A. Human development and economic sustainability. World Dev. 2000;28(12):2029–49.
Business Wire. PureAgro creates largest U.S. supplier of urban agriculture and hydroponics technologies and equipment: consolidation of retail and wholesale operations positions company for growth [Online]; 2016. http://www.businesswire.com/news/home/20161101005244/en/PureAgro-Creates-Largest-U.S.-Supplier-Urban-Agriculture. Accessed 19 Feb 2017.
Byrne D, Eno B. Once in a lifetime—Talking Heads song (Album). Compass Point Studios, Nassau Sigma Sound Studios. Philadelphia, PA: Sire Records; 1980.
Campbell RH, Skinner AS, editors. An inquiry into the nature and causes of the wealth of nations by Adam smith (1776). Oxford: Clarendon Press; 1976. http://files.libertyfund.org/files/220/0141-02_Bk.pdf. Accessed 2 Mar 2017.
Campbell RH, Skinner AS. Adam smith. New York: St. Martin's Press; 1982.
Campbell-Hyde B. ICE Case 254: breaking ground: environmental and social issues of the Three Gorges Dam in China; 2012. http://mandalaprojects.com/ice/ice-cases/china-dam-impact.htm. Accessed 14 Sept 2017.
Checkley W, et al. Managing threats to respiratory health in urban slums. Lancet. 2016;4:852–4. https://doi.org/10.1016/S2213-2600(16)30245-4.
Chetty R, et al. Where is the land of opportunity? The geography of intergenerational mobility in the United States. Q J Econ. 2014;129:1553–623.
Chowdhury S. Financial burden of transient morbidity: a case study of slums in Delhi. Econ Polit Wkly. 2011;46:59.
Costantini V, Monni S. Environment, human development and economic growth. Ecol Econ. 2008;64(4):867–80.
Dewan S, Min C. The substitution of information technology for other factors of production: a firm level analysis. *Manag Sci.* 1997;43(12):1660–75. Frontier Research on Information Systems and Economics
Ezeh A, et al. The health of people who live in slums 1: the history, geography, and sociology of slums and the health problems of people who live in slums. Lancet. 2016;389(10068):547–58. https://doi.org/10.1016/S0140-6736(16)31650-6.
Fiedler BA. Environment, human development and economic growth. Presentation at the University of Central Florida, PAF7315, 24 March; 2009.
Garrett J. Rawls' mature theory of social justice: an introduction for students; 2005. http://people.wku.edu/jan.garrett/ethics/matrawls.htm. Accessed 14 Sep 2017.
Green Jobs & Career Network. 2017. https://www.linkedin.com/grps?careerDiscussion=&gid=77194. Accessed 20 Feb 2017.
Holcombe RG. Entrepreneurship and economic growth. QJAE. 1998;1(2):46–62. https://mises.org/library/entrepreneurship-and-economic-growth. Accessed 14 Sep 2017
Katikireddi SV. Economic opportunity: a determinant of health? Lancet. 2016;1:1–2. https://doi.org/10.1016/S2468-2667(16)30004-4.
Kim K. Adam Smith's theory of economic history and economic development. EJHET. 2009;16:141–64. http://www.tandfonline.com/doi/full/10.1080/09672560802707407
Lilford RJ, et al. The health of people who live in slums 2: improving the health and welfare of people who live in slums. Lancet. 2016;389:1–11. https://doi.org/10.1016/S0140-6736(16)31848-7.
Meadows DH, et al. The limits to growth. New York: Universe Books; 1972.
Napoletano E. Blockchain: a primer and promises for the future of payment tech [online]; 2016. https://www.discovernetwork.com/en-us/business-resources/articles/blockchain-a-primer-and-promises-for-the-future-of-payment-tech?cmpgnid=ps-dnw-google-cpc-search-Content-Pilot-Blockchain-Bitcoin-bitcoin. Accessed 14 Sep 2017.
Ostrom E. Governing the commons: the evolution of institutions for collective action: Cambridge, Cambridge University Press; 1990.
Present Architecture. Green loop; 2013. http://presentarchitecture.com/project/green-loop/. Accessed 14 Oct 2017.
ProCon.org. 60 peer-reviewed studies on medical marijuana medical studies involving cannabis and cannabis extracts (1990–2014); 2016. http://medicalmarijuana.procon.org/view.resource.php?resourceID=000884. Accessed 14 Sept 2017.

Quest D. Fracking and Florida: the facts [online]. Energy in depth Florida; 2015. https://energy-indepth.org/florida/fracking-and-florida-facts/. Accessed 14 Sep 2017.
Rawls JA. Theory of justice, revised. The Belknap Press of Harvard University Press; 1999. Original work published on 1971.
Razorpay UPI. Unified payment interface (UPI) (https://razorpay.com/upi/); 2017. Accessed 14 Sept 2017.
Russo R, Screaton E. Should Florida 'frack' its limestone for oil and gas? Two geophysicists weigh in [online]. UF News; 2016. http://news.ufl.edu/articles/2016/05/should-florida-frack-its-limestone-for-oil-and-gas-two-geophysicists-weigh-in.php. Accessed 21 Feb 2017.
Sen AK. The impossibility of a Paretian liberal. J Political Econ. 1970;78:152–7.
Sen AK. Resources, values and development. Oxford: Blackwell; 1984.
Sen AK. Development as freedom. New York: Random House; 1999.
Sen AK. 2000. The ends and the means of sustainability. Keynote address at the international conference on transition to sustainability, Tokyo, 15 May 2000.
Sen AK. Adam smith and the contemporary world. EJPE. 2010;3(1):50–67. https://doi.org/10.23941/ejpe.v3i1.39.
Sentience Politics. Cultured meat; 2017. https://sentience-politics.org/research/policy-papers/cultured-meat/. Accessed 14 Sept 2017.
Statistics Brain Research Institute. Health care industry statistics; 2016. http://www.statisticbrain.com/health-care-industry-statistics/. Accessed 14 Sept 2017.
Statista. Real gross domestic product (GDP) growth rate in the United States from 2010 to 2020 (compared to the previous year); 2017a. https://www.statista.com/statistics/263614/gross-domestic-product-gdp-growth-rate-in-the-united-states/. Accessed 14 Sept 2017.
Statista. U.S. national health expenditure as percent of GDP from 1960 to 2014; 2017b. https://www.statista.com/statistics/184968/us-health-expenditure-as-percent-of-gdp-since-1960/. Accessed 14 Sep 2017.
Subbaraman R, et al. Off the map: the health and social implications of being a non-notified slum in India. Environ Urban. 2012;24:643–63.
The Lancet. US election coverage, 2016 [online]; 2016. http://www.thelancet.com/USElection2016. Accessed 14 Sep 2017.
United Nations Human Settlements Programme. World habitat day: Voices from slums; 2014. http://unhabitat.org/wp-content/uploads/2014/07/WHD-2014-Background-Paper.pdf. 2017. Accessed 14 Sep 2017.
United Nations Development Programme. Human development report: concept and measurement of human development; 2010. http://hdr.undp.org/en/reports/global/hdr1990. Accessed 14 Sep 2017.
United Nations Development Programme. Human development reports: what is human development? 2015. http://hdr.undp.org/en/content/what-human-development. Accessed 14 Sept 2017.
United Nations Human Settlements Programme. Report to the United Nations human settlements programme on housing and slum upgrading; 2015. https://www.amun.org/uploads/15_Final_Report/UN-Habitat-1-926.pdf. Accessed 14 Sep 2017.
Venkataramani AS, et al. Economic opportunity, health behaviours, and health outcomes in the USA: a population-based cross-sectional study. Lancet. 2016;1(1):e18–25. https://doi.org/10.1016/S2468-2667(16)30005-6.
Vitka W. China completes three gorges dam; 2006. http://www.cbsnews.com/news/china-completes-three-gorges-dam/. Accessed 14 Sep 2017.
Wadha V. What the U.S. can learn from India's move toward a cashless society. [online]; 2017. https://www.linkedin.com/pulse/what-us-can-learn-from-indias-move-toward-cashless-society-wadhwa?trk=eml-email_feed_ecosystem_digest_01-hero-0-null&midToken=AQFJG0wzikzRCA&fromEmail=fromEmail&ut=3srX-o-K1bg7E1. Accessed 14 Sep 2017.
World Bank. World development indicators [database], 2016. Washington, DC: The World Bank; 2016. http://data.worldbank.org/data-catalog/world-development-indicators. Accessed 14 Sep 2017

World Bank. World development indicators, 2017: sustainable development goals; 2017. http://datatopics.worldbank.org/sdgs/. Accessed 14 Sep 2017.
You Tube. Hard lesson in socialist schemes; 2014. http://www.ask.com/youtube?q=You+Tube+Socialism+Case+of+professor+and+same+grade&v=XDHShu1uUQ4&qsrc=472. Accessed 14 Sep 2017.
Zucman G. Wealth inequality: pathways, the Stanford center on poverty and inequality; 2016. http://inequality.stanford.edu/sites/default/files/Pathways-SOTU-2016-Wealth-Inequality-3.pdf. Accessed 14 Sep 2017.

Further Reading

American Planning Association (APA). Healthy communities through collaboration; 2017. https://www.planning.org/research/healthy/. Accessed 14 Sep 2017.
Congress of the United States Congressional Budget Office (CBO). Trends in family wealth, 1989–2013; 2016. https://www.cbo.gov/sites/default/files/114th-congress-2015-2016/reports/51846-Family_Wealth.pdf. Accessed 14 Sep 2017.
Fox AM, Meier BM. Health as freedom: addressing social determinants of global health inequities through the human right to development. Bioethics. 2009;23(2):1467–8519. https://doi.org/10.1111/j.1467-8519.2008.00718.x.
Grendz. The latest green, science and technology trends worldwide; 2017. http://grendz.com/. Accessed 14 Sep 2016.
Lee S-W, et al. Landscape ecological approach to the relationships of land use patterns in watersheds to water quality characteristics. Landscape Urban Plan. 2009;92(2):80–9.
National Association for Local Boards of Health (NALBOH). Leading through health system change-national network for public health institutes; n.d. http://www.nalboh.org/?page=OtherResources. Accessed 14 Feb 2017.
National Association of County & City Health Officials (NACCHO). Fact sheet: public health in land use planning and community design; n.d. http://archived.naccho.org/topics/environmental/landuseplanning/upload/Land-Use-Fact-Sheet6-19-03.pdf. Accessed 14 Feb 2017.
National Network of Public Health Institutes (NNPHI). Population health innovation; 2017. https://nnphi.org/focus-areas-service/public-health-innovation/. Accessed 17 Feb 2017.
Piccard D. A theory of social justice, by John Rawls; 2005. http://www.ohio.edu/people/piccard/entropy/rawls.html. Accessed 13 Feb 2017.
United Nations Development Programme. Human development report, 2015: work for human development; 2015. http://report.hdr.undp.org/. Accessed 17 Feb 2017.
van de Vijver S, et al. Challenges of health programmes in slums. Lancet. 2015;386:2114–6. https://doi.org/10.1016/S0140-6736(15)00385-2.
World Values Survey Association. World values survey, 1981–2014 longitudinal aggregate v.20150418 [database]. Aggregate File Producer: JDSystems, Madrid, Spain; 2015. http://www.worldvaluessurvey.org/wvs.jsp. Accessed 14 Sep 2017.

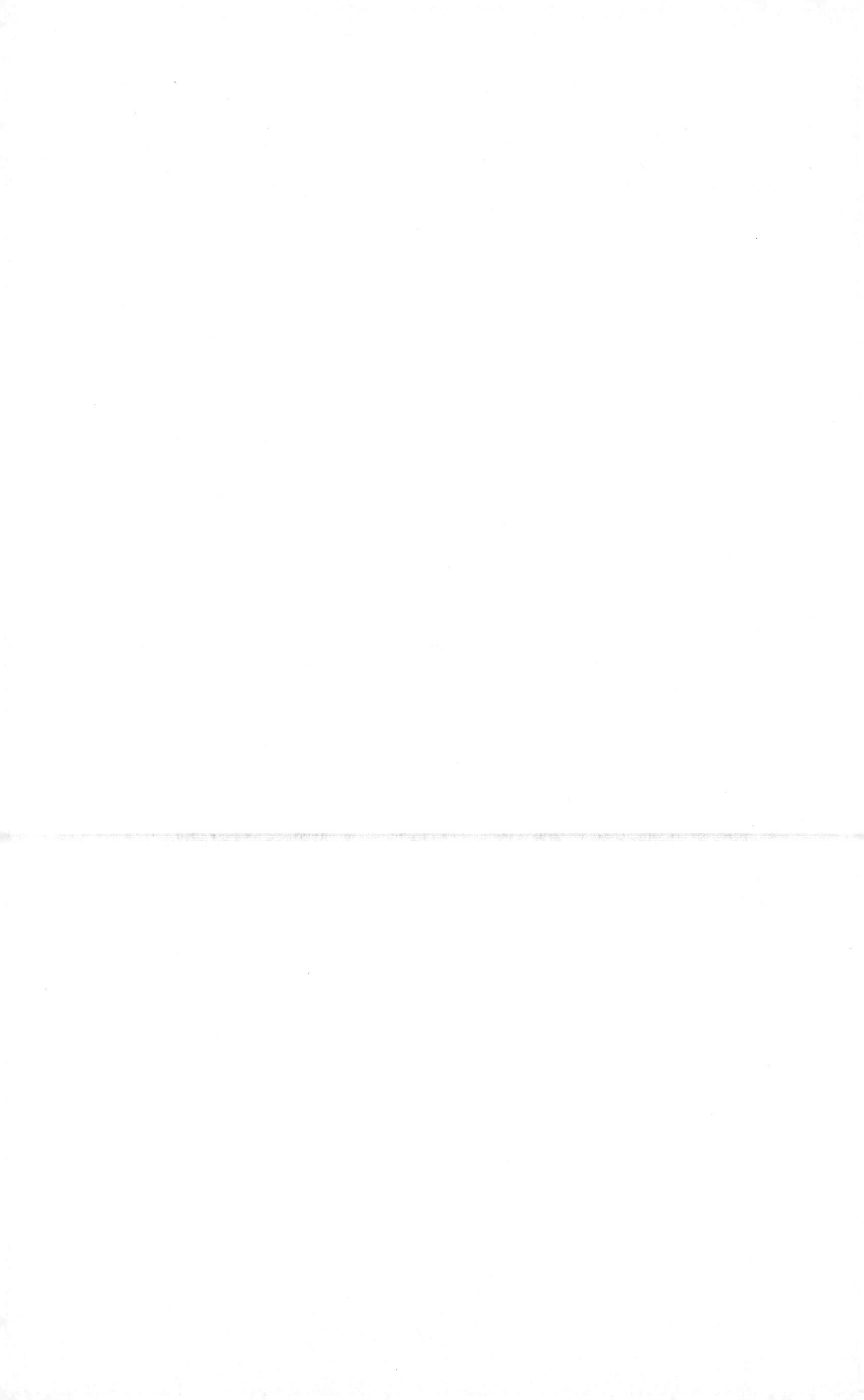

Chapter 2
Green Aid Flows: Trends and Opportunities for Developing Countries

Valeria Costantini and Antonio Mele

Abstract This chapter describes the AidData dataset (1980–2010) that collects aid flows for environmental protection, broadly defined as green aid, that are directed to developing countries. A joint analysis of historical trends and the identification of main donors and recipients reveal why green aid data must be independently gathered apart from general aid flows. The recommendation is based on evidence suggesting that disentangling the flow of different assistance can improve monitoring and performance metrics that more accurately capture the role of international transfers towards achieving global sustainable development goals. The review of specific investment domains and distribution of financing activities among recipients leads to several policy suggestions to modify the international community mechanisms that measure environmental protection and sustainability goals. General recommendations also suggest a foundation for identifying multilateral vs. green aid flow, inclusion criteria for environmental impact projects, and greater accountability stemming from improvements in data reliability.

Acronyms

ASDB	Asian Development Bank
CER	Certified Emission Reduction
CDM	Clean Development Mechanism
COP21	Conference of the Parties in Paris
EC	European Communities
EU ETS	European Union Emission Trading Scheme
GEF	Global Environmental Fund
GCF	Green Climate Fund

V. Costantini (✉) · A. Mele
Department of Economics, Roma Tre University, Rome, Italy
e-mail: valeria.costantini@uniroma3.it

B. A. Fiedler (ed.), *Translating National Policy to Improve Environmental Conditions Impacting Public Health Through Community Planning*,
https://doi.org/10.1007/978-3-319-75361-4_2

GD	Greenness degree
IFI	International financial institutions
IFAD	International Fund for Agricultural Development
IMF	International Monetary Fund
IO	International Organizations
ISDB	Islamic Development Bank
MIGA	Multilateral Investment Guarantee Agency
SDGs	Sustainable Development Goals
UK	United Kingdom
UN	United Nations
WB-CF	World Bank—Carbon Finance Unit
WB-IBRD	World Bank—International Bank for Reconstruction and Development
WB-IDA	World Bank—International Development Association
WB-IFC	World Bank—International Finance Corporation
WB-TF	World Bank—Managed Trust Funds

2.1 Introduction

The quantification of aid flows directed to developing countries to design impact assessment exercises has been addressed by several contributions in the scientific literature. These researchers demonstrate the difficulty in quantifiably differentiating and estimating aid flow that is allocated to environmental protection activities (hereafter called green aid). This problem is mainly attributed to three reasons. They are the (1) reluctance of donors to officially publish and track their financial commitments due to the lack of reliable data, (2) complex nature of determining if a single project has an environmental component embedded due to a lack of specific criteria, and (3) difficulty in identifying specific environment-related projects within total aid flows (Hicks et al. 2010).

However, a strategy to classify and thus distinguish aid flow within a specific environmental purpose presents an opportunity to individuate more precise borders improving these conditions. We draw inspiration from two ethical concepts—the ecological debt (Fenton et al. 2014; Hackmann et al. 2014; Rice 2009) and the climate justice approach (Roberts and Parks 2009). The reasoning behind these two ethical (rather than pure economic) points of view is that the combination of these perspectives provides a platform to distinguish project purpose explaining multilateral vs. bilateral green aid flows. Consequently, this information supports a method for identifying green aid, inclusion criteria for environmental impact projects, and greater accountability stemming from improvements in data reliability.

The ecological debt approach (Rice 2009) can be defined as the obligations industrialized countries owe for the uneven acquisition and exploitation of the natural resource endowments of developing countries without adequate compensation or appropriate recognition. Following this definition, some researchers within the climate change debate propose a debt relief for climate finance swaps, proposing debt-servicing payments to finance environmental projects for adaptation and mitigation (Fenton et al. 2014; Hackmann et al. 2014). This suggestion is relevant for two main reasons. First, within a budget-constrained scenario, such is the case for green aid, debt relief for climate finance swaps could provide an alternative source for financing mitigation and adaptation projects in developing countries; secondly, by financing environmental projects by means of debt-servicing payments would indirectly imply that an ecological debt exists, and the value of payments would approximate value, as perceived by developed countries.

The importance of having an alternative source for financing mitigation and adaptation projects is to increase the amount of green aid flows destined to developing countries, which are historically characterized by volatility in financial terms and geographical concentration in certain cases, and to trigger the environmental change, as recommended by Hackmann et al. (2014). Accordingly, the evaluation of green aid flows and their characteristics in terms of flow consistency, volatility, concentration, geographical distribution and project size (Denizer et al. 2013) is a necessary step both to detect if the past and current green aid flows trend is satisfactory with respect to the Sustainable Development Goals (SDGs), that the United Nations (UN) has recently declared as the new medium-term objectives of the post-2015 Development Agenda, and to determine which alternative financing sources shall be required to reach SDGs targets. Accordingly, this chapter aims at investigating selected stylized facts that can draw a complete picture of past green aid flows:

- The path of green aid flows over last decades in absolute terms to control for the total amount of the collective efforts by the developed part of the world
- The distribution of green aid flows among the recipient countries indicative of a coherent investment path with the development goals of improving equality at the intra-generational and inter-generational level
- The relative effort by major donors to investigate which investment channels should be privileged to maximize the collective efforts and which channels have not worked properly to correct market and institutional failures impeding the active participation of all suitable actors

To this purpose, in this chapter we describe an original dataset built on the project-level database AidData 2.1, which permits access to the complete list of financial bilateral aid flows from donors to recipients in accordance with the official communications given by donor governments and International Organizations (IO).

The analysis of trends over time and distribution among donors and recipients permits a basis from which to detect if such green aid flows are effective in improving the environmental performance of receiving countries. Further, the level of compliance to the two main ethical concepts mentioned above helps to present a clearer overview of resource allocation and utilization by explaining to what extent such green aid flows are effective, thus formulating more accurate assessments of reductions in ecological debt and improvements in addressing climate justice.

2.2 International Aid Flows and Environmental Protection Goals

Identifying aid flows with an environmental purpose is the first crucial problem. Multilateral donors represented by notable international institutions, such as UN agencies, international financial institutions (IFI) and the World Bank, have made the green decision an embedded part of their organizational activity, or in some cases, a priority—such as the Global Environmental Fund (GEF). The World Bank is by far the biggest multilateral donor investor in green projects, providing development assistance in the field of environmental protection through multiple channels and entities (e.g. International Bank for Reconstruction and Development (IBRD); International Development Association (IDA); International Finance Corporation (IFC); Multilateral Investment Guarantee Agency (MIGA) and GEF). Alternatively, the decision to finance and implement environmental projects is a political choice for bilateral donors—comprising donors representing country or national governments. For bilateral donors, aid flows are not always strategically oriented to development assistance and/or economic growth. The geopolitical and trade interests play a large role in determining the geographical allocation of aid flows as well as the sector relevance (Fuchs and Vadlamannati 2013; Sobis and de Vries 2009).

Various controversial positions exist with respect to the impact assessment of green aid flows on the environmental performances of the recipients. On the one hand, despite the large amount of financial support for environmental assistance, there is poor evidence to support that green aid flows have substantially improved recipient environmental performance (Buntaine and Parks 2013). One explanation for this lack of effectiveness might be found in the crucial role played by institutional quality in directing foreign aid towards fruitful environmental projects. This problem is often evident when recipients with the lowest development levels and poor institutional quality are not equipped for oversight of their environmental protection programmes.

A second correlated aspect to be considered is the volatility of the aid flow over time. Inconstant aid flows reduce the effectiveness of medium- and long-term development as well as environmental projects mainly financed in the recipient countries by aid flows due to domestic resource scarcity (Addison and Tarp 2015; Bulíř and Hamann 2008). Furthermore, aid volatility is generally higher in those countries that are most aid-dependent, which are generally the poorest and most vulnerable ones, triggering a vicious cycle (Hudson 2015).

A third explanation—flow concentration—demonstrates the general low effectiveness of green aid in improving environmental performance with respect to the amount of financial resources invested (Boyd et al. 2009; Costantini and Sforna 2014; Knack et al. 2011). In this scenario, large donors are more likely to direct aid flows in trade-related sectors to recipients where there is export competition with other donors, thus implying that the destination of such flows is often chosen under strategic criteria rather than for development or social purposes (Barthel et al. 2014).

These notable perspectives on data reliability, volatility, and flow concentration become focal points from which to generate a dataset that defines and measures the comparative efficiency and effectiveness of green aid. The necessity to rely on significant and holistic data for the correct evaluation of aid flows and the fact that the lack of comprehensive data on aid projects from both bilateral and multilateral donors are often incomplete justify the adoption of different databases per the specific investigation under scrutiny. Other investigations reveal the lack of official data and/or the use of incomplete data in aid-related analyses and studies that brought forth some uncertainty in the significance and the correctness of some empirical results (Lof et al. 2015; Röttgers and Grote 2014). Specifically, in the analysis by Lof et al. (2015) there emerge significant divergent evidences with respect to past analyses and empirical results if different databases are adopted.

Accordingly, adoption of the most complete and transparent database is necessary to reduce the risk of bias results due to subjectivity in data collection. To this purpose, the most suitable information service available in this field is the project-level database AidData 2.1 for two main reasons. First, AidData 2.1 allows reducing data inefficiencies to a minimum, and thus the second reason—the database can conceivably avoid generalizations based on incomplete information. Indeed, utilization of a complete database is paramount to optimizing results (Knack et al. 2011). Thus, AidData can be considered as the optimal choice for this purpose, since metrics include data on donors, recipients and projects obtained directly from donor agencies that were not considered in previous analyses.

2.3 Aid Flows and Green Financing in Developing Countries

AidData 2.1 provides many data allowing a deep disaggregation of sectors and activities with 93 bilateral and multilateral donors, 178 recipients, 37 sectors and years ranging from 1947 to 2012. Years selected for the sample range from 1980 to 2010, and the commitment amount is always expressed in terms of USD at 2009 constant prices and exchange rates. The disaggregation level available in AidData 2.1 allows selecting the following six green sectors, listed in the order of the AidData 2.1 code: (1) Water Supply and Sanitation (code: 14000-14082); (2) Energy (code: 23000-23082); (3) Agriculture (code: 31100-31191); (4) Forestry (code: 31205-31291); (5) Fishing (code: 31300-31391) and (6) General Environment Protection (code: 41000-41082).

According to a criterion of full availability for all the six green sectors and the time span adopted, 15 bilateral and multilateral donors have been selected: Asian Development Bank (ASDB); Denmark; European Communities (EC); Global Environment Facility (GEF); International Fund for Agricultural Development (IFAD); Ireland; Islamic Development Bank (ISDB); Italy; Netherlands; United Kingdom (UK); World Bank—Carbon Finance Unit (WB-CF); World Bank—International Bank for Reconstruction and Development (WB-IBRD); World Bank—International Development Association (WB-IDA); World Bank—International Finance Corporation (WB-IFC); World Bank—Managed Trust Funds (WB-TF). Selected donors mainly correspond to the top donors list provided by

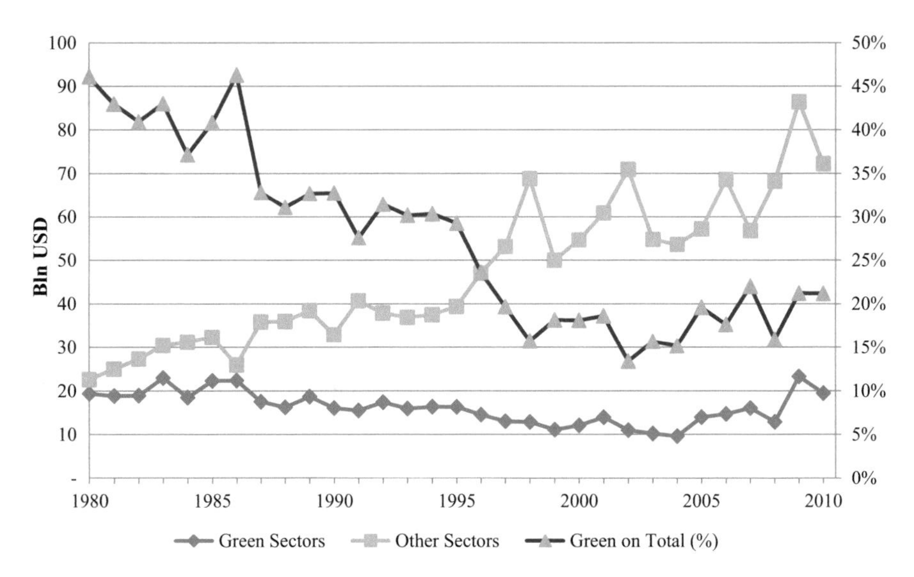

Fig. 2.1 Aid flows from selected donors to all recipients, 1980–2010

Knack et al. (2011) because of the following criteria: aid selectivity, specialization, alignment, and harmonization. Other donors, notwithstanding being very important provider of financial aids for development purposes, have not been selected for the list of selected donors because their activity does not focus on environmental schemes and logics. For example, the International Monetary Fund (IMF), which is a very important provider of financial aid to developing and poor countries, has not been included in the selected donors list because their organizational mission focuses on financial and economic supports without any green component embedded into doctrine. Contrary to donors' selection, all recipient countries available in AidData 2.1 have been included.

The general trend in the period 1980–2010 shows that the green aid flows (in terms of USD) did not increase, facing a negative peak to about 10 billion USD in 1999 and 2004 and returning to about 20 billion USD in 2010. Furthermore, the ratio between green aid flows and total aid has significantly decreased, from about 45% in 1980 to less than 25% in 2010 (Fig. 2.1).

Two dominant factors may have contributed to a portion of the misalignment of the trends related to green sectors and to other sectors approximately after 1995. First, the presence of the first severe global financial and economic crisis that most likely contributed to the increase of aid flows directed to finance development and recovery projects rather than environmental protection activities. Second, the increase in green aid flows in 2008 in absolute value might be explained by the entry into force of the second phase of the European Union Emission Trading Scheme (EU ETS) and the consequent appreciation of prices for carbon permits (Certified Emission Reduction, CER), coming from Clean Development Mechanism projects (CDM projects).

Table 2.1 Top 20 recipients for green aid flows, accumulated million USD from 1980 to 2010

Recipient	Selected donors *(A)*	Other donors *(B)*	All donors *(T = A + B)*	Selected donors on total *(D = A/T)* (%)
India	67,355	29,160	96,515	70
China	44,966	22,847	67,812	66
Indonesia	32,134	23,884	56,018	57
Brazil	25,273	5294	30,568	83
Philippines	15,600	13,954	29,554	53
Pakistan	18,501	10,983	29,483	63
Egypt	11,902	15,687	27,590	43
Mexico	19,332	3497	22,829	85
Turkey	16,942	5760	22,702	75
Bilateral, unspecified	10,209	11,985	22,194	46
Bangladesh	12,377	6339	18,717	66
Viet Nam	7349	10,000	17,349	42
Thailand	8437	7939	16,376	52
Morocco	8259	7279	15,538	53
Iraq	729	13,151	13,879	5
Kenya	5309	5619	10,928	49
Tanzania	5975	4713	10,688	56
Sri Lanka	3727	6899	10,627	35
Malaysia	4711	5565	10,276	46
Colombia	7788	1964	9752	80

This first quantitative assessment reveals that despite the growing concerns debated in the international development agenda over last decades, the degree of environmental awareness in aid investment decisions has not been increased. On the contrary, following massive changes occurring during the globalization process, most aid flows have been directed towards sectors other than the environment. This is a clear sign of institutional failure because the attention devoted to several environmental issues remained confined into theoretical declarations without translating into concrete actions.

When considering distribution patterns of aid flows across donors and recipients, noteworthy is that large countries are the main recipients of green aid flows (in absolute terms) in the whole period under consideration (here ranked in Table 2.1, Column T). Additionally, the percentage of green aid flows financed by the selected donors is a very significant part of total green aid flows received by recipients (Table 2.1, Column D). On average, selected donors contributed to 56% of the total green aid received by all recipients; moreover, the top 20 recipients received 63% of all green aid flows aimed at financing environmental protection all over the world (by all donors).

From the recipients' perspective, green aid flows in absolute terms are disproportionally oriented towards large countries such as India, China, Indonesia

Table 2.2 Top 20 green recipients ranked by GD, accumulated million USD from 1980 to 2010

Recipient	Green sectors *(A)*	Other sectors *(B)*	Greenness Degree $GD = A/(A + B)$ (%)
Niue	8	1	87
Mayotte	56	10	85
Arab Countries	4	1	81
Macao	1	0	57
Far East Asia, regional	356	341	51
Iran	1732	1788	49
Malaysia	4711	5445	46
GLOBAL	2101	2495	46
Samoa	196	242	45
Syria	1173	1477	44
Belarus	474	609	44
Micronesia, Federated States	38	49	43
Botswana	942	1269	43
South Africa	4894	6684	42
South and Central Asia	259	388	40
Palau	10	15	39
Belize	307	478	39
Egypt	11,902	18,582	39
Nauru	6	10	39
China	44,966	71,000	39

and Brazil. However, these countries are not considered as least developing countries but rather as emerging economies. This means that the environmental protection ensured by aid flows takes advantages mostly to countries better equipped in terms of economic and technological resources than poorest economies. This is a clear sign of unevenness in aid flows distribution. Considering that environmental damages and diseases directly affect human well-being and development opportunities, the poorer countries are deprived of crucial resources necessary to increase development opportunities. This unbalance is partly corrected by the facts described in terms of greenness degree (GD) quantification. While the distribution of the total amount of resources directed to green aid is strongly unbalanced favouring large (and relatively less poor) economies, the weight of green aid on total aid (here defined as greenness degree, Column GD in Table 2.2) is relatively higher for smaller and poorer countries, as shown in the table.

As shown in the table, medium and small recipient countries have a higher GD with respect to large countries. Major exception to this trend is China, which ranks number two in terms of green aid amount from selected donors (Column A in Table 2.1), and has a GD of 39%, while smaller countries tend to have higher GDs. Among the donors, GEF (93%) and the WB Carbon Fund (89%) demonstrate their higher propensity to invest in green sectors as a percent of the total aid allocated to the selected donors (e.g. Steckhan 2009, p.2, 19).

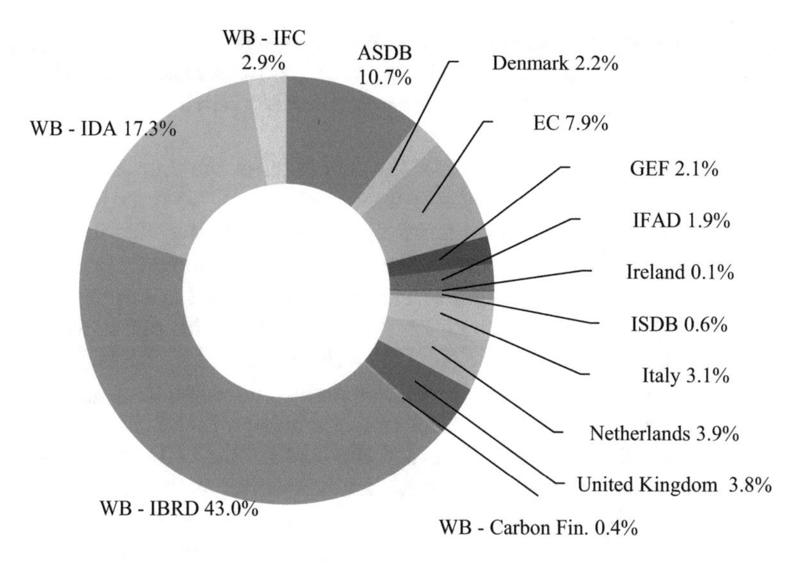

Fig. 2.2 Distribution of green aid flows across selected donors, accumulated from 1980–2010

By considering the previously mentioned UN new development agenda represented by the SDGs, the objective to meet the challenging tasks in the environmental domains emphasized in the SDG framework, (e.g. SDG 6: "Ensure availability and sustainable management of water and sanitation for all"; SDG 7: "Ensure access to affordable, reliable, sustainable and clean energy for all"; SDG 13: "Take urgent action to combat climate change and its impacts"; etc.), requires a greater attention to green aid flows distribution, which is a relevant issue to be included in the international development agenda. In addition, the amount of aid flows directed to environmental protection actions should be largely increased in accordance with the increased attention devoted to these issues by the international community. A challenging sustainable development agenda without proper financial resources specifically designed for environmental purpose could remain a visionary project without a concrete realization.

Both for green sectors and for other sectors, the World Bank Group is the most important player with about 220 billion USD financed to green sectors provided by the WB-IBRD. European Commission and the Asian Development Bank complete a framework where multilateral donors guarantee most (total and green) aid flows. Among bilateral donors selected, the United Kingdom, the Netherlands and Italy tend to be the greenest financers (Fig. 2.2).

The distribution across donors and recipients of green aid flows appears to be a crucial aspect to explore and capture some relevant information about environmental performance associated with aid projects. From the donors' side, the largest portion of green aid flows is associated with multilateral donors that have a specific environmentally oriented content in their constitutive declarations. This means that aid flows with environmental purposes might be stimulated only if such specific multilateral institutions are reinforced both in terms of financial assets, skills and competencies coherent with the increasing complexity in environmental protection actions.

One of the indicators suggested for the definition of aid specialization is the average size of project commitments (Knack et al. 2011). Accordingly, Table 2.3 reports the average project size in terms of donor commitment for the aid flows financed by the selected donors and destined to all recipients distinguished by sector. The greater selected donors as classified by Fig. 2.2 correspond to those parties financing larger projects both for green sectors and for other sectors. That also indicates that, on average, recipient countries supported by the largest donors are those receiving the larger projects in green sectors. Green sector projects tend to be slightly smaller than projects in other sectors with an average financing value to about 21 million USD for green sectors and about 24 million USD for other sectors.

However, if green sectors are disentangled, noteworthy is that the average size for energy projects is much higher than average project size for all sectors, with 36 million USD. General environmental protection projects and water projects are also very important in terms of project size, recording 28 and 23 million USD, respectively. Remaining green sectors show very different average project sizes. Also in monetary terms, the distribution of green aid flows financed by the selected donors is strongly unbalanced across the six green sectors investigated herein. The larger portions of green flows are oriented towards energy and agricultural projects (with 37% and 33% of total green flows in absolute value, respectively). Water (18%) and general environmental protection (8%) follow. Fishery and forestry projects are given markedly minor importance in terms of monetary budgets.

With respect to the general fact that the average project size in terms of total amount of financial resources invested is smaller for green sectors rather than for the other sectors, the following discussion arises. By considering the public good characteristic of environmental goods, the difficulty of assessing and quantifying the benefits deriving from environmental protection in monetary terms emerges. When facing scarce financial resources, the selection process for project financing is often oriented through a cost–benefit analysis. If the economic quantification of benefits coming from more traditional development-oriented projects is easier than in the case of environmental projects, this directly brings to a preference made by policymakers and multilateral institutions on the other sectors. The policy advice in this case is rather complex, because there is a preliminary necessary condition represented by a unanimous consensus on project evaluation methods and criteria, that is a challenging scope for the scientific and the policy communities. Secondly, other policy considerations regard the necessary coordination into multilateral donors' frameworks to gather financial assets large enough to invest in green projects that necessitate larger monetary flows. The dispersion of scarce resources across different projects might negatively influence the environmental performance of such investments, reducing the effectiveness of aid projects in achieving environmental goals.

Table 2.3 Average project size, based on accumulated million USD from 1980 to 2010

			Green sectors						
Selected donors	Total aid	Other sectors	Total	Water Supply & Sanitation	Energy	Agric.	Fores.	Fish.	General Env. Prot.
ASDB	22.49	25.32	19.65	17.79	48.74	15.11	9.29	12.38	14.61
Denmark	2.5	0.42	4.59	6.21	7.13	4.45	2.92	4.3	2.52
EC	13.38	19.46	7.3	10.19	16.83	6.18	4.57	1.84	4.16
GEF	5.45	5.85	5.06	6.75	7.33	3.62	4.3	4.84	3.48
IFAD	9.82	14.84	4.79	3.81	–	11.44	2.57	6.89	4.05
Ireland	0.16	0.19	0.12	0.25	0.04	0.23	0.03	0.09	0.09
ISDB	5.24	4.75	5.73	7.32	10.59	5.66	2.34	3.96	4.51
Italy	2.17	0.33	4.01	2.82	15.36	1.46	1.22	2.47	0.73
Netherlands	1.39	0.56	2.23	3.02	3.48	2.48	1.93	1.23	1.2
UK	2.48	1.51	3.45	2.64	9.25	3.05	2.09	1.82	1.83
WB-CF	22.06	8.62	35.51	3.73	5.68	–	1.51	–	202.16
WB-IBRD	158.56	184.54	132.57	127.91	257.01	148.88	70.3	53.04	138.29
WB-IDA	58.87	61.38	56.35	70.25	78.23	65.56	55.98	34.39	33.68
WB-IFC	30.77	29.6	31.94	77.12	71.27	15.41	15.08	5.71	7.04
WB-TF	7.32	9.82	4.81	8.57	10.92	4.6	–	2.05	2.69
Simple Average	22.84	24.48	21.21	23.23	36.13	19.21	11.61	9	28.07

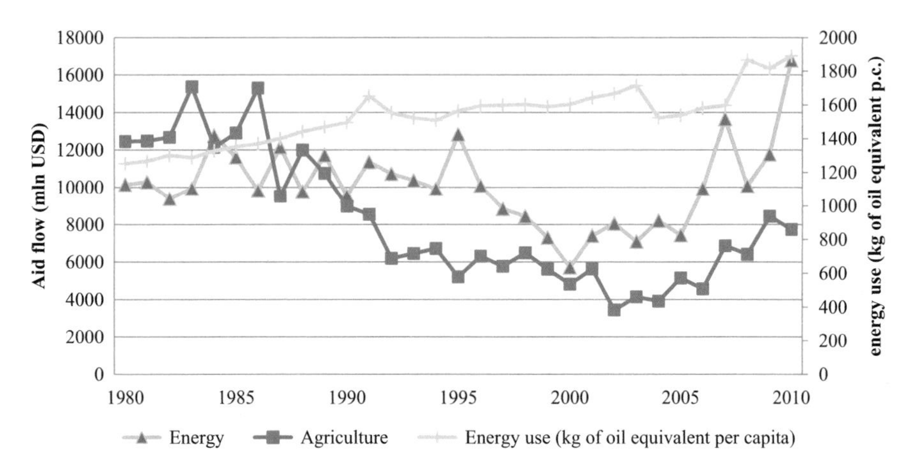

Fig. 2.3 Agriculture and energy sectors, annual total aid flows and energy use per capita from 1980 to 2010

A deeper investigation of specific green sectors allows highlighting additional stylized facts. First, green aid flows in the selected period show interesting paths especially for energy and agriculture. If monetary value of aid flows in these two sectors is compared with per capita energy use (expressed in terms of kg of oil equivalent per capita on average for the recipient countries here considered, World Development Indicators, online database), during the first decade (1980–1989) aid flows directed to agriculture are slightly higher with respect to the energy sectors (Fig. 2.3). Starting from 1989/1990, there is a clear and increasing inversion of this trend, with a relative stability for energy aid flows up to 1995/1996 (and a subsequent fall up to 2000) and a sharp fall for agricultural aids, up to 2000. On the contrary, energy use per capita reveals a stable and increasing trend over the whole period, thus explaining the growing interest in energy projects with respect to agricultural ones. In addition, aid flows in both sectors seem to have been largely influenced by the Kyoto Protocol (United Nations 2014), recording positive trends from 2006/2007 onwards.

Given the relevance of the energy sector with respect to the other green sectors and to the other sectors as emerged across the whole analysis made in this work, further information available from the database here developed with regard to the distribution across recipient countries of aid flows classified in this sector. Accordingly, the percentage of energy aid flow on total green sectors aid flows has been calculated, together with a similar percentage calculated with respect to total aid flows received by each country (Table 2.4). Countries are listed by the ranking criterion of energy aid on green aid ration, as calculated in the last Column (E/G).

The first evidence is that, apart from few exceptions (i.e. inlands and small countries), many medium size countries are in the list of top 20 energy-oriented recipients, such as South Africa, Ukraine and Pakistan. Among the top 20 recipients in terms of green aid, listed in Table 2.1, only four countries (i.e. India, Iraq,

Table 2.4 Top 20 energy recipients from all donors, accumulated from 1980 to 2010

Recipients	Total aid (million USD) *(T)*	Green aid (million USD) *(G)*	Energy aid (million USD) *(E)*	Energy aid on total aid (%) *(E/T)*	Energy aid on green aid (%) *(E/G)*
Cayman Islands	30	3	3	11.31	100.00
Hong Kong, China	54	2	2	3.62	100.00
Czech Republic	6833	549	539	7.89	98.16
South Africa	12,567	5883	4501	35.82	76.51
Tokelau	3	3	2	76.16	76.16
Libya	75	33	24	32.69	73.65
Georgia	5684	1699	1179	20.74	69.39
Estonia	907	78	53	5.81	67.54
Ukraine	28,032	2304	1526	5.44	66.21
Nauru	70	60	38	55.16	64.11
Belarus	2361	517	314	13.30	60.71
Iraq	24,306	13,879	8376	34.46	60.35
Lithuania	2004	173	104	5.19	60.27
Bahrain	136	20	12	8.72	60.00
Syria	4760	3284	1963	41.24	59.79
Malaysia	15,721	10,276	5924	37.68	57.65
Serbia	15,769	2325	1305	8.28	56.14
Pakistan	80,036	29,483	16,068	20.08	54.50
Singapore	126	12	7	5.32	53.68
India	224,767	96,515	51,728	23.01	53.60

Malaysia and Pakistan) are simultaneously present in Table 2.4, meaning that only a small portion of large recipients in terms of green sectors are energy-oriented recipients. Noteworthy is that some medium size countries have strong energy-oriented attitude even with respect to total aid flow. For instance, South Africa total aid is constituted by 35.82% of energy aid; Iraq's energy aid is 34.46% of total aid, while Syria's and Malaysia's energy aid flows are, respectively, 41.24% and 37.68% of the total aid.

This characterization of the energy sector needs further investigation. Accordingly, a selected group of oil-producing recipients has been built (formed by Algeria, Argentina, Brazil, Egypt, Indonesia, Malaysia, Mexico, Nigeria, Senegal, South Africa, Sudan) and compared with the other recipients in terms of energy aid on green aid ratio (Fig. 2.4).

The energy aid on green aid ratio is always lower for the oil-producer group. While the percentage is lower, the standard deviation assumed across the whole period is rather higher for the oil-producer group (7.2) with respect to the other recipients (5.6), revealing in the first case a stronger connection with the fossil fuel markets.

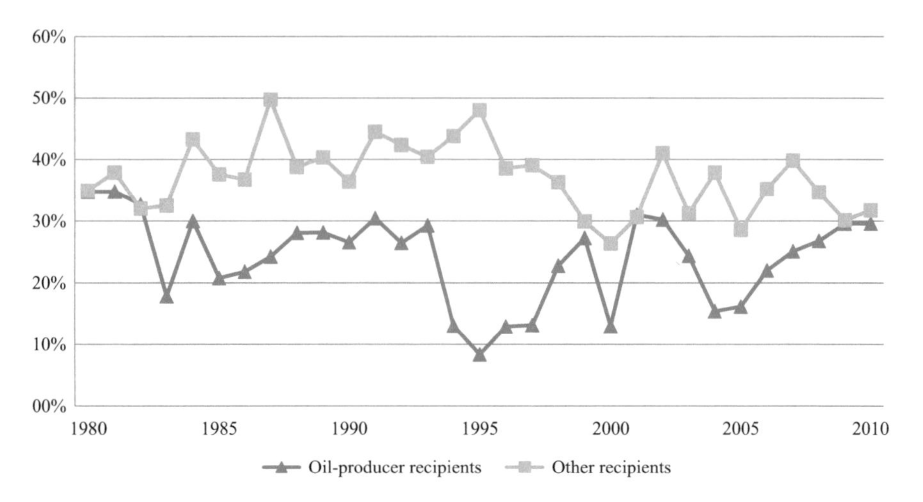

Fig. 2.4 Energy aid on green aid flows (%) for oil-producer group and other recipients

Following the description of green sectors specific paths, other interesting features appear. Starting from the early 1990s, the relative stable increase in energy-related aid flows with respect to the other green sectors is perfectly coherent with the growing consensus on the crucial role played by a secure and stable energy supply for ensuring a long-term development path. Moreover, by considering that the oil-producer recipients have a lower energy aid on green aid ratio with respect to other recipients, on average we can assume that countries that base their economic growth on oil production tend to be less active in terms of energy aid reception. This evidence is obvious from one side, since those countries obtaining from the market enough financial resources due to fossil fuel profits are less favourable to direct aid flows to the energy sector, since they can already rely on sufficient resources. On the other side, this is a clear sign of the importance of investing in the energy sector, and for those countries that cannot ensure the proper financial support thanks to domestic resources, the international aid flows represent a necessary condition for escaping energy poverty and improving the availability of a safe and affordable energy as a crucial input for dynamic development pathways.

2.4 Conclusions and Policy Implications

The descriptive analysis presented in this chapter represents a first step in the investigation on trends and causality nexus in green aid flows from donors to developing countries. Several preliminary issues arise from these results that allows formulating numerous reflections upon potential improvements in the current policy framework that could increase the effectiveness of aid flows and thus, ensure environmental protection.

First, despite the growing attention devoted by the international development agenda to environmental issues, as clearly revealed by the recent adoption of the SDGs framework by the UN, a decreasing share of global resources generally classified as aid flows has been directed towards environmental protection activities. This misalignment between the theoretical institutional framework and the practical solutions implemented at the international level should be carefully addressed in the design of future development strategies, otherwise the SDGs would remain just a dream, as exactly occurred for the Millennium Development Goals, previously adopted by the UN.

Second, there emerges that multilateral institutions are the most effective in collecting financial resources oriented towards environmental protection, while single countries represent donors with a substantially reduced capacity to collect resources oriented to environmental purposes. The direct policy implication we can draw is the necessity to increase the amount of financial resources managed by those multilateral agencies that, as the GEF or the World Bank Carbon Finance project, have in their constitutional framework the major scope of environmental protection. As an example, we can mention the vast debate arisen during last Conference of the Parties in Paris (COP21), December 2015, upon the crucial role played by the Green Climate Fund (GCF), considered as the most effective compensatory measures for climate change damages and mitigation efforts available for poor economies. While from a theoretical side the GCF is considered as an effective compensatory tool with pro-development and equality objectives, from a practical point of view GCF is considered as inconsistent in resource availability terms since the financial efforts provided by developed economies are currently well below the required investments from developing countries in a dynamic perspective (Carter et al. 2015).

Third, the uneven distribution of green aid flows among recipients, that favours medium and large economies while leaving behind those poorest countries with greater need for foreign financial resources, shows that countries where the improvement in the ecological and environmental quality is particularly challenging, due to severe underdevelopment conditions, are collecting the smallest portion of resources.

Several solutions have been discussed in this context. Researchers promote the necessity to reform the constitutional framework of several international agencies acting as multilateral donors to explicitly include in their overall scopes the environmental protection activities (Hicks et al. 2010). This will lead to increasing the number of large donors directly involved in such activities, thus collecting larger amount of financial resources for green projects.

The creation of a new World Environmental Organisation as a counterbalancing force with respect to the World Trade Organisation (Macmillan 2001), or the adoption of binding International Environmental Agreements designed as self-enforcing, with ad hoc incentives to convince countries to join or to remain part of the agreement (Fuentes-Albero and Rubio 2010), are two examples of reforming the institutional framework. Also, the adoption of specific financial instruments by existing international agencies, as for instance the release of the World Bank Green bonds (World Bank n.d.), could constitute an alternative or a complementary action that could significantly help financing green aid projects (Reiche 2010).

Finally, the financial market could be exploited. According to some researchers (Fenton et al. 2014; Hackmann et al. 2014; Stewart et al. 2009), the debt-servicing payments could be used to finance climate change actions as a form of climate finance swaps. Thus, the problem of ecological debt shall find a place within future global climate change regime, because the concept includes the historical responsibility as one of the key criteria used for distributing mitigation and adaptation costs (Gomez-Echeverri 2013; Roberts and Parks 2009).

The climate change policy regime could be a cornerstone in the direction of making greener development pathways of poor countries for three reasons. First, the descriptive statistics developed in this analysis informs that the energy sector is one of the most attractive for aid flows, revealing that it is a crucial sector for long-term development strategies. Second, given the centrality of the energy sector, the increasing attention devoted by the climate regime to technological transfer to facilitate the transition towards a low carbon energy system also in the underdeveloped world could ensure the adoption of cleaner and more efficient technologies, thus reducing those constraints associated to energy poverty. Third, the institutional framework developed over the last two decades within the UN Framework Convention on Climate Change is an example of a Grand Coalition where all countries might cooperate, which is a necessary condition for achieving a unanimous consensus on the future long-term global development vision (Bigsten and Tengstam 2015; Bourguignon and Platteau 2015; Glemarec and Connelly 2011).

Glossary

Aid flow Development (financial) aid (in form of grant or loan) provided by donor countries and international organizations to developing recipient countries with the clear aim of economic development

Bilateral green aid flow Aid flows allocated by donor countries (i.e. States) to recipient countries for environmental protection activities

Climate justice An ethical concept assessing the importance of considering historical responsibilities within climate negotiations

Donor A country (bilateral donor) or an international organization (multilateral donor) providing aid flows

Ecological debt The moral obligations industrialized countries owe for the past uneven acquisition and exploitation of the natural resource endowments of developing countries without adequate compensation or appropriate recognition

Multilateral green aid flow Aid flows allocated by international organizations to recipient countries for environmental protection activities

Recipient A country receiving aid flows

References

Addison T, Tarp F. Aid policy and the macroeconomic management of aid. World Dev. 2015;69:1–5.
Barthel F, et al. Competition for export markets and the allocation of foreign aid: the role of spatial dependence among donor countries. World Dev. 2014;64:350–65.
Bigsten A, Tengstam S. International coordination and the effectiveness of aid. World Dev. 2015;69:75–85.
Bourguignon F, Platteau J-P. The hard challenge of aid coordination. World Dev. 2015;69:86–97.
Boyd E, et al. Reforming the CDM for sustainable development: lessons learned and policy futures. Environ Sci Pol. 2009;12(7):820–31.
Bulíř A, Hamann A. Volatility of development aid: from the frying pan into the fire? World Dev. 2008;36(10):2048–66.
Buntaine MT, Parks BC. When do environmentally focused assistance projects achieve their objectives? Evidence from World Bank post-project evaluations. Global Environ Polit. 2013;13(2):65–88.
Carter P, et al. Dynamic aid allocation. J Int Econ. 2015;95(2):291–304.
Costantini V, Sforna G. Do bilateral trade relationships influence the distribution of CDM projects? Clim Pol. 2014;14:559–80.
Denizer C, et al. Good countries or good projects? Macro and micro correlates of World Bank project performance. J Dev Econ. 2013;105:288–302.
Fenton A, et al. Debt relief and financing climate change action. Nat Clim Chang. 2014;4(8):650–3.
Fuchs A, Vadlamannati KC. The needy donor: an empirical analysis of India's aid motives. World Dev. 2013;44:110–28.
Fuentes-Albero C, Rubio SJ. Can international environmental cooperation be bought? Eur J Oper Res. 2010;202(1):255–64.
Glemarec Y, Connelly C. Catalysing climate finance: a guidebook on policy and financing options to support green, low-emission and climate-resilient development. United Nations Development Programme; 2011.
Gomez-Echeverri L. The changing geopolitics of climate change finance. Clim Pol. 2013;13(5):632–48.
Hackmann H, et al. The social heart of global environmental change. Nat Clim Chang. 2014;4(8):653–5.
Hicks RL, et al. Greening aid? Understanding the environmental impact of development assistance. Oxford: Oxford University Press; 2010.
Hudson J. Consequences of aid volatility for macroeconomic management and aid effectiveness. World Dev. 2015;69:62–74.
Knack S, et al. Aid quality and donor rankings. World Dev. 2011;39(11):1907–17.
Lof M, et al. Aid and income: another time-series perspective. World Dev. 2015;69:19–30.
Macmillan F. WTO and the environment. London: Sweet & Maxwell; 2001.
Reiche D. Sovereign wealth funds as a new instrument for climate protection policy: study of Norway as a pioneer of ethical guidelines for environmental protection. Energy. 2010;35(9):3569–77.
Rice J. North–South relations and the ecological debt: asserting a counter-hegemonic discourse. Crit Sociol. 2009;35(2):225–52.
Roberts TJ, Parks C. Ecologically unequal exchange, ecological debt, and climate justice: the history and implications of three related ideas for a new social movement. Int J Comp Sociol. 2009;50(3–4):385–409.
Röttgers D, Grote U. Africa and the clean development mechanism: what determines project investments? World Dev. 2014;62:201–12.
Sobis I, de Vries MS. Technical cooperation within the context of foreign aid: trends for the CEE countries in transition (1991–2004). Int Rev Adm Sci. 2009;75(4):565–84.
Steckhan U. Financial flows for environment: World Bank, UNDP, UNEP. Washington, DC: The World Bank; 2009.

Stewart RB, et al. Climate finance for limiting emissions and promoting green development: mechanisms, regulation and governance. In: Stewart RB, et al., editors. Climate finance: regulatory and funding strategies for climate change and global development. New York: New York University Press; 2009. p. 3–34.
The World Bank (WB). World Bank green bonds. n.d. http://treasury.worldbank.org/cmd/htm/WorldBankGreenBonds.html. Accessed 13 Apr 2017.
United Nations. Framework convention on climate change: clean development mechanism. 2014. https://unfccc.int/kyoto_protocol/mechanisms/items/1673.php. Accessed 13 Apr 2017.

Further Reading

AIDDATA database. [Research Release 2.1]. http://aiddata.org/aiddata-research-releases. Accessed 1 Mar 2015.
The World Bank. Selectivity and performance: IDA's country assessment and development effectiveness. Washington, DC: World Bank Group; 2007.
The World Bank. Community development, carbon fund (CDCF): annual report. Washington, DC: World Bank Group; 2010.
The World Bank. Green bond fact sheet. Washington, DC: World Bank Group; 2013a, August 13.
The World Bank. Mapping carbon pricing initiatives: development and prospects. Washington, DC: World Bank Group; 2013b.

Chapter 3
Food Sustainability Index Report on the United States: The Good, the Bad, and the Ugly

Beth Ann Fiedler

Abstract Global concern for land use revolves around human activity, such as agriculture for food, employment, recreation, and daily sustenance (e.g., air, water, shelter). While the introduction of policy helps to abate the impact of detrimental land use practices in the United States, other national food sustainability indicators created by The Economist Intelligence Unit and the Barilla Center for Food & Nutrition (BCFN) introduce new performance metrics that inform policy. These indicators, such as the environmental impact of agriculture on natural land and water resources, provide a method to determine if key factors are being addressed or have yet to progress towards desired targets and then compare results to other nations. The Food Sustainability Index report, based on the United Nations Sustainable Development Goals and other international input such as the Milan Protocol, demonstrates the US status in the global race for improvements in diet, agricultural practices, and food waste. This brief reflects positive, marginal and poor indicators of US headway on overarching problems relating to climate change, such as food loss and waste, sustainable agriculture, and nutritional challenges impacting the ecosystem and population health. These indicators provide a baseline and progression to pinpoint areas that remain unresolved to educate, spur on innovators to pioneer solutions, and guide policymakers.

3.1 Introduction

All national contributions towards food sustainability help to advance several common targets from the United Nations Sustainable Development Goals (UN SDGs) to improve nutrition (SDG 2) and sustainable consumption and production (SDG 12) (2015). One method to achieve these and other international goals is to monitor progress on component objectives at the national level. This premise led the Barilla

B. A. Fiedler (✉)
Independent Research Analyst, Jacksonville, FL, USA

B. A. Fiedler (ed.), *Translating National Policy to Improve Environmental Conditions Impacting Public Health Through Community Planning*,
https://doi.org/10.1007/978-3-319-75361-4_3

Center for Food & Nutrition (BCFN) to create The Food Sustainability Index (FSI), "a tool designed to highlight international policies and best practices relating to global paradoxes and to the main SDGs for food, climate change, sustainable cities, responsible production and consumption, health, gender equality, education and infrastructure" (BCFN 2016a, *para* 1; United Nations 2015).

France achieved the highest overall FSI composite score (67.53) in 2016 on a scale of 100 while Japan was second overall at 66.66 followed by Canada at 64.86. France also topped two categories—(1) food loss and waste, and (2) nutritional challenges while Germany led in sustainable agriculture. The USA did not reach any top 10 categories. The highest US ranking was number 11 in food loss and waste (58.86) behind number 10 Columbia at 60.02 and narrowly edging out Ethiopia at 58.66 (BCFN 2016b).

Assessing the factors that are relevant to planetary ecosystem sustainability has continued to evolve into these new national performance measures. The Economist Intelligence Unit and the BCFN tested 25 countries in three categories—(1) food loss and waste, (2) sustainable agriculture, and (3) nutritional challenges to obtain an overall composite score in a food sustainability study. Food loss is generally defined as products that are discarded, left uneaten, or otherwise removed from the supply chain (World Resources Institute 2016), while sustainable agriculture occurs when farming methods embrace ecosystem friendly processes to avoid natural resource depletion. "The basic goals of sustainable agriculture are environmental health, economic profitability, and social and economic equity" (National Sustainable Agricultural Coalition n.d., *para* 2). Finally, the FSI incorporates the concept of nutritional challenges under the general categories of life quality (e.g., undernourishment, micronutrient deficiency), life expectancy (e.g., health impact due to nutritional deficiencies), dietary patterns such as the purchasing power for fresh food and diets high in sugar content, and policy (BCFN 2016b).

However, the grading scale reflects just how much more work is needed to reach acceptable levels of food sustainability across the globe. Scores 67+ that are approaching 100 reflect a positive direction for existing policy and practices. However even the best overall nations, such as France (67.53), barely squeaked into top category indicating that room for improvement is consistent across all nations undergoing the analysis. Marginal progress towards sustainable practice in individual and overall categories is indicated by scores ranging from 34 to 67 while scores ranging from 0 to 33 reflect little or no progress towards end goals.

"The Milan Protocol promotes healthy lifestyles to fight famine and obesity, sustainable agriculture and a 50% reduction in food waste by 2020" (BCFN 2016c, *para* 4). The FSI metrics were elicited from these three overarching global paradoxes defined in the 2015 updated Milan Protocol. Specifically, these paradoxes are (1) the amount of wasted food that could be used to feed the hungry, (2) unbalanced sustainable agriculture practices versus low nutritional value/high resource cost in raising cattle, and (3) the portion of the global population that suffer from hunger while two times that number overconsume (BCFN 2015). Thus, the index focuses on climate change resulting from the impact of global practices of agricultural production, land use, and national dietary eating patterns that could be reversed through education.

While the FSI results highlight outstanding practices in the USA, such as air quality climate change mitigation, their sluggish status in the global race for improvements in some indicators of nutrition, agricultural practices, and food waste is an important pointer targeting specific areas for improvement. The index scores provide a broad sweep of the status of sustainable agriculture that demonstrates the need for a cultural shift away from poor dietary habits reflected in a disproportionate consumption of unhealthy food products (e.g., high sugar, fast food) and general overconsumption combined with low physical activity levels. This brief reflects positive, moderate and negative indicators of progression to help educate, and perhaps formulate, innovative solutions.

3.2 United States Food Sustainability

The USA remains dedicated to improving climate change in building design standards (GAO 2016a), providing tools to communicate the environmental impact of climate change on public health (CDC 2017), and addressing the agricultural conservation through various programs including revisiting the agricultural impact of renewable biofuels on the environment (GAO 2016b, 2017a; von Witzke and Noleppa 2014). A considerable number of resources across dozens of agencies contribute to climate change resolution from the ocean floor—National Oceanographic Atmospheric Administration (NOAA), to the sky—National Aeronautics and Space Administration (NASA), and everything in between (GAO n.d.).

(GAO n.d., *para* 1):

> Federal funding for climate change research, technology, international assistance, and adaptation has increased from $2.4 billion in 1993 to $11.6 billion in 2014, with an additional $26.1 billion for climate change programs and activities provided by the American Recovery and Reinvestment Act in 2009.

The total amount of funds allocated to various agencies to address climate change should be considered in the wake of disapproval of President Trump's proposed budget reduction for the US Environmental Protection Agency (EPA) (GAO 2016c). Further, that the budget may not reflect assumed national disinterest in climate change but instead, the redistribution of funds to the many agencies engaged in climate change activities (GAO n.d.).

Table 3.1 demonstrates the positive results stemming from extensive agency investment and resource allocation towards policy development in the areas of food loss and general dietary patterns affecting public health. Food loss policy is one of two fully sustainable ratings for the USA based on the US Department of Agriculture ongoing recommendations (USDA n.d.). The other is air quality, measured in greenhouse gas (GHG) emissions, through a US EPA Agency policy platform that monitors emissions and targets specific areas to reduce emissions (EPA 2017). US plans

Table 3.1 The good: positive results of the United States Food Sustainability Index Report, 2016 (The Economist Intelligence Unit and the Barilla Center for Food & Nutrition 2016b)

Categories	United States	Food loss and waste	Sustainable agriculture	Nutritional challenges
Food Loss	Food Loss	93.58		
	Policy response to food loss	100		
	Causes of distribution-level loss	75		
	Solutions to distribution-level loss	74.93		
End-User Waste	Policy response to food waste	78.95		
Water Resources	Water Scarcity		83.33	
Land	Land ownership		71.04	
	Environmental biodiversity		94.22	
	Productivity		67.51	
Air	Climate change mitigation		100	
Life Quality	Prevalence of under-and malnourishment			98.77
	Micronutrient deficiency			88.31
Life Expectancy	Life expectancy			82.12
	Impact on health of nutritional deficiencies			99.34
Dietary Patterns	Purchasing power for fresh food			72.74
Policy response to dietary patterns	Policy			100

Note: Scale 67+ positive direction for existing policy and practices; 34–67 Marginal progress; 0–33 reflect little or no progress towards sustainable practices

to further reduce emissions by 2025 to levels 26–28% below 2005 levels were announced in the Intended Nationally Determined Contribution (INDC) following the United Nations Convention on Climate Change (UNFCCC 2015).

Environmental biodiversity—the variety of species and organisms in an ecosystem—is the strongest US indicator of positive land use (94.22) but how the nation uses land in terms of productivity barely moved beyond marginal measures (67.51). The USDA considers the protection of natural resources (e.g., farmlands, wetlands, forests, flood plains) important to the nation's water supply and an economic asset as raw material for production and agriculture (USDA 1983). Therefore, continuous attention is afforded to land policy use to secure these assets.

3.3 United States Environmental Land Use

The seven major land uses in conjunction with environmental protection are well-known having been reported in many USDA and EPA publications. They include physical resource management, waste disposition, transportation, urbanization, agriculture, wilderness, and recreation. However, the volume of US land dedicated

Table 3.2 The bad: marginal results of the United States Food Sustainability Index Report, 2016 (The Economist Intelligence Unit and the Barilla Center for Food & Nutrition 2016b)

Categories	United States	Sustainable Agriculture	Nutritional Challenges
Water Resources	Sustainability of water withdrawal	61.50	
	Waste management	50.00	
Land	Environmental impact of agriculture on land	36.99	
	Animal welfare policies	57.14	
	Diversification of agricultural system	58.92	
	Quality of R&D and innovation	55.48	
Air	Environmental impact of agriculture on the atmosphere	59.07	
Life Quality	Ecological efficiency of supporting people's well-being		37.30
	Healthcare expenditure and costs		39.61
	Ecological efficiency of supporting people's well-being		37.30

Note: Scale 67+ positive direction for existing policy and practices; 34–67 Marginal progress

to agricultural purposes makes the topic of sustainable agriculture important to the vitality of the nation.

The USDA compiles US Census of Agriculture reports reporting land use details in conjunction with information supplied by the Economic Research Services (ERS) since the mid-twentieth century. Alaska contains the principal portion of forest land while grassland pasture and range are prominent in the contiguous 48 states accounting for approximately 52% of the US land base in 2012 was "used for agricultural purposes, including cropping, grazing (on pasture, range, and in forests), and farmsteads/farm roads" (USDA 2017, *para* 1). The total US land area approximates 2.3 billion acres (USDA 2017).

Table 3.2 reflects marginal progress on several aspects of land use that continue to be problematic for the USA despite concerted efforts in agricultural conservation (GAO 2017a). Not surprisingly, these challenging activities are based on agricultural use causing environmental impact on the land (36.99) and the atmosphere (59.07).

While US food sustainability policy has positively addressed some aspects of food loss, dietary patterns, and climate change mitigation for air quality, the FSI indicates that the nation has not sufficiently advanced in the development of instruments, programs, or tools to address other specific elements related to land use. Weaknesses in policy and long-term implications for quality of life are inherent in several factors. For example, Native American tribal land use including road access, transportation and consequent education benefits (GAO 2017b), protection of drinking water sources (GAO 2016d), and rural water infrastructure (GAO 2015) contaminated with farming pesticides are among some of the topical areas of concern. Further, they demonstrate the wide array of technical proficiencies and collaboration between and among multi-sectoral agencies to address the complex nature of land use problems that are slowly improving over time.

3.4 United States Environmental and Nutritional Challenges

While the impact of agriculture on water resources (2.48), animal feed and aggressive biofuel policies (2.43) (GAO 2016b, 2017a) present obstacles to national policy, poor personal food selection of products high in sugar and fat are leading challenges for Americans (BCFN 2016c). Heart disease continues to be at the top leading causes of death for Americans despite a reported 61% decline between 1975 and 2015 from 431.2 to 168.5 deaths per 100,000 population; however, an uptick between 2014 (167.0) and 2015 (168.5) represents reason for pause for the persistent health problem (National Center for Health Statistics, 2017, p.4).

Table 3.3 reflects insufficient progress reflected in nutritional challenges including dietary patterns with high sugar diets (0) and too much access to fast food with little nutritional value (0). Further, the combination of poor food intake and low physical activity (10.91) and prevalence of overnourishment (14.90) reduces life quality and expectancy (BCFN 2016b).

Table 3.3 The ugly: poor progress results of the United States Food Sustainability Index Report, 2016 (The Economist Intelligence Unit and the Barilla Center for Food & Nutrition 2016b)

Categories	United States	Food Loss and Waste	Sustainable Agriculture	Nutritional Challenges
End User-Waste	Food loss at end user	9.34		
Water Resources	Environmental impact of agriculture on water		2.48	
Land	Impact of land of animal feed and biofuels		2.43	
	Land use		30.82	
	Land users		31.44	
	Agricultural subsidies		0	
Life Expectancy	Prevalence of over nourishment			14.90
	Physical activity levels			10.91
Dietary Patterns	Prevalence of sugar in diets			0
	Number of people per fast food restaurant			0

Note: Scale 67+ positive direction for existing policy and practices; 34–67 Marginal progress; 0–33 reflect little or no progress towards sustainable practices

3.5 Summary

This chapter introduces some of the persistent and emerging topics of environmental conditions impacting public health, such as food sustainability and land use, posing areas for improvement demonstrated in the Food Sustainability Index (FSI). While this chapter focused on US results, the FSI serves as an international performance metric developed by the Barilla Center for Food & Nutrition. The FSI objective is to determine national progress on three facets of climate change—food loss and waste, sustainable agriculture, and nutrition on the global ecosystem. International comparisons demonstrate that despite superior ratings in some areas, such as food loss and air quality policy, the USA is lagging other nations in land, life quality, and life expectancy. However, the FSI report indicates that all 25 countries in the study have challenges to progress in a positive direction for multiple existing policy and practices. This chapter also provides additional recommended resources to enrich the foundation of public and international law.

Glossary

Environmental biodiversity The variety of species and organisms in an ecosystem

Food loss Products that are lost along the food supply chain for various reasons including spoilage and retail requirements for display

Land use Linked to several major areas of public administration such as natural resource management, waste disposal, transportation, urbanization, agriculture, recreation, and forest

Sustainable agriculture Environmentally friendly agriculture methods with the objective to preserve an ecological balance by avoiding natural resource depletion

References

Barilla Center for Food & Nutrition (BCFN). Food sustainability index. 2016a. https://www.barillacfn.com/en/food_sustainability_index/. Accessed 6 Aug 2017.

Barilla Center for Food & Nutrition (BCFN). Food sustainability index: country ranking. 2016b. http://foodsustainability.eiu.com/country-ranking/. Accessed 6 Aug 2017.

Barilla Center for Food & Nutrition (BCFN). Dissemination. 2016c. https://www.barillacfn.com/en/dissemination/. Accessed 6 Aug 2017.

Barilla Center for Food & Nutrition Foundation (BCFN). The Milan protocol on food and nutrition. 2015. https://www.barillacfn.com/media/pdf/MilanProtocol_en.pdf. Accessed 6 Aug 2017.

National Center for Health Statistics. Health, United States, 2016: with chartbook on long-term trends in health. Hyattsville, MD; 2017. https://www.cdc.gov/nchs/hus/index.htm. Accessed 19 Aug 2017.

National Sustainable Agricultural Coalition. What is sustainable ag? n.d. http://sustainableagriculture.net/about-us/what-is-sustainable-ag/. Accessed 6 Aug 2017.

United Nations. Sustainable development goals. 2015. http://www.un.org/sustainabledevelopment/sustainable-development-goals/. Accessed 7 Aug 2017.

United Nations Framework Convention on Climate Change (UNFCCC). INDCs as communicated by parties. 2015. http://www4.unfccc.int/submissions/indc/Submission%20Pages/submissions.aspx. Accessed 19 Aug 2017.

United States Centers for Disease Control and Prevention (CDC). National environmental public health tracking. Climate change communication tools. 2017. https://ephtracking.cdc.gov/showClimateChangeCommunicationTools.action. Accessed 7 Aug 2017.

United States Department of Agriculture. Selected new and ongoing USDA food loss and waste reduction activities. n.d. https://www.usda.gov/oce/foodwaste/usda_commitments.html. Accessed 19 Aug 2017.

United States Department of Agriculture (USDA). Departmental regulation 9500-003: land use policy. 1983. https://www.ocio.usda.gov/sites/default/files/docs/2012/DR9500-003.htm. Accessed 19 Aug 2017.

United States Department of Agriculture (USDA). Economic Research Service. Major land uses. 2017. https://www.ers.usda.gov/topics/farm-economy/land-use-land-value-tenure/major-land-uses/. Accessed 24 Jul 2017.

United States Environmental Protection Agency. Greenhouse gas (GHG) emissions. 2017. https://www.epa.gov/ghgemissions. Accessed 19 Aug 2017.

United States Government Accountability Office (GAO). Rural water infrastructure. Federal agencies provide funding but could increase coordination to help communities. Statement of Alfredo Gomez, Director, Natural Resources and Environment Team. Testimony Before the Subcommittee on Environment and the Economy, Committee on Energy and Commerce, House of Representatives, GAO-15-450T. 2015. http://www.gao.gov/products/GAO-15-450T. Accessed 19 Aug 2017.

United States Government Accountability Office (GAO). Climate change funding and management. n.d. https://www.gao.gov/key_issues/climate_change_funding_management/issue_summary. Accessed 30 Jul 2017.

United States Government Accountability Office (GAO). Climate change. Improved federal coordination could facilitate use of forward-looking climate information in design standards, building codes, and certifications. Report to the Honorable Matthew Cartwright, House of Representatives, GAO-17-3. 2016a. http://www.gao.gov/products/GAO-17-333SP. Accessed 30 Jul 2017.

United States Government Accountability Office (GAO). Renewable fuel standard: low expected production volumes make it unlikely that advanced biofuels can meet increasing. Targets, GAO-17-108. 2016b. http://www.gao.gov/assets/690/681256.pdf. Accessed 7 Aug 2017.

United States Government Accountability Office (GAO). Declining resources: selected agencies took steps to minimize effects on mission but opportunities exist for additional action, GAO-17-79. 2016c. http://www.gao.gov/assets/690/681736.pdf. Accessed 28 Aug 2017.

United States Government Accountability Office (GAO). Drinking water: EPA needs to collect information and consistently conduct activities to protect underground sources of drinking water. 2016d. http://www.gao.gov/assets/680/675690.pdf. Accessed 19 Aug 2017.

United States Government Accountability Office (GAO). Agricultural conservation. USDA's environmental quality incentives program could be improved to optimize benefits. Report to the Honorable Bob Gibbs House of Representatives, GAO-17-225. 2017a. http://www.gao.gov/assets/690/684401.pdf. Accessed 30 Jul 2017.

United States Government Accountability Office (GAO). Tribal transportation: Better data could improve road management and inform Indian student attendance strategies. Report to the Ranking Member, Committee on Transportation and Infrastructure, House of Representatives, GAO-17-423. 2017b. http://www.gao.gov/assets/690/684809.pdf. Accessed 19 Aug 2017.

Von Witzke H, Noleppa S. Biofuels: Agricultural commodity prices, food security, and resource use. Agripol–network for policy advice GbR, Agripol research paper 2014-02. 2014. http://www.agripol-network.com/wp-content/uploads/2014/07/agripol_rp022014_2014.pdf. Accessed 20 Aug 2017.
World Resources Institute. Food loss & waste protocol: food loss and waste accounting and reporting standard, version 1. 2016. http://www.wri.org/sites/default/files/REP_FLW_Standard.pdf. Accessed 6 Aug 2017.

Further Reading

Cornell Law School, Legal Information Institute. Land use: an overview. n.d. https://www.law.cornell.edu/wex/Land_use. Accessed 24 Jul 2017.
Food and Agricultural Organization (FAO) of the United Nations. Our strategic objectives. 2017. http://www.fao.org/about/en/ Accessed 19 Aug 2017.
Food Tank. 12 ways the tech industry is hacking food waste. 2017. https://foodtank.com/news/2017/08/food-waste-technologies/ Accessed 25 Aug 2017.
Intergovernmental Panel on Climate Change (IPCC). Climate change 2014: synthesis report. Contribution of Working Groups I, II and III to the Fifth Assessment Report of the Intergovernmental Panel on Climate Change [Core Writing Team, R.K. Pachauri and L.A. Meyer (eds.)]. IPCC, Geneva, Switzerland, 151 pp.; 2014.
Milan Center for Food & Policy. Right to food map. 2015. http://rtfmap.milanfoodlaw.org/. Accessed 6 Aug 2017.
US Department of the Interior. Bureau of land management, featured topics. n.d. https://www.blm.gov/. Accessed 17 Jul 2017.
United States Centers for Disease Control and Prevention (CDC) [internet]. Diet/nutrition. 2017. https://www.cdc.gov/nchs/fastats/diet.htm. Accessed 19 Aug 2017.
United States Government Accountability Office (GAO). Climate change: selected governments have approached adaptation through laws and long-term plans. Report to the Honorable Matthew Cartwright, House of Representatives, GAO-16-64. 2016. http://www.gao.gov/assets/680/677230.pdf. Accessed 7 Aug 2017.

Chapter 4
Planning Healthy Communities: Abating Preventable Chronic Diseases

Arthi Rao and Catherine L. Ross

Abstract While creating healthy communities through built environment interventions became an objective of international health organizations, such as the World Health Organization since the mid-twentieth century, abating preventable chronic diseases continues to be a global concern. Consequently, there are few examples of mainstream application of local policy to include health priorities explicitly into community planning. This chapter discusses the case of Atlanta, Georgia, as a demonstration for prioritizing health and utilizing a health impact assessment in the region's long-term comprehensive plan. PLAN 2040 envelopes key elements of the built environment (e.g., land use, transportation, access to health) known to impact population health. Further, the Atlanta Regional Commission incorporated economic development and sustainability principles to positively influence these factors as social determinants of health outcomes. The chapter introduces foundational definitions and philosophical frameworks to illuminate the legal basis for health inclusive community planning in Atlanta and discusses relevant frameworks for future application.

4.1 Introduction

Over the course of the last two centuries, population health trends have shifted from a focus on infectious disease to an epidemic of chronic diseases. Heart disease, cancer, and diabetes figure prominently as the leading causes of death and share many risk factors including obesity, physical inactivity, and unhealthy diets. Following this pattern, health research has cycled through social and individual models to explain risk factors and develop therapeutic regimens. Communities, jointly defined by their physical and social components, are recognized in current scientific investigation as prominent barriers or enablers of healthy lifestyles which can influence the health trajectories of community residents.

A. Rao (✉) C. L. Ross
Center for Quality Growth and Regional Development, College of Design, Georgia Institute of Technology, Atlanta, GA, USA
e-mail: arthir@gatech.edu; catherine.ross@design.gatech.edu

B. A. Fiedler (ed.), *Translating National Policy to Improve Environmental Conditions Impacting Public Health Through Community Planning*,
https://doi.org/10.1007/978-3-319-75361-4_4

The fields of public health and urban planning have intertwined histories in their mission to create healthy communities. Despite the awareness of the role of the physical and social environments in influencing health outcomes, health priorities are rarely incorporated in an explicit way into community planning. However, recent scientific paradigms (such as sustainability), legislative trends, and political affirmations have created policy levers that provide opportunities to consciously pursue health priorities in planning processes. Comprehensive planning, often legally required at multiple scales through multi-organizational coordination, provides a systemic approach to address health through numerous community elements such as land use and transportation. Health Impact Assessment (HIA), derived from the federally mandated environmental impact assessment process, is another method that can be used to analyze the health impacts of policies, plans, and projects, especially those where health is not the primary target of decision-making. Recommendations from the HIA process can be valuable in mitigating negative health impacts from policy decisions outside of the health sector. Collectively, these two mechanisms provide useful practice-based approaches to creating healthy communities where making healthy choices are default choices. Stakeholder involvement is strongly encouraged if not required in both tools, making it an ideal platform for urban planners and public health practitioners to worth together in creating a joint vision for community health and disease prevention.

This chapter describes the elements of community planning and the various pathways along which these elements influence human health. The focus is on the physical elements of a healthy community which is collectively referred to as the built environment. The chapter begins with defining a healthy community and the role of the built environment as acknowledged in these definitions. The next section focuses on the profession of urban planning and its historical connections with the public health profession. The comprehensive planning process is then discussed, as an example of the legal basis to influence health outcomes. The chapter concludes with an examination of the Regional PLAN 2040 that includes the Health Impact Assessment of PLAN 2040, showcasing a regional comprehensive planning process where health was considered an integral part of the planning objectives. Unlike most health impact assessments which are local, the PLAN 2040 HIA represents one of the first HIAs to be conducted at the metropolitan scale. The analytical framework and recommendations adopted a multiscale approach, examining local implications of regional decisions.

4.2 Theoretical Frameworks for Defining Healthy Communities

The role of communities in the development of healthy communities is important because they act as a social and physical foundation for citizens to engage in positive activities. The inclusive nature of local policy facilitating social and physical engagement can promote long-term benefits that improves the health and well-being

Table 4.1 Elements of healthy communities (Foley 2013)

Healthy community characteristics	Healthy community processes
• Equity (lack of disparities) • A strong economy and employment opportunities (lack of poverty) • Education • Healthcare and preventive health services • A stable, sustainable ecosystem and environment • Housing/shelter • Healthy public policy • Access to healthy food • Safety • Opportunities for active living • Transportation • Empowered population • Healthy child development	• Civic engagement • Inclusive, equitable and broad community participation • Employ environmental strategies • Engage multi-sector participation • The capacity to assess and address their own health concerns • Collaboration between partners • Use data to guide and measure efforts

of the general population as well as discourages the onset of debilitating disease. Therefore, healthy communities can be defined based on three specific philosophical and methodological traditions discussed in this section.

4.2.1 *Defining Healthy Communities*

Two broad elements that define a healthy community emerge from a comprehensive review of current literature. Healthy communities are characterized by (1) healthy community characteristics and (2) healthy community processes (Foley 2013). For example, desirable community characteristics include opportunities for employment, equitable distribution of funds, and the ability to access basic needs such as healthy food, shelter, and healthcare. Further, these characteristics must be supported by processes embedded in local policy, community involvement, and self-empowerment (Table 4.1).

While the table describes a potentially universal definition of healthy communities, several parallel theoretical frameworks have contributed to this definition. They are discussed in the succeeding sections.

4.2.2 *Philosophical and Methodological Role of Communities in Determinants of Health*

Communities play a significant social and physical role as determinants of health, well-being and conversely disease. These are highlighted in philosophical and methodological traditions such as the Ottawa Charter, the Salutogenic Model, and the Socioecological model of public health. The roots of these paradigms can be traced back to the public health phase of "non-specific immunization" where infectious diseases were ameliorated with vaccination protocols and were no longer the main causes of death (Duhl and Sanchez 1999). Thus, these models reflect the transition to the population health impact of non-communicable diseases, such as diabetes, cancer, heart and respiratory conditions, and how the social and physical environment contributes to the onset of these chronic conditions. These transitioning philosophies and health conditions have led global organizations to promote the concept of health as a basic human right.

(WHO 2006, p.1):

> Health is a state of complete physical, mental and social wellbeing and not merely the absence of disease or infirmity. The enjoyment of the highest attainable standard of health is one of the fundamental rights of every human being without distinction of race, religion, political belief, economic or social condition.

4.2.2.1 Ottawa Charter for Health Promotion

The Ottawa Charter for Health Promotion set a new course for public health theory and practice. Discourse and practice on health revolved around pathogenesis and disease prior to the Charter's enactment in 1986. The Charter reified the definition of health as set forth in the initial Constitution of the World Health Organization in 1948, "as a state of complete physical, mental and social well-being." Health promotion strategies were operationalized into the five domains of building healthy public policy, creating supportive environments, strengthening community action, developing personal skills, and reorienting health services.

The Ottawa Charter presented two significant innovations with respect to defining healthy communities. First, the Ottawa Charter redefined health as a positive objective to pursue rather than the avoidance of negative outcomes. Consequently, the document highlights the role of peoples' living environments and daily interactions in the production of a healthy state. Second, the Charter's strategies and domains of action suggest that the pursuit of health extends well beyond the reach of the healthcare sector (Potvin and Jones 2011).

The charter outlines the role of the physical and social environment as critical components of supporting the fundamental prerequisites for health. These health prerequisites include peace, shelter, education, food, income, a stable ecosystem, sustainable resources, social justice and equity. To date, social epidemiologists continue to conceptualize the processes associated with the physical and social environment to formulate the most inclusive definition and methodological operationalization of the connection between human health and the environmental envelope.

4.2.2.2 The Salutogenesis Model

Parallel with the principles in the Ottawa Charter and in pursuit of an inclusive definition is the *Salutogenesis* model by Aaron Antonovsky in 1979. A central tenet of the salutogenic model is the "sense of coherence" or the ability to "mobilize resources to cope with stressors" (Mittelmark and Bauer 2017, p.7). The modern application adapts this model to communities and neighborhoods. Referring to an asset-based orientation, Vaandrager and Kennedy describe resources as factors embedded in communities that help individuals and populations sustain health and well-being (2017). These assets can be social, physical, financial, or environmental factors that operate along numerous pathways.

Two aspects of the physical environment—the natural and built environment—collectively create a shared geographic identity providing potential opportunities to participate in physical activity and other health-promoting behaviors. Thus, the physical attributes in a community play a large role in defining individual/collective identities and in shaping the experience or sense of community.

Social resources are often measured through aspects such as neighborhood cohesion and social capital. A healthy community is considered to have high levels of social cohesion and community attachment which are influenced by characteristics such as residential stability, social ties, and rates of public participation. The salutary effects of social cohesion operate at the community or ecological level by creating strong social networks and trust that facilitate cooperation for mutual benefit. This lays a strong foundation for community resilience and collective action. In other words, communities with high levels of social capital are more resilient to adversity and are better able to advocate for themselves due to shared interest and vision.

4.2.2.3 Social Epidemiology

Social epidemiology explores how the built environment is an expression of or reinforces social phenomena such as socioeconomic status, racism, social support, and stress, thus mediating the relationship between health and place (CSDH 2007; Krieger 2001). Ecosocial theory or the social-ecological systems perspective analyzes population health on a continuum of biological, ecological, and social factors (e.g., cell, organ, organism/individual, family, community, population, society, ecosystem). Krieger (1994) aptly characterizes the socioecological system of the production of disease and health as the web of causation. The focus is on understanding the complex and potentially non-reductionist interactions between all the levels and can be considered a more comprehensive theory that incorporates the first two. An important concept in this approach is embodiment. Embodiment involves how the human body biologically incorporates material and social environments to create different pathways between exposure, susceptibility, and resistance (Krieger 1994).

Examples of the generation of different pathways relevant to healthy communities include residential segregation/exclusionary zoning policies and how they affect health outcomes differentially among population sub-groups. Residential segregation leads to higher rates of economic deprivation among African-Americans who also face extended consequences from this condition. For example, African-Americans living in poorer communities whose neighborhoods do not have access to grocery stores offering healthy foods, have higher exposures to environmental toxins such as lead paint in older homes, and greater proximity to waste facilities. Poor nutrition (high fat, high sodium foods, and low vegetable consumption) at the individual level increases risk for obesity. Further, both poor nutrition and environmental toxins are significant determinants of hypertension and chronic kidney disease.

Multiple community level factors impact health outcomes (Fig. 4.1). Nested within macrosocial factors (upstream determinants), the physical/built environment is further categorized into key traditional domains of operation for urban planners (Northridge et al. 2003). While land use and transportation planning in many ways can be the main or founding domains, other domains include environmental planning, economic development, and housing.

Figure 4.1 is particularly useful in providing an operational model of socioecological systems theory as it highlights the community level factors and the causal pathways along which these factors operate (proximate level) to influence health outcomes at the individual and population levels.

4.3 Urban Planning and Public Health

The common roots of the urban planning and public health professions can be traced back to the late eighteenth and early nineteenth century, a time of rapid industrialization and urbanization. Urban living was characterized by pathogenic sociological (e.g., crime, loose morals) and environmental elements (e.g., industry, poor housing conditions, improper sanitation, marshes, cemeteries). The prevalent miasma theory of disease hypothesized that effluents released from these pathogenic environmental elements caused infectious disease epidemics. From a health equity perspective, these epidemics disproportionately affected poor immigrant and minority populations that mostly comprised the working class. Overcrowding and slum-like conditions where the working class resided contributed to poor health outcomes, whereas the wealthy avoided most ill health because they could afford to live in more salubrious neighborhoods (Freudenberg et al. 2006).

The 1848 Sanitary Reform and the 1878 Housing Reform Movements in Chicago succeeded by the City Beautiful Movement in the late 1890s were the first collaborative efforts between city planning and public health professionals representing physically deterministic interventions to solve public health problems (Corburn 2004, 2007; Duhl and Sanchez 1999; Ross et al. 2014; Szczygiel and Hewitt 2000; Verbeek and Boelens 2016). Collectively they generally included modifying the physical form of densely populated cities by reconfiguring sanitation and sewer systems, revamping building codes, and creating urban parks to support public recreation, moral rejuvenation, and mental health.

The germ theory redefined disease causation in the late nineteenth century. The focus shifted from environmental hazards to identifying infectious microbial agents and treating the associated specific diseases. The change in epidemiological thought led to the divergence between urban planning and public health and a concurrent

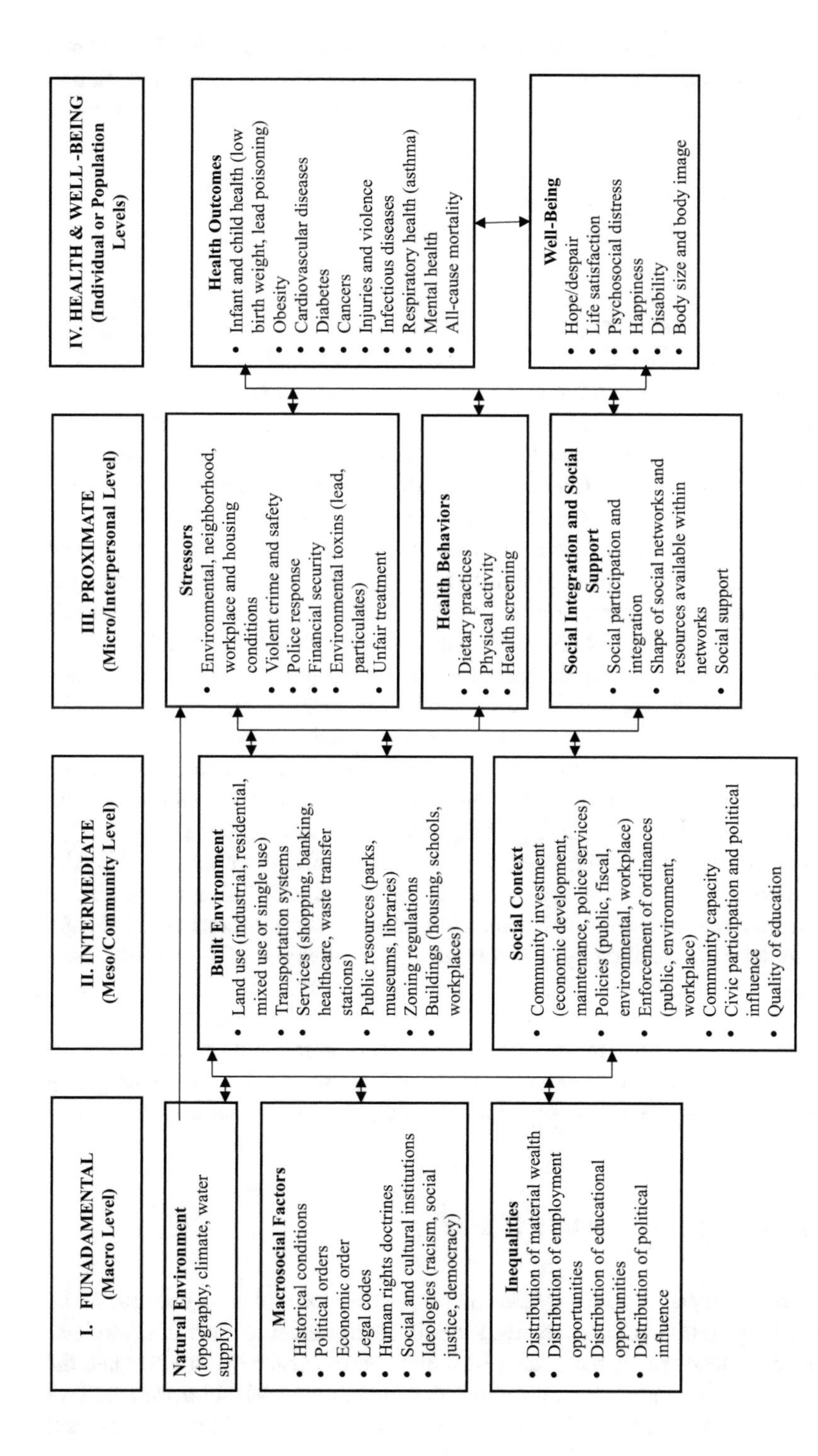

Fig. 4.1 Social determinants of health and environmental health promotion, a model developed by AJ Schultz and ME Northridge (Northridge et al. 2003, p.559, Used with Permission)

separation between social and medical causes of disease (Corburn 2007; Duhl and Sanchez 1999). Therapeutic protocols focused on vaccination and immunization as well as the modification of individual risk factors (e.g., diet, exercise, substance abuse). Non-biological factors as mediators of pathogenic conditions were dismissed and the medical profession took on a more reductionist approach to curing disease (Hewa 2015; Verbeek and Boelens 2016).

However, a significant development for the urban planning profession was the passing of zoning ordinances as the primary instrument for regulating land uses. Zoning targets the separation of undesirable uses of the land (industrial areas, cemeteries, and other sources of toxic odors and emissions) from desirable ones (homes and schools) (Cullingworth and Caves 2008; Verbeek and Boelens 2016). The biomedical model heralded a formal separation between planning and public health professionals. Planners now turned their attention to economic development efforts through large infrastructure and transportation related projects. The nationwide implementation of zoning ordinances gradually led to the development of low-density residential areas separated from other types of land uses.

Prior to the development of effective medications, researchers in the 1940s were finding that improvement in nutrition, living conditions and other environmental factors were associated with declines in mortality rates. Social epidemiologists were introducing the concepts of multi-causality and general susceptibility which provided a more complete explanation of disease causation and the differential distributions of mortality rates across groups with different demographic and social profiles. In summary, these epidemiological models establish that disease causation was the result of complex interactions between disease agent, human host, and the environment. Also, environmental conditions and social ties were important mediators in determining the susceptibility of the host to infectious agents (Hewa 2015).

The new definition of health as put forth by the constitution of the World Health Organization and the Ottawa Charter in the 1980s coupled with a resurgence of ecosocial epidemiology in the 1990s heralded a renewed connection between health and the social, cultural and physical context of the individual. The transition from infectious diseases to chronic diseases as the leading causes of morbidity and mortality makes this connection apparent. The inability of the biomedical model to explain chronic disease and mortality due to social and community factors prompted this reconsideration of the established notions of health and disease, reenergizing the symbiotic relationship between urban planning and public health.

4.4 Contemporary Urban Planning

Saelens and Handy define the physical environment as that which "is constructed by human activity" (2008, p.2). Generally, the built environment consists of the following elements: "land use patterns, the distribution across space of activities and the buildings that house them; the transportation system, the physical infrastructure of roads, sidewalk, bike paths, etc., as well as the service this system provides; and urban design, the arrangement and appearance of the physical elements in a community" (Saelens and Handy 2008, p.2). In the present-day context, the profession of Urban Planning and planning practitioners play a primary role in designing and managing the built environment in collaboration with other urban design professionals such as architects, landscape architects, civil engineers, and other allied professionals.

The American Planning Association (APA) (https://www.planning.org/) and the Association of the Collegiate Schools of Planning (ACSP) are the two primary professional organizations for urban planning in the United States. The APA is a platform for professional engagement around the topics of ethics, professional development, planning education, and the standards of planning practice that also governs the American Institute of Certified Planners (AICP) certification. The ACSP is the APA equivalent for planning academicians. Planning is a "systematic, creative way to influence the future of neighborhoods, cities, rural and metropolitan areas, and even the country and the world" (ACSP n.d., *para* 1).

In the ACSP vision, urban and regional planners use their professional skills to serve communities facing social, economic, environmental, and cultural challenges (http://www.acsp.org/). They advocate and facilitate collaboration between community residents, government officials, and business leaders to achieve the following:

- preservation and enhancement of their quality of life
- protection of the natural and built environment
- identification of policies to promote equity and equality
- improvement of services to disadvantaged communities through designed programs
- effectively deal with growth and development using a variety of methods

While the definitions of planning described above are only representative samples, they clearly signal a primary role for planners in healthy community planning. In fact, the APA runs the Planning and Community Health Center as an integral part of its applied research departments. The purpose of this center is to help communities address and advance health goals using planning strategies. Primarily through planning practice, this center has played a pioneering role in reconnecting planning's purpose with public health through capacity building, tool development, education and professional guidance (APA 2017).

A similar trend reveals itself in the scientific literature around planning healthy communities. The topic of built environment and health currently occupies a formal position of academic inquiry within both the fields of public health and planning. Ten years since the American Journal of Public Health first published its special issue on this topic, the reconvergence between planning and public health is cemented and growing (Jackson et al. 2013). This research paradigm is firmly embedded in the socioecological model or the notion that the health status of an individual is simultaneously produced by individual biology and the surrounding physical, social, cultural, and political environment. Collectively termed the "social determinants of health," these are known to influence individual health as well as the differential distribution of health outcomes among populations (health disparities). The rise of chronic conditions as leading causes of mortality and morbidity are harsh reminders that the biomedical model is truly anachronistic. Risk factors such as obesity are considered the underlying causes of these conditions and have acquired "epidemic" status. The design of the built environment is a key barrier or enabler of healthy behaviors such as healthy eating and active living.

4.5 The Legal Basis for Comprehensive Planning

Comprehensive planning is the process by which a community collectively envisions future physical development (Cullingworth and Caves 2008; Godschalk et al. 2006). The Comprehensive Plan, synonymous with Master Plan, General Plan, or Municipal Development Plan, serves as a foundation or policy document to guide growth and physical development in an area. One of the key purposes of a Comprehensive plan is to guide land use decision-making. Comprehensive planning is legally mandated or incentivized in most states. The agency responsible (planning commission, local government) for developing a comprehensive plan can vary state by state (Cullingworth and Caves 2008; Godschalk et al. 2006).

States also regulate the contents of the comprehensive plan by prescribing the required and optional elements to be included in the plan. True to the name, the plan addresses multiple areas that can influence the growth and development of a community. These include population, demography, land use, traffic circulation and transportation, parks and open space (natural resources), housing, utilities and services, urban design, community facilities, economic development, historical preservation, and other elements. States may also have requirements to address unique geographical attributes. For example, California requires a safety element in their comprehensive plans to address seismically induced (earthquakes) and geological hazards (flooding, wildfires) (Cullingworth and Caves 2008).

Many states require citizen participation during the comprehensive planning process. This allows for a diverse representation of community stakeholders to participate in developing a shared vision of the comprehensive plan. Multiple techniques are used to garner public involvement including public hearings, surveys, mailings and establishing public committees. Adopting the comprehensive plan also requires local resolution which is generally coordinated through a public process involving public hearings, recommendations, and votes from the planning commission and city council. Several tools and techniques are used to implement the plan which may or may not be regulatory. Common techniques include zoning, historic preservation and design review ordinances. Mandatory public participation in the plan-making process builds healthy communities' processes such as civic engagement, community empowerment, and collective efficacy.

The American Planning Association (APA) (2016) recently published the document "Health Impact Assessment Toolkit for Planners." In the document, they illustrate ways in which health priorities can be introduced into the various phases of developing a comprehensive plan at any geographic scale. The health impact assessment process is discussed later in this chapter, but the diagram on page 13 of the APA resource (https://planning-org-uploaded-media.s3.amazonaws.com/document/HIA-Toolkit.pdf) demonstrates systematic opportunities to integrate health priorities and evaluate a comprehensive plan for health impacts.

The comprehensive plan provides an inherently multidisciplinary, systems-based approach to planning healthy communities. This chapter focuses on land use planning, transportation planning, and zoning. Rossen and Pollack (2012) suggest the following ways in which zoning can support healthy communities:

- Support urban farms and agriculture, community gardens, or farmers' markets by allowing for these land uses in certain areas.
- Bring supermarkets to underserved areas or food deserts by removing zoning barriers such as lot size requirements.
- Use conditional use permits to regulate availability of healthy food choices at corner/grocery stores, within specified distances of schools and other ways to incentivize consumption of healthier foods.
- Encourage active transportation (i.e., walking or biking) through complete streets, sidewalks, bike paths, and street connectivity.
- Facilitate access to open spaces, parks, and playgrounds for active play.
- Limit availability of liquor or tobacco retail outlets within a certain distance of child-centered spaces (e.g., schools, recreation centers, playgrounds).
- Mitigate the effects of climate change by increasing tree canopy, greenspace, and access to public transportation.
- Reducing traffic to decrease pollution and other hazards such as injuries.
- Increase access to healthcare facilities.
- More equitably distribute resources to address health disparities by race and ethnicity or income.
- Create or preserve mixed-use and mixed-income neighborhoods.

4.5.1 Comprehensive Planning in Georgia

Comprehensive planning in Georgia is regulated by the Georgia Planning Act of 1989 (O.C.G.A. 45-12-200, et seq., and 50-8-1, et seq.) and administered by the Department of Community Affairs (DCA). The legislation considers "coordinated and comprehensive planning by all levels of government within the State of Georgia is of vital importance to the state and its citizens." Promoting, developing, and maintaining coordinated and comprehensive planning by all levels of government is considered of primary interest to the state. Under the direction of the Governor, coordination of planning is required by departments, agencies, commissions, and other institutions of the state.

The Georgia Planning Act authorized the creation of 12 Regional Commissions across the state to "develop, promote and assist in establishing coordinated comprehensive planning in the state." The DCA works closely with the Regional Commissions to coordinate and implement regional and local planning. The DCA also sets standards for the plan contents and requires at a very minimum for plans to include elements related to transportation, housing, economic development, and land use with stakeholder/community participation at every stage (Georgia DCA 2014).

4.5.2 The Atlanta Regional Commission and Planning

The Atlanta Regional Commission (ARC) is designated as a Metropolitan Planning Organization (MPO) by the U.S. Department of Transportation (USDOT), as well as a Metropolitan Area Planning and Development Commission and Regional Commission under the laws of the State of Georgia.

As the regional planning and intergovernmental coordination agency, ARC is the forum through which officials of local governments in the Atlanta region confer to solve mutual problems and decide issues of region-wide importance. ARC serves a 10-county development planning area, an 18-county (and partial county) transportation planning area, and a 20-county federal air quality nonattainment area, as well as providing some support for the 28-county Consolidated Statistical Area as designated by the U.S. Census Bureau. While most of the work of ARC is in planning and policy-making, ARC generally does not implement plans. As such, ARC's regional planning may exert significant influence over health outcomes associated with transportation, land use, and other planning activities. State and local government also plays a key role in implementation of plans and projects, particularly in project management, design, and operation/maintenance.

4.5.3 Health in PLAN 2040

PLAN 2040 is the long-range plan for the Atlanta metropolitan region and is the first ever integrated transportation and land use plan in the region prepared by the Atlanta Regional Commission (ARC) (http://atlantaregionsplan.org/). The plan represents an unprecedented opportunity to influence the long-term health, sustainability, and prosperity of the region. The integration of land use and transportation policies permits evaluating the impact of various land use scenarios on transportation systems during the planning process. The plan was officially adopted in July 2011 after an extensive review process by diverse stakeholder groups.

As the MPO for the Atlanta region, ARC is required by the U.S. Department of Transportation (USDOT) to develop a fiscally constrained long-range (minimum 20-year span) Regional Transportation Plan (RTP) as well as a short-range (minimum

4 years) Transportation Improvement Program (TIP). ARC must update the RTP at least every 20 years while they must update the corresponding TIP at least every 6 years based on the region's changing vision, demographics, development, and funding. Amendments to the plan and program may be made between updates. The TIP serves as the prioritized first 4 years of the RTP, and is subject to more specific, annual fiscal constraint requirements. In an air quality nonattainment area like Atlanta, a conformity determination report must also be prepared to document that the transportation plan will not cause or contribute to worsened air quality.

Any project seeking federal transportation funds, or any project of regional significance (regardless of fund source) in an air quality nonattainment area, must be channeled through ARC's transportation planning process. ARC conducts the regional land use planning process, but approved projects, development decisions, and zoning are implemented by city and county governments. Of notable importance is that projects falling on local and collector streets are largely excluded from regional plan process because they typically do not require Federal funds or are not considered regionally significant. This is important because many of the types of transportation improvements that are necessary to influence health outcomes are very local in nature and may not be captured in RTP/TIP process directly.

PLAN 2040 generates demographic and employment forecasts through the year 2040 and uses these forecasts as a basis for infrastructure and service demand on a regional scale. The region is projected to grow by approximately 3 million people to a total of 8.3 million by 2040 (Atlanta Regional Commission 2009, p.1). Job growth projections are slower, growing from 2.7 million in 2010 to 4.5 million by 2040 after declining during the period 2005–2010 (Atlanta Regional Commission 2009, p.7). Overall, the labor participation rate is expected to decline from almost 70% in 2010 to just 62% in 2040 (Atlanta Regional Commission 2009, p.2). Much of this decline is attributed to the growing proportion of senior citizens while some decline may be directly related to economic or other factors. Regardless of the causes, the decline in the rate of labor participation raises questions about the functionality or sustainability of a region with relatively low workforce participation.

The Atlanta Regional Commission has already embraced health as an essential element of a thriving and productive region in several important ways. Specifically, many of ARC's activities deal with the social determinants of health in indirect ways when visioning development, planning communities, and extending public services. They achieve this by considering sustainability, equity, aging, housing, transportation, land development, energy, and many other topics also touch on the elements of a complete, healthful community.

4.5.4 Health and Outreach in PLAN 2040

PLAN 2040 was built on ARC's ongoing efforts to plan and evaluate by educating citizens about the planning process, engaging businesses and residents to reveal their needs and desires, and capturing the long-term changes that the region could or should experience. ARC began to address topics such as health, equity, aging, sustainability, and livability during PLAN 2040 development using six online public meetings, information from previous regional visioning initiatives such as the Fifty Forward and Civic League forums, and numerous meetings with stakeholder groups. Stakeholder groups that participated in the process included ARC's standing social equity advisory committee, bicycle and pedestrian task force, a transit operators committee, and many others. Feedback from participants emphasized economic prosperity, equity, environmental quality, sustainability, walkable communities and nodes, and many references to healthy communities.

Based on inputs from the public engagement process, ARC developed three overarching goals and five objectives for PLAN 2040.

(Atlanta Regional Commission 2011):

Goals:

- Lead as the global gateway to the South.
- Encourage healthy communities.
- Expand access to community resources.

Objectives:

- Increase mobility options for people and goods.
- Foster a healthy, educated, well-trained, safe, and secure population.
- Promote residential choices in locations that are accessible to jobs and services.
- Improve energy and resource efficiency, while preserving the region's environment and critical assets.
- Identify innovative approaches to economic recovery and long-term prosperity.

The objectives are meant to provide guidance towards measurable outcomes. Increased mobility options can lead to less travel time, more physical activity, more leisure time, and better air quality, all of which can have a positive impact on health. Increased residential choices can lead to reduced commute times and increased social capital and quality of life. Introducing health into the planning discussion and the multi-dimensional goals and objectives in the region-wide strategy is suitable for a diverse metropolitan area. The operationalization of these objectives through the planning process was instrumental in the formation of the core assessment strategy for the health impact assessment.

4.5.5 The PLAN 2040 Health Impact Assessment

The World Health Organization defines Health Impact Assessment (HIA) as "a combination of procedures, methods, and tools by which a policy, program, or project may be judged as to its potential effects on the health of a population, and the distribution of those effects within the population" (WHO 1999, p.4). HIA is a key mechanism to reveal the health impacts of policies, programs, and projects especially where health is not their primary target (Ross et al. 2014). The aim of the HIA is to promote healthy decision-making built on the premise of "health in all policies" or the underlying notion that all modifications to the physical, natural, social, or political environment can impact human health.

The goal of the PLAN 2040 HIA was to lay out an evidence-based framework for assessing the health impacts of a large, complex, long-range plan encompassing multiple jurisdictions and unknown future variables. The first steps in the HIA process for PLAN 2040 were to identify regional health priorities to assess and to identify potential stakeholder concerns relating to health. The initial scoping of this HIA was based on reviewing stakeholder feedback from various public forums including over 100 public meetings, three online public meetings, and collaboration with the HIA advisory committee made up of 16 individuals representing different stakeholder groups. The ARC's public involvement process was based on the larger PLAN 2040 approach that did not explicitly address health. However, the feedback brought up many issues that are directly related to health. Stakeholders expressed their need for more transportation options in the region, housing options where employment was available, increasing amount and better-connected greenspace, choices in housing location and type, and expansion in existing development and infrastructure. They also expressed their concern about the aging of the population and their ability to access public services.

The HIA team conducted extensive outreach efforts through workshops and team meetings throughout the HIA process. Attendees included representatives from ARC, local governments, representative from various departments of public health, and other stakeholder associations. Over the course of two meetings, the group developed a list of primary health concerns, including their potential impacts related to regional planning and the distribution of impacts. Feedback was sought around the categories of access and social equity, spatial mismatch, and active transportation and mobility.

After initial priorities and concerns were outlined, current health research was reviewed to generate a list of potential indicators that represent information about health determinants or health status. Potential health indicators to assess in PLAN 2040 were outlined, based on the literature review, including safety/security, access to services, economic development, physical activity, and air quality. Next, PLAN 2040 was reviewed to provide an overview and synopsis of the background and plan. Planning scale, from regional to the neighborhood level, was an important consideration. The substantive elements of the plan (i.e., transportation, land use) as well as the types of analysis used in the planning process also underwent review.

From these analyses, health indicators were selected to assess health trends on a regional scale. Active living health indicators, such as obesity, other chronic disease rates, and methods of commuting by alternative modes, were assessed. In analysis of these regional health indicators, attention was paid to spatial variation within region and variation between subpopulations as determined by socioeconomic status, ethnicity, etc. Several case studies were examined to identify and appraise representative cases used to drill down health impacts to specific scales and plan elements. These case studies include a variety of transportation issues ranging from freight to bike and pedestrian planning.

Primary methodologies include document analysis and spatial analysis using geographic information systems, among others. The results of the assessment are categorized into "Transportation" and "Land Use" with corresponding recommendations on how each component can better mitigate negative health impacts and health disparities while maximizing health benefits in PLAN 2040.

4.5.6 Transportation

Physical activity levels are inversely associated with the incidence of cardiovascular disease, stroke, obesity, high blood pressure, and diabetes. A transportation system that provides alternatives to the automobile and promotes connectivity can lead to increased levels of daily physical activity for improvements in health outcomes and lower incidences of these health problems. The Atlanta region is one of the most congested in the nation. Additionally, development in many areas did not incorporate paths to promote walking or biking between destinations contributing to a lack of physical activity.

According to PLAN 2040 survey responses, 75% of the region's residents have no transportation option other than driving (Ross et al. 2012, p.57). There is a need to connect not only jobs and housing, but also greenspace, various modes of transportation, and the various city centers that are located throughout the region.

Socioeconomic and other demographic information further interact with environmental factors to influence health. For example, there are many areas of the Atlanta region that have large populations living in poverty and the region is aging. In an area dominated by car travel, many of these groups are limited in their mobility, particularly when they live in the suburbs and exurbs. These groups have poor access to social services, jobs, and healthy foods. "Food deserts" are areas characterized by shortage of healthy food availability (such as retail grocery stores) and can increase the risk of diet-related health problems. For vulnerable populations, this translates to a higher risk of obesity-related chronic disease conditions.

While evaluating the transportation plan, evaluating multimodal transportation and its ability to support active living was emphasized. The following recommendations were made.

(Ross et al. 2012):

- Clear standards should be developed for the funding of pedestrian and bicycle projects to incorporate new local and regional guidelines such as "Complete Streets" policies.
- Improvements in the Atlanta Region Bicycle Transportation and Pedestrian Walkways Plan should explicitly aim to increase Level of Service scores for the bicycle and pedestrian networks. Examples of such improvements include creating a regional bicycle network, bicycle access to schools and activity centers and

increasing transportation choices. Local zoning ordinances should also be updated to synchronize with these improvements and collectively enable active transportation.

- Non-motorized travel modes and public transport show positive correlations with physical activity, safety, emissions, social interaction, and household travel cost. Transportation-related social externalities such as these should be included in the RTP and TIP performance measures, as they are fundamental to achieving the overarching planning goals of health, safety, equity, and economic vitality.
- Congestion-related externalities should be mitigated through enhanced street network connectivity which improves accessibility and provides alternative routes to prevent. From a safety perspective, encourage the control of speed and conflict points to improve the pedestrian and bicycle environment as well as design intersections to serve all types of users.
- Higher-density and mixed land use should be promoted to increase the number of destinations in walking or bicycling distance. Create pedestrian-friendly environments with urban design features such as wide sidewalks, planting or furniture zones between the vehicle lanes and the sidewalk, benches, waste and recycling receptacles, shade trees, sidewalk-oriented building frontage and design, street and sidewalk lighting, and pleasant streetscape.
- Project selection should balance interests of the region and the local community. Project selection should address equity concerns for communities with carless households, disabled/aged populations, or households with low income and high potential transportation costs, and areas lacking in transportation alternatives. Some census tracts with over 30% carless households, such as those in northwest City of Atlanta, have roadway capacity projects programmed or in the long-range list, but no transit or non-motorized facilities (Ross et al. 2012, p.150). Some roadway projects may routinely include pedestrian and bicycle facilities.
- Current modeling tools are a barrier to evaluating project costs and benefits across diverse transportation modes and do not include positive social externalities. Projects such as Livable Centers Initiative (LCI) investments may outperform capacity projects in terms of economic development, access, and air quality, but never have a chance to compete on those grounds. Metrics that make performance and benefit-cost comparable across classifications should be included to clarify the complete regional costs of project prioritization.
- Encourage state and local governments to identify where maintenance projects may incorporate bicycle and pedestrian accommodations (if not routine), to improve accessibility and reduce motor vehicle speeds.
- The regional planning process is where the costs and benefits of current transportation funding and scoring become apparent. This provides a prime opportunity to advocate for better planning and resource allocation to pedestrian, bicycle, and transit projects, ensure adequate maintenance and operations, manage land use, and offer coordinated programs.

4.5.7 Land Use

The Regional Development Guide (RDG) and Unified Growth Policy Map (UGPM) (http://atlantaregionsplan.org/regional-development-guide-unified-growth-policy-map/) developed by ARC identify many types of centers and corridors including those that are participating in the Livable Centers Initiative Program described below (Ross et al. 2012). These various centers—Regional Centers, Community Activity Centers, Regional Town Centers, Town Centers, Village Centers, and Crossroads Communities—represent different categories of urban forms characterized by different development densities, land use configurations, etc. The RDG effectively captures the wide range of forms that higher-density centers can take, from small villages and neighborhood business districts to the regional core.

The Atlanta Regional Commission describes the Livable Centers Initiative (LCI) as a "grant program that incentivizes local jurisdictions to re-envision their communities as vibrant, walkable places that offer increased mobility options, encourage healthy lifestyles and provide improved access to jobs and services." The LCI has also helped to recast activity centers in the region.

The 2011 LCI Implementation Report found that LCI studies had influenced 88% of comprehensive plans, 64% of zoning codes, and 28% of policies for senior and affordable housing (Ross et al. 2012, p.175). ARC's project criteria currently include implementation of the goals of the lifelong communities' initiative and are making progress towards policies for senior housing. In the implementation report, the livability survey showed increases in walking and bicycling, which means an increase in physical activity and social interaction, and possibly a decrease in vehicle miles traveled (VMT).

The LCI program is likely creating a healthier environment for regional residents and workers, but the project selection methodology could be updated. The distribution of LCI zones is based on local initiative as well as eligible centers identified by the UGPM. Additional measures, such as environmental justice and other such measures of vulnerable populations, should help guide the geographic distribution of these zones to reduce health disparities. A spatial analysis also revealed that majority of LCI initiatives were in high-risk areas from a health perspective (Ross et al. 2012). Other recommendations for land use planning are as follows:

- The Regional Development Guide identified many types of activity nodes, or Places, which correspond with many of the characteristics that support good health—unique nodes where a range of residences, jobs, and services are concentrated to improve access to daily needs, reduce travel distance, support transportation alternatives, and create and support communities. Planning that emphasizes these places along with the existing LCI would likely promote health. Additionally, guidance on growth or conservation in areas not designated as Places might need to be strengthened (Ross et al. 2012).
- Contextually appropriate density and zoning standards should be developed. Underperforming areas and gaps in the urban fabric that are suitable for immediate infill should be deprioritized for redevelopment. Transportation corridors and

centers, especially with existing or planned quality transit, should take the highest-density development. Any redevelopment should occur gradually with considerations for the conservation of agriculture, greenspace, or general conservation. Accommodations for public and private gardens, farm stands, and farmers markets are also recommended (Ross et al. 2012).

- Diversity in housing should be incentivized. A wide range full of housing sizes, prices, and terms should be permitted relative to regional household types, life phases, and incomes. Senior housing opportunities, including retirement and assisted care facilities to encourage development of lifelong communities, should be included (Ross et al. 2012).
- Opportunities to develop expedited assessment for small transportation projects that use LCI funding should be pursued with Federal Highway Administration and GDOT. Funding opportunities to build, operate, and maintain LCI enhancements through community improvement districts and tax allocation districts should be continuously pursued (Ross et al. 2012).
- Land conservation targets should be explicitly identified in addition to rural areas and greenspace. Areas that are best suited for increased development intensity, development expansion, preservation, or reclamation (conversion from development back to agriculture or greenspace) should be identified locally based on infrastructure, soil quality and other ecological factors, and spatial distribution (Ross et al. 2012). Conservation corridors should be integrated into the region's core, to create wildlife corridors, potential greenways, and access to greenspace and urban agriculture for residents of the core counties (Ross et al. 2012).

4.5.8 *PLAN 2040 Regional Transportation Plan Performance Framework*

The PLAN 2040 RTP utilizes a multi-step decision framework for project selection and resource allocation, based on performance criteria. The four key decision points (KDP) framework was developed as a tool to help organize and guide various steps of the transportation plan development process (ARC 2011). Each KDP defines a step in the process where resource allocation decisions are informed by technical or policy evaluation and highlight which steps are supported through performance assessment. For example, KDP 1 is to do a scenario analysis and determine available funding across various transportation programs. The allocation of funds at this step forms a critical first link between stated PLAN 2040 policy and RTP development objectives. The focus at this stage, however, is to determine funding distribution for maintaining or preserving existing transportation infrastructure. The performance measurement framework was reviewed, and recommendations were made regarding the incorporation of health-related priorities into the metrics.

A key finding of the HIA was that Plan Level Performance Measures did not adequately measure pedestrian access, bicycle access, transportation cost, multimodal access for children and seniors, transportation costs, or other important health impacts. The performance measures rely on traditional metrics, such as car and transit travel time, crash rates, regional emissions modeling, and driving speed. Impact on community and environment was measured through regional emissions. While the metrics that were used can be elements of a healthy, thriving region, other key measures are essential to the overall quality of life, social justice, and economic productivity of the region and should be used for project prioritization as well.

4.6 Discussion

The previous sections discuss the history and theoretical foundations between urban planning and public health. The chapter then demonstrates the practice of healthy urban planning through the lens of regional comprehensive planning and health impact assessment. This final section discusses the larger implications and research gaps to the practice of urban planning and health.

4.6.1 *Current Frameworks for Incorporating Health into Urban Planning Practice*

The connection between the urban planning practice and public health fields is emphasized in a few select approaches. Two popular frameworks are discussed in this chapter—Comprehensive Planning and Health Impact Assessment. While certainly not the only frameworks, most of the activities that interface between the two fields occur in these two arenas.

As the MPO for the Atlanta region, the Atlanta Regional Commission provides an example through the Regional Transportation Plan (RTP). The RTP is an integral part of the region's Comprehensive Plan (PLAN 2040). A central tenet of this plan is to create healthy, livable communities and the RTP is considered a key component in achieving this goal. Several elements of the plan address this connection through safety, accessibility, physical activity, and air quality. While these are traditionally quantifiable measures, less quantifiable externalities of transportation planning are equally important for health and quality of life. Land use planning is also core to these aspects but is primarily a means to the objectives stated above.

Health Impact Assessment (HIA) is another framework that aims to create synergies between urban planning and public health. Firmly embedded in the socioecological model of public health, HIA is simultaneously holistic and reductionist.

Screening is the first step in the HIA process and involves a preliminary determination of potential positive and negative impacts that a policy, program, or project can have on area (Ross et al. 2014). In the PLAN 2040 HIA discussed above, the assessment of health was done only after the plan was proposed. However, the understanding and consideration of health prior to plan formulation can present a truly prospective approach and a continuous awareness of health at the regional scale. Regional transportation planning already provides a strong existing knowledge-seeking framework within which to integrate health concerns. Procedures such as extensive data collection and coordination (from other state agencies) regarding health as well as stakeholder involvement that includes explicit approaches to understanding health could aid this approach. Local knowledge also helps elucidate unique local interactions between social and built environment attributes and provide insights into various causal mechanisms that impact health.

Scoping establishes the study area boundaries, identifies possible consequences, and determines a management approach for the HIA (Ross et al. 2014). At the regional scale, it can imply establishing geographic boundaries around areas of health-based concerns identified from the screening process for future planning and monitoring. For example, the establishment of Equitable Target Areas (ETAs) in PLAN 2040 was not prospectively included in the planning process but was only used for assessment post-planning. Furthermore, the ETA indicator does not include health-based metrics. The inclusion of these metrics could point to cumulative health risks and vulnerable populations. The scoping process can also help determine a roadmap for all collaborative efforts that need to be initiated so that health can be effectively considered in the planning process. These include partnerships with state and local health departments to access data as well as coordination with local jurisdictions for plan implementation.

In HIA, the assessment stage considers the nature, magnitude, and direction of health impacts and the affected population (Ross et al. 2014). At the regional scale, this can be redefined to mean a prioritization of health impacts and corresponding interventions. It can also be a determination of all potential existing policy levers that can be utilized to better address health in the regional planning process, making health-based considerations upfront.

Post appraisal, a HIA process suggests changes to the policy, program, or project based on the assessment findings. Within the context of regional planning and the ARC, it can involve clarifying regulatory, advisory, and advocacy roles for implementation of health-based goals. The ARC already has a strong program-based framework for sustainability initiatives throughout the region. These include Community Choices, Green Communities, Lifelong Communities, and the Livable Centers Initiative. The LCI program was discussed in prior sections of the chapter. Other programs incorporate achieving measurable sustainability goals within communities. However, most of these programs are voluntary and involve community entrepreneurship. This points to an advocative and advisory role for regional commissions and MPOs nationwide in incentivizing the incorporation of health metrics within sustainability goals as well as overseeing the distribution of location and funding for these programs to enable health equity in the region. Regarding transportation planning, the ARC may have more regulatory powers to enforce health-based considerations.

In an HIA, the dissemination phase involves the circulation of the results of the HIA to decision-makers, individuals implementing the plan/policy, and community stakeholders. Within the ARC regional planning process, this can involve the integration of public health departments, hospitals, community health centers, and other health-based organizations within information and policy networks.

In HIA, monitoring and evaluation involve both short-term process evaluation and long-term evaluation of the policy-program/project to monitor the accuracy of HIA predictions as well as detect unintended consequences. This stage is the least well-developed of all the other stages and is an active topic of discussion in the HIA literature. In contrast, the monitoring and evaluation tend to be the best developed in the regional planning process due to the presence of transportation planning. Even within the ARC process, stakeholders continue to discuss health metrics in the context of monitoring and evaluation of transportation projects. This existing evaluatory infrastructure can be expanded to include both individual and systemic health indicators to monitor health impacts over time.

Planning agencies (such as the ARC) and planning organizations (such as the American Planning Association) have used or recommend using HIAs to study the impact of planning decisions on community health (APA 2016). HIAs such as those conducted on the Atlanta Beltline evaluate the multifactorial impact of urban renewal projects on physical activity, social capital, and economic development. However, the very definition of HIA treats policies, programs, and project as separate entities. In reality, they form a hierarchical continuum and incorporate valuable synergies that may be missed when evaluated separately (Rao and Ross 2014). HIAs are also often piecemeal, retrospective, and not legally mandated. Their impact on decision-making and continued monitoring/evaluation is, at best, inconsistent.

While both are valuable frameworks as a starting point for including health into urban planning decisions, they have theoretical and methodological limitations. While the transportation frameworks can inform health, the conversation revolves around measures that enable active transportation, access, and air quality as an important externality. Health impact assessment is usually applied to individual projects, whereas regional applications are starting to be explored (such as the HIA of the PLAN 2040). In summary, we see fragmented methods at different spatial and temporal scales.

4.6.2 Envisioning Future Potential for a Preemptive Approach

In epidemiology, the practice of disease surveillance is to monitor the spread of disease and identify patterns of progression. The main role of disease surveillance is to predict, observe, and mitigate the negative impacts of disease outbreaks. Another key role is to also identify risk factors that contribute to the prevalence, incidence, and spread of disease. While health risk behaviors and some environmental factors are tracked for chronic disease surveillance, the built environment is not explicitly included. Moreover, surveillance systems reside in public health agencies.

From the purview of community health, urban planning agencies can offer a much wider conception of health and well-being. The "exposome" concept highlights environmental exposures as an important component of chronic disease causation (Buck Louis and Sundaram 2012; Wild 2005) from a life-course perspective. The exposome includes the measurement of the totality of sources of environmental exposures throughout an individual's lifetime.

The physical and social environment domains of a community contribute to this exposome. These conditions highlight the role of neighborhood deprivation—a multidimensional proxy measure for socioeconomic processes, and certain land uses in disease causation. This puts planning agencies in a primary role in their ability to track and potentially mitigate certain disease conditions.

The notion of land use as exposure reconceives and expands the framework currently used to examine built environment and health relationships. Sprawl, physical activity, and other existing transportation frameworks are potentially applicable to a limited spectrum of health outcomes and determinants such as those strongly linked with obesity. However, socioeconomic characteristics of communities emerge as strong predictors of mortality from a variety of causes and can potentially be viewed as universal indicators (Messer et al. 2006; Stimpson et al. 2007).

Different diseases have different epidemiological mechanisms and thus need different sets of metrics that link them to environmental exposures. From a surveillance perspective, future research necessitates a framework for a comprehensive, cohesive, and holistic approach for synthesizing theory, data, and methods in a way that allows planning organizations to monitor disease because of built and social environments. Combining techniques from urban planning with other disciplines, such as Landscape Epidemiology and Social Epidemiology, provides great promise in setting the foundation for such a framework at different temporal and spatial scales. It also provides for sub-system monitoring as would be required to distinguish between chronic and infectious diseases.

Applying cutting-edge machine learning and predictive modeling techniques to temporal data can result in the selection of leading indicators incorporated into a signaling system that prospectively portends changes in health outcomes based on changes in urbanization patterns. In the era of big data, such data intensive techniques are entirely feasible. Additionally, planning agencies are beginning to develop internal capacity for sophisticated data analytics and modeling.

In the hierarchy of epidemiological research, ecological research typical of built environment and health studies serve as the foundation for defining and testing new conceptual frameworks. Further refinements to research design are implemented once significant correlations are observed. Overcoming the limitations of cross-sectional research would also greatly enhance the potential for predictive modeling. Understanding time lags between land use changes and their corresponding impact on changes in health outcomes is an important longitudinal aspect that must be considered. Several statistical techniques for classification and regression can calculate probabilities for disease based on a set of environmental predictors. These probabilities, when mapped, help visualize risk surfaces spatially. Incorporating methodological improvements suggested previously can result in the creation of predictive risk maps that can further inform practice and policy-making.

Similar approaches are used in remote sensing techniques for the surveillance of zoonotic diseases such as malaria and lyme disease (Dambach et al. 2012; Midekisa et al. 2012). The variety of disease causing mechanisms and the spectrum of analytical methods in epidemiological research demonstrates that a "one size fits all" approach might not be the most appropriate one. Indeed, a systems-based surveillance structure would be able to mesh and utilize these frameworks as appropriate. This approach adds a new way of conceptualizing healthy/unhealthy communities and thus significantly expands built environment and health research (Rao 2016).

4.7 Summary

The chapter demonstrates the potential for urban planning to influence the creation of healthy communities through the comprehensive planning process. A discussion of current practice frameworks such as health impact assessment was also included. Current frameworks such as plan performance metrics and HIA tend to be retrospective and consider health on a case-by-case basis. A more prospective and comprehensive approach is suggested. This approach addresses the fragmentation in metrics and methods that currently persists in the research and practice of healthy places. The most important takeaway is that urban planning agencies can play a primary role in influencing the development of healthy communities. Planners are trained to be systems-based practitioners and researchers where interdisciplinary approaches are the norm rather than the exception. From a translational perspective, planners play a key role in converting critical health research to the three-dimensional reality of space and place.

Glossary

Built environment The built environment from an urban planning perspective consists of the land use and transportation systems that influence the patterns of human activity across space and time as well as the arrangement and appearance of the physical elements in a community, such as buildings, parks, and other infrastructural elements; referred to as the physical environment or that which is constructed by human activity

Complete streets A combined urban design and transportation policy approach for street design that can accommodate users of all ages, abilities and transportation mode; ideally allows for various traffic such as driving, pedestrian, cycling, and public transportation

Effluents Gases/pollutants emanating from water, land, or other sources

Embodiment The physical manifestation of abstract factors; the concept in this chapter explains how the human body "soaks up" the social and physical environment surrounding it and health outcomes become a physical expression of these environments

Exposome The sum of all exposures (physical and social environments) accrued by an individual from conception through death, their interaction with genetic and biological factors and the related health outcomes

Exurbs Regional designation of an area outlying the suburban limits of a city; often inhabited by individuals and families with high socioeconomic status

Local or collector streets Streets are assigned a hierarchy based on their functions, capacities, and speeds in transportation and urban planning; local and collector streets occupy the lower levels of the hierarchy as they have lower volumes of traffic and lower speed limits

Miasma theory of disease The predominant theory of disease causation in the early to mid-nineteenth century espousing that disease was caused by foul air/gases produced from decaying organic matter

Neighborhood cohesion (social cohesion, social capital) A characteristic of communities with a strong, trusting network of social relationships where residents have shared values and norms leading to social networks that can facilitate cooperation—a collective action within and among groups; social epidemiologists has shown that neighborhood cohesion is an important determinant of overall health and well-being

Social determinants of health (SDOH) The social and economic conditions of the places in which individuals live, work, and play can influence their health outcomes as well as the distribution of these outcomes among various population scales such as local, national, or global; often characterized on a spectrum of macrosocial (e.g., culture, mass media, political systems, the economy, climate change, and migration) to microsocial determinants such as community-level conditions in a neighborhood or county

Socioecological model (SEM) A theoretical model for understanding the multilevel and interactive effects of personal and environmental factors that determine individual-level health behaviors and outcomes; a typical SEM model has five nested levels: individual, interpersonal, community, organizational, and policy/enabling environment; can also identify behavioral and organizational leverage points for public health interventions

Spatial mismatch Spatial mismatch generally refers to the geographical discordance between the location of low-income communities and spatial access to employment opportunities.

The germ theory The germ theory of disease causation succeeded the miasma theory of disease towards the late nineteenth century. The germ theory postulated that infectious diseases were caused by microorganisms called pathogens.

Upstream determinants See Social Determinants of Health and macrosocial factors.

References

American Planning Association (APA). Health impact assessment toolkit for planners. 2016. https://www.planning.org/media/document/9112967/. Accessed 21 Aug 2017.

American Planning Association (APA). Planning and community health center: Plan4Health. 2017. https://www.planning.org/nationalcenters/health/. Accessed 16 Oct 2017.

Association of Collegiate Schools of Planning (ACSP). What is planning? n.d. http://www.acsp.org/page/CareersWhatis. Accessed 16 Oct 2017.

Atlanta Regional Commission (ARC). PLAN 2040 RTP—Chapter 3: plan development framework. 2011. http://documents.atlantaregional.com/plan2040/docs/tp_PLAN2040RTP_ch3_072711.pdf. Accessed 10 Oct 2017.

Atlanta Regional Commission. Regional snapshot: ARC's 20-county forecasts: what the future holds. 2009. www.atlantaregional.com/regionalsnapshots. Accessed 16 April 2018.

Buck Louis GM, Sundaram R. Exposome: time for transformative research. Stat Med. 2012;31(22):2569–75. https://doi.org/10.1002/sim.5496.

Commission on Social Determinants of Health (CSDH). A conceptual framework for action on the social determinants of health. World Health Organization; 2007. http://www.who.int/social_determinants/resources/csdh_framework_action_05_07.pdf?ua=1. Accessed 10 Aug 2017.

Corburn J. Confronting the challenges in reconnecting urban planning and public health. Am J Public Health. 2004;94(4):541–9.

Corburn J. Reconnecting with our roots. Urban Aff Rev. 2007;42(5):688–713.

Cullingworth JB, Caves RW. Planning in the USA: policies, issues and processes. London: Routledge; 2008.

Dambach P, et al. Utilization of combined remote sensing techniques to detect environmental variables influencing malaria vector densities in rural West Africa. Int J Health Geogr. 2012;11:8.

Duhl LJ, Sanchez AK. Healthy cities and the city planning process: a background document on links between health and urban planning. European Health Target 13, 14. Copenhagen, Denmark: WHO Regional Office for Europe; 1999.

Foley J. Defining healthy communities. Health Resources in Action. 2013. https://hria.org/wp-content/uploads/2016/10/defininghealthycommunities.original.pdf. Accessed 9 Jul 2017.

Freudenberg N, et al. Cities and the health of the public. Nashville: Vanderbilt University Press; 2006.

Georgia Department of Community Affairs (DCA). Minimum standards and procedures for local comprehensive planning. 2014. http://www.dca.state.ga.us/development/planningquality-growth/DOCUMENTS/Laws.Rules.Guidelines.Etc/DCARules.LPRs.pdf. Accessed 21 Aug 2017.

Georgia Planning Act of 1989. Official Code of Georgia Annotated (O.C.G.A.) 45-12-200; O.C.G.A 50-8-1 https://www.dca.ga.gov/development/PlanningQualityGrowth/DOCUMENTS/Laws.Rules.Guidelines.Etc/GAPlanningAct.pdf. Accessed 16 Oct 2017.

Godschalk DR, et al. Urban land use planning. Urbana: University of Illinois Press; 2006.

Hewa S. Theories of disease causation: social epidemiology and epidemiological transition. Galle Med J. 2015;20(2):26–32.

Jackson R, et al. Health and the built environment: 10 years after. Am J Public Health. 2013;103(9):1542–4.

Krieger N. Epidemiology and the web of causation: has anyone seen the spider? Soc Sci Med. 1994;39(7):887–903.

Krieger N. Theories for social epidemiology in the 21st century: an ecosocial perspective. Int J Epidemiol. 2001;30(4):668–77.

Messer L, et al. The development of a standardized neighborhood deprivation index. J Urban Health. 2006;83(6):1041–62.

Midekisa A, et al. Remote sensing-based time series models for malaria early warning in the highlands of Ethiopia. Malar J. 2012;11(1):165.

Mittelmark M, Bauer G. The application of salutogenesis in communities and neighborhoods. In: Mittelmark MB, et al., editors. The handbook of salutogenesis. Switzerland: Springer International Publishing; 2017. p. 159–70. https://link.springer.com/content/pdf/10.1007%2F978-3-319-04600-6.pdf. Accessed 13 Jul 2017.

Northridge ME, et al. Sorting out the connections between the built environment and health: a conceptual framework for navigating pathways and planning healthy cities. J Urban Health. 2003;80(4):556–68. https://doi.org/10.1093/jurban/jtg064.

Potvin L, Jones C. Twenty-five years after the Ottawa Charter: the critical role of health promotion for public health. C J Public Health. 2011;2(4):244–4.

Rao A. Landscape anthropometrics: a multi-scale approach to integrating health into the regional landscape. Dissertation, Georgia Institute of Technology; 2016.
Rao A, Ross CL. Health Impact Assessments (HIAs) and healthy schools. J Plan Educ Res. 2014;34(2):141–52. https://doi.org/10.1177/0739456X14531488.
Ross CL, et al. Health impact assessment of Atlanta regional PLAN 2040. Center for Quality Growth and Regional Development. Atlanta, GA: Georgia Institute of Technology; 2012.
Ross CL, et al. Health impact assessment in the United States, Springer, New York; 2014. Available from ProQuest Ebook Central. [6 October 2017].
Rossen L, Pollack K. Making the connection between zoning and health disparities. Environ Justice. 2012;5(3):119–27.
Saelens BE, Handy SL. Built environment correlates of walking: a review. Med Sci Sports Exerc. 2008;40(7 Suppl):S550–66. https://doi.org/10.1249/MSS.0b013e31817c67a4.
Stimpson J, et al. Neighborhood deprivation and health risk behaviors in NHANES III. Third national health and nutrition examination survey. Am J Health Behav. 2007;31(2):215–22.
Szczygiel B, Hewitt R. Nineteenth-century medical landscapes: John H. Rauch, Frederick Law Olmsted, and the search for salubrity. B Hist Med. 2000;74(4):708–34.
Vaandrager L, Kennedy L. The application of salutogenesis in communities and neighborhoods. In: Mittelmark MB, et al., editors. The handbook of salutogenesis. Switzerland: Springer International Publishing; 2017. p. 159–70. https://link.springer.com/content/pdf/10.1007%2F978-3-319-04600-6.pdf. Accessed 13 Jul 2017.
Verbeek T, Boelens L. Environmental health in the complex city: a co-evolutionary approach. J Environ Plann Man. 2016;59(11):1913–32. https://doi.org/10.1080/09640568.2015.1127800.
Wild C. Complementing the genome with an "exposome": the outstanding challenge of environmental exposure measurement in molecular epidemiology. Cancer Epidem Biomar. 2005;14:1847–50. https://doi.org/10.1158/1055-9965.EPI-05-0456.
World Health Organization (WHO). Constitution of the World Health Organization. In: WHO basic documents, 45th edn, Supplement. Geneva: World Health Organization; 2006. http://www.who.int/governance/eb/who_constitution_en.pdf. Accessed 16 Oct 2017.
World Health Organization (WHO) European Centre for Health Policy. Health Impact Assessment: main concepts and suggested approach. Gothenburg consensus paper. Brussels, Belgium: WHO European Centre for Health Policy; 1999. http://webarchive.nationalarchives.gov.uk/20170106084428/http://www.apho.org.uk/resource/item.aspx?RID=44163. Accessed 10 Oct 2017.

Further Reading

National Academy of Sciences. Improving health in the United States: the role of health impact assessment. Washington, DC: The National Academies Press; 2011. https://www.ncbi.nlm.nih.gov/books/NBK83546/pdf/Bookshelf_NBK83546.pdf
Robert Wood Johnson Foundation and The Pew Charitable Trusts. Health impact assessment legislation in the States. 2015. http://www.pewtrusts.org/~/media/assets/2015/01/hia_and_legislation_issue_brief.pdf. Accessed 18 Sept 2017.
The Pew Charitable Trust. Atlanta Regional PLAN 2040. 2017. http://www.pewtrusts.org/en/multimedia/data-visualizations/2015/hia-map/state/georgia/atlanta-plan-2040. Accessed 18 Sep 2017.
United States Center for Disease Control and Prevention (CDC). Health impact assessment resources. 2015. https://www.cdc.gov/healthyplaces/hiaresources.htm. Accessed 18 Sept 2017.

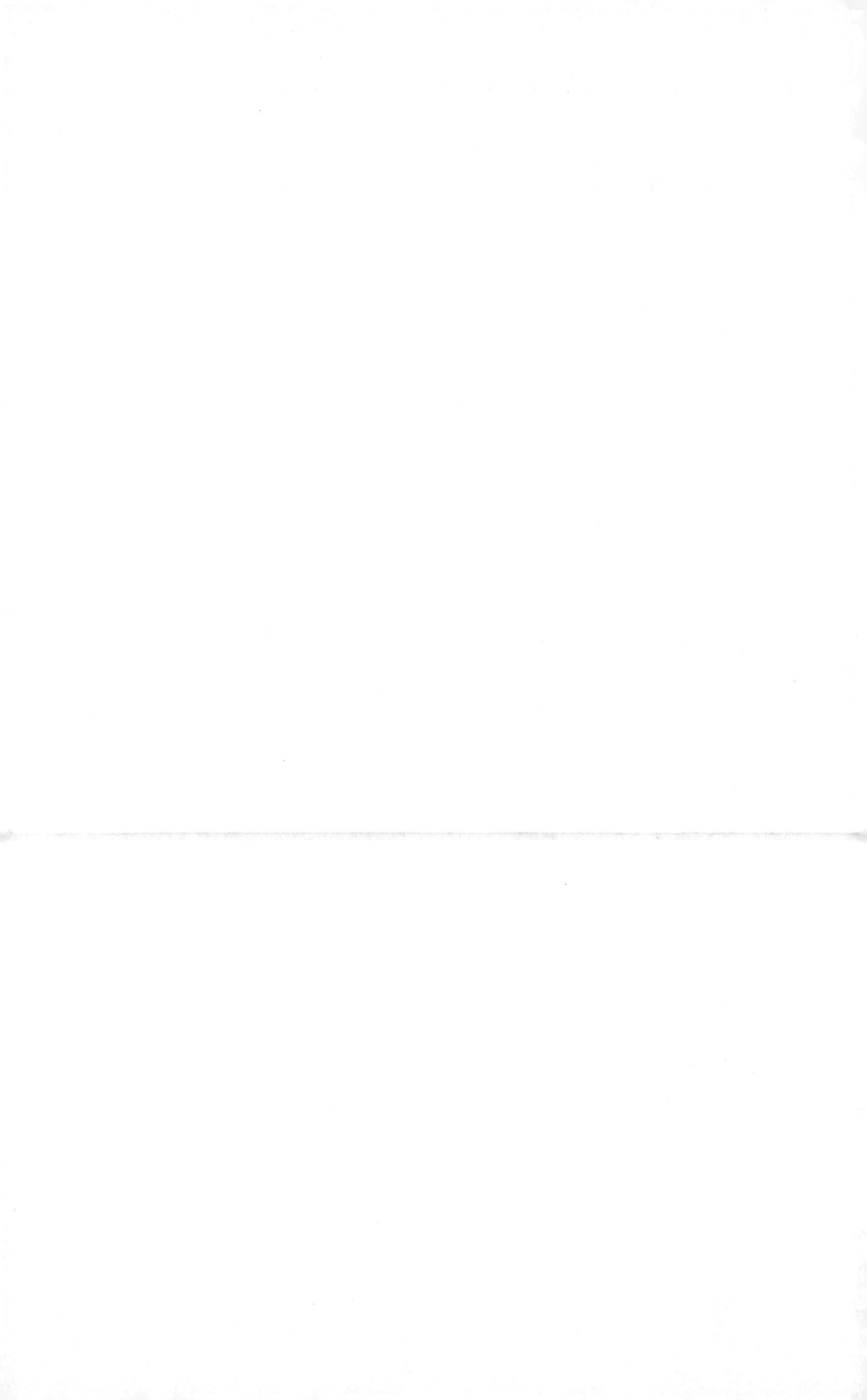

Chapter 5
A Regulatory Primer of International Environmental Policy and Land Use

Beth Ann Fiedler

Abstract A review of international environmental regulation and land use in action establishes the high-level legal foundation of regulatory guidelines to define concepts, highlight important areas of law to promote fundamental understanding, create general discourse, address existing conditions, and prioritize ecosystem destruction avoidance from common ground. The analysis discusses natural resources, land use, and economic development on a global scale guiding the reader through high-level international environmental policy with a focus on land use and land degradation. The chapter demonstrates the overarching role of international environmental policy and land use in the development of policy at subsequent levels of government—national, state, or local—shaping land use policy and decision-making that can incrementally contribute to overall improvements to the global landscape, and thus population health.

5.1 Introduction

The topic of land use spans the gamut from the international land governance in global organizations such as the Organization for Economic Cooperation and Development (OECD) to requesting local permits to construct an addition to your home according to your local zoning ordinance. Land use is diverse and linked to several major areas of public administration. They include transportation, agriculture, recreation, and forests but also natural resource management, waste disposal, and urbanization (USDA 2016). Efforts to address various problems often result in a conflict of authority impeding resolution because of the intersection of these many activities often resulting in a land use imbalance. The subsequent disparity is a global problem demonstrated by the inability of the ecosystem to naturally dissipate extreme heat in concrete and pavement laden cities or to purify ground water sources that are bombarded with agricultural runoff in rural areas. The impact of human

B. A. Fiedler (✉)
Independent Research Analyst, Jacksonville, FL, USA

B. A. Fiedler (ed.), *Translating National Policy to Improve Environmental Conditions Impacting Public Health Through Community Planning*,
https://doi.org/10.1007/978-3-319-75361-4_5

development and production, natural disasters, and others combine to hinder the natural process of corrective action resulting in land degradation.

> (INTOSAI 2013, p.12; United Nations 1997):
> Land degradation is "the reduction or loss of the biological or economic productivity and complexity of rain-fed cropland, irrigated cropland, or range, pasture, forest or woodlands resulting from natural processes, land uses or other human activities and habitation patterns such as land contamination, soil erosion and the destruction of the vegetation cover."

Deforestation, biodiversity loss, soil erosion, and desertification are the primary types of land degradation that impact the quality of air and water as soil becomes contaminated from waste, mining, or because of public services (INTOSAI 2013). The Food and Agricultural Organization (FAO) of the United Nations reports that 25% of the globe is designated as highly degraded land requiring immediate remediation (FAO 2011, p.18). However, the persistent rate of decline is most evident in areas of high levels of poverty precluding the capacity to respond with the amount of financial investments required to make improvements. "The rate of socio-economic change and the accumulation of environmental problems have outpaced institutional responses" (FAO 2011, p.21) resulting in less positive impact in developing regions that often require the most attention.

Recognizing that there exist physical and human contributions to the designation of land use as a stressed resource consequent to human activity and production (INTOSAI 2013) is key to developing solutions. Therefore, every community planning decision and valuation of the existing landscape is critical to halting the further destruction of the planet's natural capacity to support life and to rectify degrading conditions.

The relationship between and among the environment (e.g., natural resources, land use) and economic development is inherently embedded in the four levels of environmental law discussed herein. Focusing on environmental problems that converge on land use and land degradation, this chapter will review the complex nature of international law from these perspectives. The nuances of the convergence of environmental and public health policy are most apparent in the implementation, policy strategy, and enforcement at the local (e.g., state, city) levels of government. However, international regulations act as fundamental guidelines and frameworks driving national and thus local policy implementation. Therefore, we begin by introducing international environmental policy.

5.2 International Environmental Policy

How we use land effects everyone. "Land use matters for many of the most important policy questions of our time: environmental sustainability, CO_2 emissions and biodiversity, and public health" (OECD 2017b, p.9). Deforestation and forms of land degradation through the built environment, such as urbanization and road construction, can directly impact air quality and access to clean water. The long-term

Table 5.1 Primary international environmental agreements for natural resource conservation, particularly contributing factors leading to land and water preservation

Treaties	Brief description	Find more information
1972 United Nations (UN) Convention on the Human Environment[a]	Recommends an international framework for environmental action and the creation of a UN Environmental Organization	http://staging.unep.org/Documents.multilingual/Default.asp?DocumentID=287
1992 United Nations Conference on Environment and Development (UNCED), which produced the Rio Declaration[a]	Global environmental integrity; Led to 1994 UN Statement of Forest Principles	http://wedocs.unep.org/bitstream/handle/20.500.11822/19163/Rio_Declaration_on_Environment_and_Development.pdf?sequence=1&isAllowed=y
1997 Kyoto Protocol, enacted 16 Feb 2005[a]	National commitment to reduce carbon dioxide and other greenhouse gas emissions; engage in "carbon trading" to offset inability to reduce emissions	http://unfccc.int/resource/docs/convkp/kpeng.html
2002 World Earth Summit[a]	Sustainable development	http://www.earthsummit2002.org/Es2002.pdf
United Nations (UN) Sustainable Development Summit, enacted[a] Jan 2016[b]	Sustainable development goals 2030	http://www.un.org/sustainabledevelopment/sustainable-development-goals/

Source: [a]Cornell University Law School, Legal Information Institute (n.d.); [b]United Nations (2017)

global implications of decreasing forest and plant life are important. Reduction in these natural resources equates to less capacity to perform oxygen-producing photosynthesis and to provide root systems to stabilize ground water, cover to protect fresh water systems from evaporation, and impede against natural disasters such as landslides, avalanches, and coastal erosion. Thus, these and other human altered environmental conditions "can directly impose health risks or impair ecosystem services that subsequently influence health" (Myers et al. 2013, p.18756). International agreements (Table 5.1) represent an overarching method to manage natural water resources (e.g., oceans, fisheries, polar ice caps) and atmospheric conditions by monitoring and reducing carbon emissions and other airborne particulates (Cornell University n.d.).

The Rio Declaration captures the important nature of preserving natural forests and recommending the utilization of environmental impact assessments to limit the impact of development while the Kyoto Protocol is particularly concerned with reducing carbon emissions. Both are important to human health having direct and indirect impact on air and water quality. While the international declarations include overlapping ideologies to protect natural resources, they also generate a framework for cooperative action to prompt national governments to build environmental governance into policy directives. INTOSAI recommends that achieving this objective requires that all nations pool resources and share knowledge to effectively implement global initiatives towards sustainable resource management (2013).

Consequently, these international treatises must trickle down to national objectives in which the general framework is applied to conditions specific to each country. Taking into consideration such information as production activity, population growth, population movement, current land use, natural resources, and national policy will eventually form planning systems and new policy to address these and other environmental conditions (Choi and Lee 2016).

Regional policy (e.g., states, multi-national) and local governments further build upon this framework to make local government environmental and land use decisions encompassing a wide array of guidance and public law. Subsequently, variance in land use strategies is inherently different even within national boundaries due to several factors. They include dynamic conditions, such as population or demographic changes, but also the level of cooperation, types and number of institutions, roles of leadership defined in statutes and development of partnerships embedded into the political structure and policy development process (OECD 2017a, 2017b).

Other key factors to consider include, "the types of actors involved in land use governance and even the levels of social trust in a society, which affects relationships between and among residents, businesses, governments and non-governmental groups" (OECD 2017b, p.15). Determining the project scale and the span of cooperation and collaboration between and among the economic regions will help to streamline the number of spatial planning stakeholders making success feasible through improved coordination and monitoring of multi-sourced funds (Cheshire 2007; Institute for Spatial and Landscape Development 2008; Tudor 2014; Turkoglu et al. 2012).

Access to land has extended socioeconomic consequences in addition to the impact of land use on environmental conditions due to the high value placed on land, built environment, and property. Notable is that land use decisions can increase land value impacting other areas of quality of life, such as housing affordability, and the subsequent impact on economic growth and production (OECD 2017b). These disparities are in direct contrast to the United Nations (UN) Sustainable Development Goals (SDGs) emphasizing economic opportunity (Goal 8), reduced inequalities (Goal 10), and sustainable human settlements (Goal 11) (UN 2017).

The regional capacity to promote clean air and retain ground water sources through natural plant life and vegetation found in forest areas and a strong agricultural presence is important to elevating populations out of poverty, providing a healthier environment, and increasing quality of life. On the other hand, the problem of the impact of agriculture on natural resources and the environment remains a dilemma because of ecosystem destruction. Following international guidelines has led to the introduction of various instruments (e.g., regulatory and economic) as well as collaborative arrangements to control agricultural expansion to limit natural habitat encroachment. They include national regulation in Brazil, community-based partnerships in Australia, and economic instruments in the United States that have achieved moderate success but not without pitfalls (Tanentzap et al. 2015). Researchers demonstrate that local obstacles exist to policy implementation (e.g., enforcement, implementation cost); social rewards for local partnerships may limit long-term, national solutions; and the problematic nature of environmental outcomes as an incentive as opposed to economic benefits in the long-term sustainability of individual farmers (Tanentzap et al. 2015).

To further complicate the matter, some of the land required by farmers and cattle ranchers has been at the expense of forests. Examples include the development of oil palm plantations in the lowland rainforests of Indonesia, cattle ranches established on the savanna of Brazil, and soybean production in parts of the Amazon rainforest (McClellan 2017). "Primary forests account for 80% of land biodiversity" and "exchange of carbon between vegetation, soil and atmosphere" (INTOSAI 2013, p.50). The destruction of these habitats often releases plant, animal, and insect life into foreign areas unable to contain the unique protective balance within the natural ecosystem (Ostfeld 2017a). "The destruction of forest habitats for many species facilitates the transmission of infectious diseases to humans through contact with mosquitoes, monkeys, virus- and bacteria-carrying rodents that are potentially hazardous to humans" (INTOSAI 2013, p.50). The persistence of malaria and the introduction of the Zika Virus are two examples of the public health consequences of the transition from forest to agricultural areas (Robbins 2016).

Therefore, developing ways to counter this effect is important to maintaining biodiversity and abating infectious and zoonotic disease. Environmental research institutions, such as the Stanford Woods Institute for the Environment, report that one way to responsibly expand agriculture with less environmental impact is to clear forests along the outer perimeter versus cutting out tracts within forest boundaries (Chaplin-Kramer et al. 2015; Jordan 2015; Solie 2015). Chaplin-Kramer's et al. method of spatially implicit analysis and planning optimizes large-scale land mass conversion focusing on how land is converted and not just the prevailing system of analysis that relies on the total quantity of land slated for conversion (2015). This novel perspective that values nature reports the impact on the whole system by reducing total potential deforestation impact (e.g., biodiversity loss, carbon storage) and enveloping community, social development and economic sustainability.

Nonetheless, food demand and living space for a growing population often require hard tradeoffs apparent in the national socioeconomic status of a country and lack of policy limiting deforestation for agriculture, building materials, fuel, and other uses (Table 5.2). Despite forest losses reported in low and lower middle-income countries whose citizens depend on these resources or daily needs, many governments have not enacted a quota or provide best practice methods to educate citizens to follow that could limit destruction.

Table 5.2 demonstrates that while low-income countries have gained 647,126 km^2 (249,857 mi^2 or about 1916 mi^2 less than the size of Afghanistan in 2013) of land used for agriculture from 2000 to 2014, they have simultaneously lost about 252,280 km^2 (97,406 mi^2 or 2480 mi^2 more than the size of Guinea in 2013) of natural forest land from 2000 to 2015. On the other hand, high-income countries have

Table 5.2 The World Bank world development indicators for forest and agricultural land use, square kilometers (km^2) based on country socioeconomic status[†††]

Socioeconomic Status[†]	Agriculture[a] km^2		% Land Area[d††] Agriculture		Forest[b] km^2		% Land Area Forest[c††]	
	2000	2014	2000	2014	2000	2015	2000	2015
High Income	13,510,032	12,748,640	38.56	36.41	9,994,008	10,090,494	28.56	28.85
Upper Middle Income	20,236,524	20,454,795	34.84	35.16	20,234,599	20,174,822	34.77	34.68
Middle-Income Aggregate[‡]	31,027,899	30,653,799	38.19	37.69	26,479,802	26,071,323	32.55	32.06
Lower Middle Income	10,791,375	10,199,004	46.62	44.07	6,245,203	5,896,501	26.98	25.48
Low Income	4,888,131	5,535,257	36.53	39.23	3,990,720	3,738,440	29.82	27.40

Source: [a]The World Bank (2017a); [b]The World Bank (2017b); [c]The World Bank (2017c); [d]The World Bank (2017d). All based on most recent complete available data.
Notes: [†]Socioeconomic status is based on the 2015 Gross National Income (GNI) per capita defined as the average income per citizen. Low-income economies was \$1025 or less such as Haiti, Tanzania, Senegal, and Cambodia; Lower middle income between \$1026 and \$4035 such as Cambodia, Cameroon, and Kenya; ‡Middle-income aggregate between \$1026 and \$12,475 combines the categories of Lower Middle Income and Upper Middle Income; Upper middle income between \$4036 and \$12,475 such as China, Egypt, Nigeria, Jordan, or Ecuador; and High income was \$12,476 or more such as Singapore, Luxembourg, and the United Arab Emirates; [††]rounded to two decimal places; [†††]Multiple # of km^2 × 0.38610216 = # square miles (mi^2). Find the international list of the World Bank GNI per capita at https://data.worldbank.org/indicator/NY.GNP.PCAP.CD?year_high_desc=true.

lost 761,392 km^2 (293,976 mi^2 or about 2046 mi^2 more than the size of Chile in 2013) of agricultural land and 96,486 km^2 (37,253 mi^2 or 1334 mi^2 more than the size of Hungary in 2013) of forest. Of course, the impact of decreasing agricultural space is more easily offset by higher income nations than lower income nations because of their greater capacity to import goods. (Country land area to provide readers with a spatial reference of these losses and gains in this and following paragraphs were obtained from Compare Infobase, Ltd. 2017; NationMaster 2013.)

However, a compelling item in Table 5.2 is the Middle-Income Aggregate of the Lower Middle-Income and Upper Middle-Income countries. In this socioeconomic national status, we find losses in both land for agriculture (−341,100 km^2 or 131,699.45 mi^2 or 1100 mi^2 more than the size of Finland in 2013) and forest (−408,479 km^2 or 157,715 mi^2 or 667 mi^2 more than the size of the nation of Paraguay). The losses of agriculture and forest land in lower income nations, −592,371 and −348,702 km^2, respectively, negate the positive improvements in Upper Middle-income nations, +218,271 and +59,777 km^2, respectively. If not offset by the Upper Middle-Income nations, the lower middle-income losses would have been comparable to agricultural loss slightly less than the size of Madagascar and forest loss approaching the size of Germany.

Yet, there is a turn towards national resource conservation based on empirical evidence linking environmental conservation to health benefits. For example, Cambodian policymakers can now make an informed decision to support tropical forest conservation there based on research conducted by the National University of Singapore revealing the negative impact on children's morbidity and mortality (e.g., diarrhea, fever, and acute respiratory infection) linked to deforestation (Ostfeld 2017b; Pienkowski et al. 2017).

The tradeoff between increasing agricultural land at the expense of forests is not without hazard to natural habitats and public health. The next section relays the problem of land use imbalance and the global consequences to public health.

5.3 Balancing Urgent Global Population Needs Against Long-Term Global Population Health

> Even though land use planning is primarily a local task and concerns local issues, it has consequences for issues of national global importance: the long-term stability of ecosystems, social justice, food and energy security, long-term economic growth, housing costs, and the mitigation of and adaption to climate change. Planning also has a crucial role to play to accomplish 6 of the 17 UN Sustainable Development Goals. (OECD 2017b, p.14)

The role of international treatise embedded in the UN SDGs is important to a global approach to a multiplicity of environmental and population health concerns. Table 5.3 demonstrates that land use planning and implementation plays a pivotal role towards achieving overall objectives. The difficulty in simultaneously achieving balance in global population needs for quality of life, environmental protection, and population health with more than one-third of the SDGs emanating from land use planning is daunting. This statement is based on the inherent nature of multiple government functions embedded in the topic of land use and the potential

Table 5.3 United Nations sustainable development goals prominent in planning (United Nations 2017)

	Goal brief	Objective(s)
7	Affordable and clean energy	Ensure access to inexpensive, reliable, and sustainable energy
9	Industry, innovation, and infrastructure	Foster innovation to bring forth sustainable industrialization and resilient infrastructure
11	Sustainable cities and communities	Plan inclusive human settlements and cities factoring in safety, resilience, and sustainability
13	Climate action	Prioritize climate change remediation
14	Life below water	Develop seascapes using sustainable development
15	Life on land	Remediate land degradation through restoration and incorporating sustainable management practices for new land development to protect, halt, and reverse degradation and biodiversity loss

for conflict between and among sectoral government objectives. But with growing recognition of the link between man and nature and cooperative response, we would add that the task, though daunting, is not impossible.

Unprecedented global land use planning and resource management may be the necessary step in balancing these variety of outputs with limited natural resource inputs. While the OECD Land-Use Governance Survey conducted in 2015–2016 across the 32 OECD nations reports that "all levels of government use spatial and land-use plans as instruments to shape land use" (OECD 2017a, p.9), spatial or strategic planning and policy is emphasized by national governments while land use objectives are determined locally for most nations with some exception. However, large municipalities with dense population, overlapping regions, or overlapping national boundaries may require a regional plan and coordination (Institute for Spatial and Landscape Development 2008; Tudor 2014; Turkoglu et al. 2012). "Spatial plans aim to structure the general pattern of human activity across space without necessarily determining land use at any given location" while "land-use plans aim to prescribe particular land used for specific locations" (OECD 2017a, p.9).

Clearly the role of land use planning and resource management must continue to morph and stretch beyond current limitations to achieve global objectives inclusive of public health. Novel policy development, critical thinking on the dual nature of environmental and public health, and innovation in the research community may be a good place to start.

New policy development, though sometimes seen as the slow road to resolution, is certainly important as a guide to national and lesser levels of government to plan, budget, and to obtain resources to implement policy instruments able to define and address national problems contributing to global environmental decay. However, what is often overlooked is the impact of current policy on the forward motion of novel legislation. Existing land use policies detail "how land is permitted to be used" based on environmental regulations, building codes, spatial and land use planning while nonspatial policies (e.g., tax codes, agriculture, energy policy) impact "how individuals and businesses want to use land" sometimes deterring development (OECD 2017b, p.75). The problematic conflict between spatial and nonspatial regulation is that land use decisions stemming from these separate restrictions result in "how land is [actually] used" (2017b, p.75) versus potentially advantageous positioning of new development (e.g., transportation, housing, grocery store, bike path, industry). This regulatory gap, if you will, presents another problem—"how to ensure that national objectives are represented in local land-use regulations" (OECD 2017a, p.10). How land is used comes into sharper focus considering this perceptive observation bringing forth "the question of how to provide clear and unambiguous regulations, while at the same time leaving lower levels of government and private actors sufficient flexibility" (OECD 2017a, p.10). Targeting policy in answer to this question provides a starting point for application of international environmental and public health objectives embedded in the UN SDGs.

Other approaches to problem resolution offer new opportunities to utilize critical thinking, science, and technology to balance environmental health with public health. First, Richard Ostfeld of the Cary Institute of Ecosystem Studies in Millbrook, NY has considered the dual concern for environmental and public health proposing to formulate new policy under the umbrella of planetary health (2017a). "Careful analysis of the mechanisms that underlie co-benefits to environmental and human health, could uncover key principles and inform new applications, while providing concrete options for policy and management" (Ostfeld 2017a, p.e2). Ostfeld proposes key metrics, such as species diversity and risk of exposure to zoonotic diseases, that concurrently afford the opportunity to gauge impact on both environmental and human health, respectively (2017a). Second, other research proposes scientific approaches to mitigating some of the environmental impact on respiratory health by increasing the land use land cover (LULC) in critical areas. Rao et al. (2017) suggest increasing the tree canopy by 5% can reduce the concentrated amount of ambient air pollution in critical areas by 6%, and thus improve respiratory health in those locations with benefits to the entire city. The introduction of metric development and scientific research to address concurrent environmental and health problems through critical thinking, research design, modeling, and simulation promises to substantiate a common interest towards balancing both components.

5.4 Summary

This chapter generally introduces the primary treatises of international environmental law and land use offering several resources for further exploration. These international laws provide the foundation for national, regional, and local policy. Focusing on two major areas of land use: (1) agriculture land 2000–2014 and (2) forest land 2000–2015, global dynamic changes in natural resources are categorized according to their socioeconomic status. Selection of representation of the data in this fashion emphasizes the global distribution of these natural resources, their change in availability, and the capacity of nations to address environmental destruction based on their financial capacity. The impact of forest loss is particularly hard felt in low and lower middle-income nations with significant impact to health. However, the introduction of critical thinking and scientific research to address concurrent environmental and health problems promises to substantiate a common interest towards balancing both components.

Acknowledgements The author would like to thank the Legal Information Institute at Cornell University Law School for their commitment to open access of legal topics and associated law in their online directory. Also, the Organization for Economic Cooperation and Development for thought-provoking content and forward-thinking research. Finally, The World Bank in cooperation with the Food and Agriculture Organization of the United Nations and the United Nations for access to their consistent and reliable data. Dissemination of this information is the sole responsibility of the author and utilization of this material does not imply legal advice or endorsement.

Glossary

Biodiversity The number of different species contained within specific ecosystems

Biodiversity loss A consequence of land degradation; when species are lost to an ecosystem due to deforestation and other human activity

Deforestation A consequence of land degradation; when human activity strip forests without concern for the long-term consequences of land and water quality

Desertification One consequence of land degradation; when a region that is already characterized as being dry with relatively less precipitation or naturally occurring bodies of water, plants, and animals suffers losses from human activity, weather, and other conditions

Environmental impact assessments Analyzing various effects on social, economic, environmental conditions and taking measures to minimize impact of new development

Land degradation When land is unable to produce natural resources (e.g., crops, wilderness, grazing areas) due to overuse, contamination or other causes elicited from human activity and production

Land use Linked to several major areas of public administration such as natural resource management, waste disposal, transportation, urbanization, agriculture, recreation, and forest

Land use planning Task of local governments to utilize national or regional spatial planning guidance to formulate specific land use

Malaria Dangerous disease transmitted when an infected mosquito bites several humans; impacts human red blood cells that, in turn, impact organs such as the brain, kidneys, and liver

Soil erosion A consequence of land degradation; when human activity removes soil stabilizing canopies that protect water resources and soil fertility is lost as weather (e.g., wind, rain, direct sunlight) removes top soil rendering it useless for crops

Spatial planning A task of national governments to determine the potential general structure of human activity to guide local planners on specific land use

Zika Virus Spread by infectious mosquitoes; particularly harmful to fetus development

Zoonotic disease The transmission of infectious diseases in animals to humans caused by a variety of pathogens including viruses (e.g., rabies, HIV, and Ebola), bacteria (anthrax found in soil consumed by goats, sheep; bartonella from cat scratches), fungi (dermatomycoses from rats), or parasitic activity (Trichinella found in cows and pigs)

References

Chaplin-Kramer R, et al. Spatial patterns of agricultural expansion determine impacts on biodiversity and carbon storage. P Nat A Sci. 2015;112(24):7402–7.

Cheshire PC. Identifying principles for spatial policy: levels of intervention. Portuguese J Reg Stud. 2007;13:55–65. http://www.apdr.pt/siteRPER/numeros/RPER13/13.4.pdf. Accessed 2 Sept 2017.

Choi H-S, Lee G-S. Planning support systems (PSS)-based spatial plan alternatives and environmental assessment. Sustain For. 2016;8:286. https://doi.org/10.3390/su8030286.

Compare Infobase, Ltd. World interactive map. 2017. https://www.mapsofworld.com/world-map-viewer.html. Accessed 3 Sept 2017.

Cornell Law School, Legal Information Institute. International environmental law. n.d. https://www.law.cornell.edu/wex/International_environmental_law. Accessed 24 Jul 2017.

Food and Agricultural Organization (FAO) of the United Nations. The state of the world's land and water resources for food and agriculture. FAO Rome. 2011. http://www.fao.org/docrep/015/i1688e/i1688e00.pdf. Accessed 27 Aug 2017.

Institute for Spatial and Landscape Development, ETH Zurich. Spatial planning and development in Switzerland; observations and suggestions from the international group of experts, Swiss Federal Office for Spatial Development (ARE). 2008.

International Organization of Supreme Audit Institutions (INTOSAI) Working Group on Environmental Auditing (WGEA). Land use and land management practices in environmental perspective. 2013. http://www.environmental-auditing.org/LinkClick.aspx?fileticket=NiwOS89K5Jk%3D&tabid=128&mid=568. Accessed 24 Jul 2017.

Jordan R. Agriculture and deforestation: how to reduce impacts. Stanford Wood Institute for the Environment. 2015. https://woods.stanford.edu/news-events/news/agriculture-and-deforestation-how-reduce-impacts. Accessed 3 Sept 2017.

McClellan R. Farming: habitat conversion & loss. 2017. http://wwf.panda.org/what_we_do/footprint/agriculture/impacts/habitat_loss/. Accessed 3 Sept 2017.

Myers SS, et al. Human health impacts of ecosystem alteration. Proc Natl Acad Sci U S A. 2013;110(47):18753–60.

NationMaster. Country land area. 2013. http://www.nationmaster.com/country-info/stats/Geography/Land-area/Square-miles. Accessed 2 Sept 2017.

Organization for Economic Cooperation and Development (OECD). Executive summary. In: Land-use planning systems in the OECD: country fact sheets. OECD Publishing, Paris; 2017a. https://doi.org/10.1787/9789264268579-2-en. Accessed 14 Sept 2017.

Organization for Economic Cooperation and Development (OECD). The governance of land use in OECD countries: policy analysis and recommendations. Paris: OECD Publishing; 2017b. https://doi.org/10.1787/9789264268609-en. Accessed 20 Jul 2017

Ostfeld RS. Biodiversity loss and the ecology of infectious disease. Lancet Planet Health. 2017a;1(1):e2–3.

Ostfeld RS. Tropical forests and child health. Lancet Planet Health. 2017b;1(5):e164–5.

Pienkowski T, et al. Empirical evidence of the public health benefits of tropical forest conservation in Cambodia: a generalised linear mixed-effects model analysis. Lancet Planet Health. 2017;1:e180–7.

Rao M, et al. Assessing the potential of land use modification to mitigate ambient NO_2 and its consequences for respiratory health. Int J Environ Res Public Health. 2017;14(7):750. https://doi.org/10.3390/ijerph14070750.

Robbins J. How forest loss is leading to a rise in human disease. 2016. https://e360.yale.edu/features/how_forest_loss_is_leading_to_a_rise_in_human_disease_malaria_zika_climate_change. Accessed 3 Sept 2017.

Solie S. How valuing nature is transforming decisions. 2015. https://woods.stanford.edu/news-events/news/how-valuing-nature-transforming-decisions. Accessed 14 Sept 2017.

Tanentzap AJ, et al. Resolving conflicts between agriculture and the natural environment. PLoSBiol. 2015;13(9):e1002242. https://doi.org/10.1371/journal.pbio.1002242.
The World Bank. Agricultural land (sq km) [Data source Food and Agriculture Organization]. 2017a. https://data.worldbank.org/indicator/AG.LND.AGRI.K2?view=chart. Accessed 31 Aug 2017.
The World Bank. Forest land (sq km) [Data source Food and Agriculture Organization]. 2017b. https://data.worldbank.org/indicator/AG.LND.FRST.K2?view=chart . Accessed 31 Aug 2017.
The World Bank. Forest land (% of land area). [Data source Food and Agriculture Organization]. 2017c. https://data.worldbank.org/indicator/AG.LND.FRST.ZS?view=chart. Accessed 1 Sept 2017.
The World Bank. Agriculture land (% of land area) [Data source Food and Agriculture Organization]. 2017d. https://data.worldbank.org/indicator/AG.LND.AGRI.ZS?view=chart. Accessed 1 Sept 2017.
Tudor CA. How successful is the resolution of land use conflicts? A comparison of cases from Switzerland and Romania. Appl Geogr. 2014;47:125–36.
Turkoglu H, et al. A participatory spatial planning process: the case of Bursa, Turkey. 48th International Society of City and Regional Planners (ISOCARP) Congress, Perm, Russia, 10–13 September. 2012.
United Nations (UN). Glossary of environment statistics, studies in methods, Series F, No. 67. 1997. New York: United Nations.
United Nations (UN). Sustainable development goals. 2017. http://www.un.org/sustainabledevelopment/sustainable-development-goals/. Accessed 1 Sept 2017.
United States Department of Agriculture (USDA) Economic Research Service. Major land uses. 2016. https://www.ers.usda.gov/topics/farm-economy/land use-land-value-tenure/major-land uses/. Accessed 24 Jul 2017.

Further Reading

American Society of International Law. Electronic information system for international law (EISIL). 2013. http://www.eisil.org/index.php?sid=478272769&t=sub_pages&cat=18. Accessed 28 Aug 2017.
Hennig B. Views of the world: ecological footprints. 2015. http://www.viewsoftheworld.net/?p=4639. Accessed 14 Sept 2017.
Oldekop JA. 100 key research questions for the post-2015 development agenda. Dev Pol Rev. 2016;34(1):55–82.
Norton RK, Bieri DS. Planning, law, and property rights: a U.S.-European cross-national contemplation. 2014. http://david-bieri.com/docs/NB_PlanningLawPropertyRights_IPS14.pdf. Accessed 18 Sept 2017.
OpenLandContracts.Org. An online repository of open land contracts. n.d. http://openlandcontracts.org/. Accessed 27 Aug 2017.
Organization Economic Cooperation and Development (OECD). Search 'land use planning'. [Online]. 2017. http://www.oecd-ilibrary.org/. Accessed 14 Sept 2017.
The Center for Climate & Security. Exploring the security risks of climate change. 2017. https://climateandsecurity.org. Accessed 24 Jul 2017.
The World Bank Group. Data catalog. 2017. http://data.worldbank.org/data-catalog/. Accessed 28 Aug 2017.
Werrill C, Femia F. Chronology of military and intelligence concerns about climate change. 2017. https://climateandsecurity.org/2017/01/12/chronology-of-the-u-s-military-and-intelligence-communitys-concern-about-climate-change/#more-11797. Accessed 24 Jul 2017.

Chapter 6
A Regulatory Primer of United States Multisectoral Land Use and Environmental Policy

Beth Ann Fiedler

Abstract A broad sweep of multitiered government policy in the United States (e.g., federal, state, and city) provides a scale view of land use and environmental regulation. Establishing the legal foundation of regulatory guidelines helps to define concepts, highlight important areas of law to promote understanding, create general discourse, address existing conditions, and prioritize avoidance of ecosystem destruction to facilitate population health. The analysis introduces the interdependent role of natural resources, land use, and economic development embedded in three levels of environmental law through overviews of U.S. national policy, the State of California, and the City of Chicago, Illinois. The intent of aligning subordinate law with higher levels of law is an important objective but analysis reveals the challenges in overlapping ideologies in relation to proximity of development impact and positional perspective. Therefore, defining the role of each level of policy demonstrates the complexity of establishing policy by identifying local obstacles, environmental conditions, and their health consequences in diverse populations even while sharing the same national boundaries.

6.1 Introduction

United States land use has historical roots emanating from colonization, westward expansion, and the relatively recent shift to urban expansion. The overabundance of land meant few regulations for over one hundred years. Guidelines that did exist, starting in 1862 with the Homestead Act, had a focus on land and resource exploitation versus protection. That is, until utilization of natural resources (e.g., forest, gold, oil, minerals) and railroad access began to steer policy development in the latter part of the nineteenth century. Then, urban development was the next impetus for regulation in the early twentieth century appearing in the form of zoning

B. A. Fiedler (✉)
Independent Research Analyst, Jacksonville, FL, USA

B. A. Fiedler (ed.), *Translating National Policy to Improve Environmental Conditions Impacting Public Health Through Community Planning*,
https://doi.org/10.1007/978-3-319-75361-4_6

regulations empowering local municipalities to control housing, commerce, and industrial development. (Brugger 2017; Cornell Law School, Legal Information Institute n.d.-c; Gates 1976; Nolon 2008).

A small number of federal laws, or lack thereof, play a key role in the development of state and municipal regulations for land use and environmental policy. The Clean Air Act of 1970—an air quality and environmental law, and National Environmental Policy Act (NEPA) are modern applications of environmental regulation authorizing federal and state legislation to prevent and take corrective action on environmental conditions. However, environmental land regulation was not implemented until the 1976 Federal Land Policy and Management Act emerging several years after NEPA became federal law. Environmental decay, population growth, and competition for prime real estate development also birthed the enactment of the U.S. Environmental Protection Agency (EPA) and additional legislation, such as the Environmental Quality Improvement Act and the National Environmental Education Act. (Cornell Law School n.d.-b; Gates 1976; U.S. Department of the Interior, Bureau of Land Management n.d.). But the convergence of land use planning and environmental policy was an important step in federal statutes guiding the formation of state statutes and local municipal ordinances for implementation of corrective action.

Ironic is the basic purpose of NEPA "to force governmental agencies to consider the effects of their decision on the environment" (Cornell Law School, Legal Information Institute, n.d.-b, *para* 3; Nolon 1996), while the U.S. struggles with 28 areas of environmental contamination emanating from legacy land use decisions by federal agencies (GAO 2017, p.i). Since 1994, the U.S. Government Accountability Office (GAO) recommends that offending agencies should remove harmful toxins and other dangerous substances left in the environment because of direct and indirect operations; compliance with GAO recommendations is less than half (13/28) to date (GAO 2017, p.i). Two U.S. Government agencies: (1) the Department of Energy (83%), and (2) the Department of Defense (14%) in 2016 accounted for nearly all the government environmental liabilities estimated at $447 billion more than doubling the 1997 estimate (GAO 2017, p.i).

Other controversial U.S. environmental topics include the continued lack of support by the U.S. Senate for international environmental treaties such as the Kyoto Agreement (UNFCCC 2014) due to the economic burden that unnecessarily inhibits business operations. While previous Presidential Administrations fought to join the international agreements, President Donald J. Trump's Energy Independence Executive Order strives to address legislation brought forth by the Obama Administration, such as the Clean Power Act (CPA) of 2015. The CPA of 2015 was vehemently opposed by most of the states, trade associations, and labor unions. Amidst political opposition that the public health is endangered by repealing such items as the CPA (Hultman 2017), the reality is that a bipartisan majority of the U.S. Congress already disapproved the CPA in December 2015 less than two months after enactment. This activity made way for the actual Proposal to Repeal the Clean Power Plan and the Regulatory Impact Analysis that paints a different picture in favor of CPA modification (EPA 2017). Proposed changes to the CPA will return to the “best system of emission reduction” for each source item of emission instead of the cost prohibitive facility-based solution. President Trump’s directive with EPA modifications will focus attention on cleaning the used coffee cup versus the intent of the initial CPA in October 2015 that instructed to wash all your clean dishes every time there was a cup in the sink. The U.S. remains diligent in forest restoration by increasing the 1990 total of 3,024,500 km^2 of forest by adding more than 76,450 km^2 reaching 3,100,950 km^2 in 2015 (World Bank 2017a) and substantially reducing carbon emissions (Boden et al. 2014, 2017; World Bank 2017a). Nevertheless, forest use and croplands have generally declined from 1959 to 2012 while grasslands and urban areas have gained larger land mass (USDA 2016).

This chapter focuses on providing a synopsis of overarching federal legislation and the problematic nature of legacy development decisions. Then, we drill down to specific environmental areas of concern to public health in the State of California and then the City of Chicago. Together, they represent the local development of land use and environmental policy in relation to the limited national land use policy (developed in the mid-nineteenth century) and national environmental policy (developed in the mid-twentieth century). The analysis does not include an example of county-level jurisdiction but demonstrates the difficulty in addressing multisectoral land use and environmental policy within national boundaries from a national, state and city perspective.

6.2 National Land Use and Environmental Policy

National policy tools in the form of “regulatory instruments, such as legislation, regulations, permits, licenses, bylaws, and ordinances), and economic instruments such as subsidies, incentives, taxes or grants” represent the primary tools of government to manage land and to limit environmental harm by engaging in “conservation, prevention, protection, restoration, and mitigation” (INTOSAI 2013, p.7). Public policy tools grant authority to create new agencies or task existing agencies to infuse sustainable objectives of environmental protection into land use decisions. These activities include monitoring, legal authority to fine, and to establish standards providing that the policy receives economic and political feasibility by including transparent accountability and other factors to achieve support and full implementation (Salamon 2002).

NEPA is an overarching framework for procedural review requiring “consideration” for mitigation and alternative measures but does not have the authority to halt development or require implementation of those alternatives. Thus, this groundbreaking legislative action is not without certain limitations. Often the NEPA requirement for the conduct of an Environmental Impact Assessment (EIA) to minimize environmental impact is not a preplanning element and can be bypassed apart from two conditions. First, the project is considered a major federal action (40 Code of Federal Regulations § 1508.18); second, the project may affect human health

Table 6.1 Key United States federal laws regarding land use

Policy	Brief description	Find more information
1862 Homestead Act[1]	Gave those who lived in the U.S. at least 5 years incentive to migrate West providing settlers 160 acres of public land	https://www.ourdocuments.gov/doc.php?flash=true&doc=31
1872 Mining Act[1]	Guides transfer of rights to mine metals and minerals on federal land	https://www.perc.org/articles/mining-law-1872-0
1920 Mineral Leasing Act,[1] as amended July 26, 2005	Governs leasing of public lands for developing hydrocarbons (e.g., coal, petroleum, natural gas), sodium and others	https://www.onrr.gov/Laws_R_D/PubLaws/PDFDocs/MineralLeasingAct1920.pdf
1877 Desert Lands Entry Act[2]	Prompted economic development for individuals to reclaim the (semi)arid public lands of the Western states through irrigation/cultivation	http://what-when-how.com/the-american-economy/desert-land-act-1877/
1934 Taylor Grazing Act,[1] grazing now managed by Bureau of Land Management	Regulates grazing on public lands except Alaska	http://plainshumanities.unl.edu/encyclopedia/doc/egp.ag.071
1960 Multiple Use Sustained Yield Act,[1] Public Law 86-517, as amended December 31, 1996, Public Law 104–333	National forests "renewable surfaces" used for recreation, natural resources, wildlife, and watershed	https://www.fs.fed.us/emc/nfma/includes/musya60.pdf
1976 Federal Land Policy and Management Act, as amended May 7, 2001, Public Law 94-579[3a]	Establish and administrate federal land policy assigning Bureau of Land Management as Director	https://www.blm.gov/or/regulations/files/FLPMA.pdf

Source: [1]National Youth Advisory Board (1974), p.ii; [2]Vincent et al. (2017); [3]US Department of the Interior, Bureau of Land Management and Office of the Solicitor (2001)
Note: [a]Instrumental in federal land use planning (OECD 2017, p.222)

(e.g., hazardous substances, pollutants, safety, radiation, contamination) and must undergo review by other federal agencies (42 U.S. Code § 4332; NEPA § 102(2) c).

U.S. national land use and environmental policies developed in the nineteenth and twentieth centuries represent an antiquated perspective in the overall schema of land use (Table 6.1) and land use planning (Table 6.2). Nevertheless, from the Homestead Act of 1862 that incentivized migration to the western U.S. to the subsequent development of a population safety-motivated national highway system nearly a century later, these policies are the building blocks for public administration. But changes in the international geopolitical fabric and global climate conditions suggest a review to further accommodate avoidance of natural disasters, emergency response, and other safety concerns.

Further, each item in Table 6.2 represents an obstacle for decisions of the built environment that would disturb the natural habitats of endangered animals, disrupt

Table 6.2 Key United States federal laws affecting land use planning and convergence with environmental policy (OECD 2017, p.222)[1]

Policy[1]	Brief description	Find more information
Federal Highway Act of 1956	Initiated the construction of a national highway system to address safety, emergency routes, allow faster travel	http://www.history.com/topics/interstate-highway-system
National Flood Insurance Act of 1968 Public Law 90-448	National Flood Insurance Program; provides government backed mortgage insurance to protect homeowners from flood loss	https://www.fema.gov/media-library/assets/documents/7277
National Environmental Policy Act of 1969 Public Law 91-190	Established a council to create harmony between man and nature; environmental protection	https://www.fws.gov/r9esnepa/RelatedLegislativeAuthorities/nepa1969.PDF; https://ceq.doe.gov/
Clean Water Act of 1972 (Water Pollution Control Act of 1948)	Standard for controlling pollutants discharged into waterways; regulates water standards	https://fas.org/sgp/crs/misc/RL30030.pdf
Endangered Species Act of 1973	Provides protection for natural habitats and species that are endangered with extinction or are threatened with potential for extinction	https://www.fws.gov/endangered/laws-policies/
Energy Policy Act of 2005 Public Law 109–58	Energy efficient production, conservation measures, and funding for technology to abate environmental damage	https://www.epa.gov/laws-regulations/summary-energy-policy-act

the safety of the national water supply, pollute air, or otherwise introduce a hazard into a community. Others, such as the national highway system or access to mortgage insurance that protect citizens and homeowners from natural disasters, are also influential in land use planning to protect communities from loss. The introduction of the Land Policy and Management Act of 1976 (Public Law 94-579) delineated administration and planning of federal lands for conservation and other government agency land use. These overarching laws represent a strong influence on state and local decision-making and, as such, a source of land use conflict.

The primary concerns of land use conflict consist of the long-term impact to the environment and human health from land use decisions where land is degraded, polluted, or otherwise unusable. However, less daunting aesthetic considerations include retaining the historical look of a neighborhood, moderating nuisances that may develop if an airport or tavern is poorly situated causing noise disturbances, or the delegation of land to one industry (e.g., agriculture, forest) over others (e.g., manufacturing, tourism).

Perspective and proximity (e.g., developer vs. community resident; state rates of unemployment vs. potentially hazardous local business development) play a large role in the utilization of natural resources. Balancing the advantage of development, such as economic growth and employment opportunities, against the potential for environmental degradation is where the federal legislation often defers to state governance. While Article I, § 8 of the U.S. Constitution (https://usconstitution.net/xconst_A1Sec8.html) establishes regulatory power of the federal government in interstate commerce (Nolon 2008), the problematic nature of these examples becomes evident upon discovery that state governments have concurrent power in this area (Nolon 1996). However, this hurdle can be overcome in many cases when state government officials appoint and confirm a governance board to address environmental protection of natural resources in a significant portion of the state. (See St. Johns River Water Management District at https://www.sjrwmd.com/governing-board/ for further information about the volunteer Governing Board representing several counties in northeast Florida.)

There are also similarities in land use and environmental policy that span the various levels of government leading to "overlapping regimes, with all three levels of government establishing rules for some matters, such as wetlands and habitat protection, preservation of natural resources, transportation development, and prevention of environmental pollution" (Nolon 2008, p.1). Consequently, the historical development of various multisectoral legislation requires two key responses: (1) integration of diverse legislation optimizing natural resources for land use, and (2) eliminating redundancy while capitalizing on a flexible approach to the geographic specificity of multisectoral goals (Nolon 2008). Coordination between levels of state government is also problematic (Nolon 2008; OECD 2017) but important to resolving the noted response actions.

The role of each level of government is an important dimension to understanding land use and environmental policy. The protection of property rights is a shared U.S. Constitutional provision to both the federal and state governments while national governments are given the authority to tax and allocate funds, delegate powers to the states, and protect individual freedoms (Nolon 1996; OECD 2017). The role of the state government in the U.S. Constitution is centered on the protection of natural resources, environment, religious freedoms, and the ability to "police" citizens (Killenbeck 2002). Local municipalities focus on development of land use plans that conserve local resources through zoning ordinances and other construction regulation (Nolon 1996; OECD 2017).

Clearly, municipalities are a driving force behind local conservation, but collaborative efforts of the federal/state governments may not be as visible. Federal agencies were enacted to provide states with minimum standards of safety in toxicology levels for various substances to inform their policymaking decisions (HHS 2017; OECD 2017). For example, The Comprehensive Environmental Response, Compensation, and Liability Act of 1980 (CERCLA), established the Agency for Toxic Substances and Disease Registry (ASTDR) under the U.S. Department of Health and Human Services (HHS) to facilitate standards and local policy implementation (HHS 2017). The ASTDR is instrumental in the conduct of health assessments, investigates reports of potential environmental contaminants, and is driven by their mission to protect population health.

The U.S. federal government also impacts federal land use directly and non-federal land use indirectly through legislation by empowering states with the authority for land use regulation. But there are gaps in multisectoral conditions that require attention and we mention two here. First, the conflict between concurrent federal and state autonomy is a major hurdle in conditions where natural resources span multiple jurisdictions. What, if any, federal or state-to-state mechanisms are in place when a natural resource, such as a watershed, cross state borders? Second, many are familiar with the concept of "use it or lose it" when it comes to government budgets. What mechanisms are in place to ensure that conservation funding held in trust can be exempt from reallocation when budgets go virtually untouched during the extensive amount of time it takes to site and acquire land? The Florida Forever Act 259.105 of the Florida Statutes, a program of the Florida Department of Environmental Protection, is a directive to conserve natural fauna and flora receiving funding under 259.1051 Florida Forever Trust Fund. But the effort for the state to protect natural resources is succumbing to financial pressure to divert funds to other projects. State conservation projects, such as Forever Florida, are susceptible to traditional government accounting measures because they hold money in accounts while time-consuming land deals are developed. Even as states have primarily given regulatory authority to local municipalities (http://www.ushistory.org/gov/12.asp) through statutes embedded in state constitutions, they also maintain some level of control with funding allocation and various limits on utilization of policy tools (Cornell Law School, Legal Information Institute n.d.-d; OECD 2017). While local municipalities in proximity to proposed development with foreseeable hazards can actively engage in assessments and thwart controversial development, they are often at the mercy of allocated state funding to do so. Thus, there is a notable hierarchy between national, state, and local regulation; but there is also a requirement that subordinate plans must not conflict with higher levels of legislation (OECD 2017). In the next section, we demonstrate how California environmental policy struggles against subordinate status to NEPA.

6.3 State of California Environmental and Public Health Policy CEQA vs. NEPA

The State of California, where the discovery of gold, introduction of agriculture and federal utilization of land for conservation (e.g., forest, wildlands) and national defense drove policy, is one example of a western U.S. state that typically has a higher percentage of federally owned and managed land versus other areas in the nation. In 2015, nearly half (45.9%) or 46,000,329/100,206,720 acres (Vincent et al. 2017, p.7) of the total acreage in California is federally owned by the Department of Defense (DOD) and four primary federal agencies. Slightly more than 95% of the estimated 640 million acres owned by the federal government, most of which is in the west, is managed by the four primary federal agencies: (1) Bureau of Land Management—248.3 million acres, (2) Forest Service—192.9 million acres, (3) Fish and Wildlife Service—89.1 million acres, and (4) National Park Service—79.8 million acres (Vincent et al. 2017, p.ii). Common use of federal land is dedicated to wilderness preservation, recreational activities, natural resource development and military installations. These conditions and the implementation of the California Environmental Quality Act of 1970 (CEQA), almost concurrently with NEPA makes this state of interest from a policy perspective and in the ongoing problem of abating health problems emanating from environmental conditions.

Environmental contaminants that are particularly harmful to children in the development stage has been the focus of a report by the California Environmental Health Tracking Program (CEHTP 2015). Lead exposure, environmental toxins causal to cancer, and air pollution that exacerbate asthma demonstrate a significant long-term cost to the health system and health burden of individuals and their family members concurrently experiencing poverty and racial disparities (CEHTP 2015). Their objective to reduce environmental hazards is shared as related studies on cancer using "California-specific exposure prevalence estimates to calculate hazard-specific environmental attributable fractions (EAFs)" (Nelson et al. 2017, *para* 2) concur with the CEHTP report. "Reducing environmental hazards and exposures in California could substantially reduce the human burden of childhood cancer and result in significant annual and lifetime savings" (Nelson et al. 2017, *para* 4).

Two suggested methods that could effectively reduce health risks associated with environmental conditions include (1) improvements in balancing land development and conservation (Santos et al. 2014), and (2) recognizing the health co-benefits of emphasizing intersectoral collaboration of climate change and public health experts (Gould and Rudolph 2015). First, recalling the concurrent capacity for both the state and federal government to regulate interstate commerce, environmental and conservation policy helps to place the Santos et al. (2014) position in perspective. For example, they reason that since "land use planning is by definition based on the parcelizing [sic] of land for development … done by cities," that this represents a considerable obstacle with "conservation need and habitats [that] do not observe political boundaries" (Santos et al. 2014, p.7; Schrag 1998). This example also represents a prime example of the problem of perspective and proximity. Further, Santos et al. consider the cost of land acquisition to be a topic of considerable innovation since conventional conservation funding sources have dried up (2014). The political barrier demonstrated by Santos et al. may find a solution by determining "shared root causes of climate change and health inequities" in the second method (Gould and Rudolph 2015, p.15649). Gould and Rudolph propose climate change strategies that envelope problematic social determinants of health (e.g., race, poverty, cumulative environmental exposures) (2015). Given the common objective, this option may have the capacity to cross intersectoral boundaries into political feasibility.

CEQA being substantive—having authority to halt development if the assessment provides reason to determine that mitigation will not reduce potential harm, may additionally benefit from the concept of overcoming multisectoral policy by enacting legislation that enfolds conservation with the concept of climate change to benefit health outcomes. CEQA's conduct of an environmental impact report (EIR) early in the planning process as opposed to the conditional NEPA EIS provides the public visibility and opportunity to engage a larger span of stakeholders in the process. Finally, other states may consider developing a similar approach to facilitate coordination first among state levels of government and eventually between states.

6.4 City of Chicago, Illinois CMAP

The consequences of local municipalities in land use planning is recognizable on a global scale taking into consideration "the long-term stability of ecosystems, social justice, food and energy security, long-term economic growth, housing costs, and the mitigation of and adaption to climate change" (OECD 2017, p.14). Urbanization—the movement from agrarian society to concentrated metropolitan areas, is expected to increasingly impact the rate of resource consumption and production with greater amounts of harmful emissions that can cumulatively affect public health (Hancock 2017; World Bank 2017b). More than 54% of the global population in 2015 reside in an urban area with greater than 10% growth projections by 2050 (United Nations 2017, p.e93). Population growth places the onus on cities to take a radical assessment of their long-term planning in relation to land use decisions. The long history and legal framework of legacy decisions represent a continuous battle to address notable problems still echoing the truth of decades past that the "current built environment does not promote healthy lifestyles" (Perdue et al. 2003, p.1390). So too are looming challenges to cities to overcome massive reductions in the stream of federal funding, deteriorating infrastructure, and sweeping changes in the demography of urban residents (Security & Sustainability Forum, National League of Cities 2017). Therefore, cities across the globe must develop long-term plans that improve environmental conditions and thus, address the growing public administration and population health needs of urban dwellers.

The requirement to improve conditions has been federally mandated in U.S. cities. Thus, planning must address the long-term goals of remediating existing conditions by optimizing current assets against future needs. One example is the enactment of Chicago Metropolitan Agency for Planning (CMAP) under Public Act 94-0510 in 2005 to represent seven counties in northeast Illinois as their metropolitan planning organization (MPO). These counties include Cook nestled on the southwest section of Lake Michigan, McHenry and Lake to the north, DuPage and Kane to the west, and Kendall and Will southwest of Cook County. A comprehensive plan, by definition, is a strategic planning tool of local government used to guide development and zoning but without substantive standing (OECD 2017).

"However, adopting a *Comprehensive Plan* is a legal requirement for enacting *Zoning Ordinances* in many other states, and some states make financial support for municipal investment projects dependent on the existence of a *Comprehensive Plan*" (OECD 2017, p.222). While zoning laws have achieved some semblance of uniformity following the U.S. Commerce Department Standard State Zoning Act in

1928, there are some differences due to the specific state constitutional development, from which municipalities garner their authority, and other local factors (Fischel 1998).

GO TO 2040, CMAPs comprehensive regional plan, was adopted in 2010 and underwent further modifications in 2014 promoting the importance of investment in regional mobility and economic stability by aiming improvements in public transportation and freight logistics (CMAP 2014a). While several items are targeted by CMAP (e.g., livable communities, human capital, and efficient governance), regional mobility is a major issue in Chicago due to an anticipated 25% population increase to 11 million people by 2040 (CMAP 2014a).

In the U.S., the federal interest in freight logistics is demonstrated by the large number of people served by this industry. "The Nation's 117.5 million households, 7.4 million business establishments, and 89,500 governmental units are part of an enormous economy that demands the efficient movement of freight" (US DOT 2017, *para* 1). Generating municipal plans to accommodate the freight industry (CMAP 2014b; US DOT 2012) to supply the growing population is a key problem in addition to concern for modes of transportation for personal vehicles and activities such as pedestrian or bicycle traffic. The emerging pattern of incorporating transportation alternatives to personal vehicles is threefold in nature. First, to provide routes to obtain necessities in "urban-built environments [that] are often poorly equipped to provide stable sources of food for sustaining massive populations" (Jowell et al. 2017, p.e176); second, to increase healthy activities; and third, to reduce the environmental impact by reducing smog and greenhouse emissions. Funding for these large-scale transportation projects are scarce and proposed taxes levied on gasoline may only support small-scale projects due to the impact of increased transportation efficiency resulting in the effect of less revenue under the fuel tax model. Nevertheless, planning for problems tangential to population growth (e.g., urban supply chain; transportation logistics; health services; access to fresh food items) is necessary to promote well-rounded and inclusive solutions to common problems that require novel solutions.

Another important element in the CMAP 2040 plan is the development and implementation of qualitative regional indicators to benchmark initial conditions and assess plan implementation. While CMAP and county planners were introduced to data analysis and evaluation, the indicators were influential in the initial plan, modification, and ongoing implementation. Benchmarks were established on each of 12 recommended actions. For example, one recommendation under Regional Mobility was to "create a more efficient freight network" (CMAP 2017, *para* 8). Achieving these goals was measured against two metrics. They include tracking the target completion date of 2030 for 71 GO TO 2040 projects in the Chicago Region Environmental and Transportation Efficiency Program (CREATE)—a multisectoral collaboration with various rail partners (e.g., Metra, Amtrak) and freight railroads founded in 2003; and monitoring with intent to reduce wait times at grade rail crossing at intermediate target dates (CMAP 2014c, p.312). Expanding the capacity for advanced statistical analysis and setting intermittent goals generates an atmosphere of continuous improvement as sovereign legislation, new information, funding streams, partnerships, and other opportunities become apparent further influencing the direction of CMAP goals.

The ON TO 2050 plan, scheduled for adoption in October 2018, expands the high-level topics with examples of items garnered from community outreach shown in parenthesis such as livable communities (climate resilience); human growth (inclusive growth), regional mobility (asset management, transit modernization), and efficient governance (community capacity, shared services) (CMAP 2016, p.2). Expanding municipal planning by soliciting regional input across various jurisdictions promotes "outside the box" thinking permitting the incorporation of unfamiliar and emerging concepts into the array of traditional planning concepts.

From compact cities (Stevenson et al. 2016) to megacities (Jowell et al. 2017), city planning, and urban design is progressively being linked to preplanned transportation strategies. Strategies must continue to embed the concept of healthy lifestyles, the reduction of personal vehicle emissions by providing alternate methods of local transportation, and the effective convergence of the natural and the built environment to offset higher temperature variance in large cities. City planners must envelope the greater implications of urban development and design to offset the negative local and planetary consequences of population density and scarce resources. Addressing public transportation and the role of freight logistics is one way in which to address daily necessities (e.g., work travel, grocery shopping, physical activity) with the least environmental impact.

6.5 Summary

The multisectoral legislation of sovereign U.S. government entities (e.g., federal, state) have a significant influence on the implementation of land use and environmental policy through local (e.g., regional, municipal) public administration. Common denominators of public administration, such as healthcare and transportation, are only two factors in a long list of sectors that must be taken into consideration.

Several key factors: concurrent environmental legislative sovereignty; legacy land use; environmental impact on health; growing population; and freight logistics must be a part of community dialogues to adapt sustainable approaches, develop infrastructure for multiple goals, and achieve financing through shared resources.

Acknowledgements The author would like to thank the Legal Information Institute at Cornell University Law School and Humboldt State University Library Environmental Research Guide for their commitment to open access of legal topics and associated law in their respective online directories. Analysis and interpretation of these items is the sole responsibility of the author but is not intended to be construed as legal advice. Special thanks to Nate van Ness for helpful commentary on the final first draft.

Glossary

Biocapacity The limit of an environment measured in land and water resources to provide for daily needs such as water, construction material for housing, transportation, and waste removal; often measured in geographic regions, such as nations, to determine how life style consumption choices of available natural resources result in an ecological surplus (biocapacity creditors) or deficit (biocapacity debtors) (Global Footprint Network 2017)

Bylaws Regulatory instrument of a municipal or city government to create local law; typically called a bylaw or ordinance because the local government is empowered by the state to regulate specific items

Environmental Impact Assessment Analysis that determines economic, environmental, and political feasibility of projects prior to development to minimize environmental impact

Federal land Refers to any land owned (fee simple title) and managed by the federal government, regardless of its mode of acquisition or managing agency; it excludes lands administered by a federal agency under easements, leases, contracts, or other arrangements (Vincent et al. 2017, p.1)

Grant Economic instrument that can include money, land, or similar form of assistance

Incentives Economic instrument; reward for adhering to minimal levels of pollutants or minimizing consumption

Land degradation When land is unable to produce natural resources (e.g., crops, wilderness, grazing areas) due to overuse, contamination, or other causes elicited from human activity and production

Land use Linked to several major areas of public administration such as natural resource management, waste disposal, transportation, urbanization, agriculture, recreation, and forest

Land use planning Task of local governments to utilize national or regional spatial planning guidance to formulate specific land use

Legislation Regulatory instrument; the capacity to formulate law

Ordinances Regulatory instrument; normally a municipal-level law

Permits Regulatory instrument; to formally present a document giving permission to utilize a specific resource (e.g., construction, land use)

Public land Refers to lands managed by the Bureau of Land Management as defined in 43 U.S.C. §1702(e) (Vincent et al. 2017, p.1; Cornell Law School, Legal Information Institute n.d.-a)

Subsidies Economic instrument; a sum of money to an organization to perform a specific activity

Taxes Economic instrument; an obligation to pay a certain percentage of earned income to the government

Zoning ordinances Official designation of how property can be utilized in a given geographic location; zoned for commercial use, residential use, etc.

References

Boden TA et al. Total fossil-fuel CO2 emissions. 2014. http://cdiac.ornl.gov/trends/emis/top2014.tot. Accessed 27 Jun 2017.

Boden, T.A., G. Marland, and R.J. Andres. Global, Regional, and National Fossil-Fuel CO2 Emissions. 2017. Carbon Dioxide Information Analysis Center, Oak Ridge National Laboratory, U.S. Department of Energy, Oak Ridge, Tenn., U.S.A. https://doi.org/10.3334/CDIAC/00001_V2017.

Brugger J. Living with the environmental and social legacy of U.S. land policy in the American west. 2017, January 24. https://aesengagement.wordpress.com/2017/01/24/living-with-the-environmental-and-social-legacy-of-u-s-land-policy-in-the-american-west/. Accessed 24 Jul 2017.

California Environmental Health Tracking Program. Costs of environmental health conditions in California children. 2015. http://www.phi.org/resources/?resource=cehtpkidshealthcosts. Accessed 28 Sep 2017.

Chicago Metropolitan Agency for Planning (CMAP) Federal Agenda 2016 Go To 2040 plan materials. 2014a. http://www.cmap.illinois.gov/about/2040/download-the-full-plan. Accessed 8 Oct 2017.

Chicago Metropolitan Agency for Planning (CMAP). Freight policy and funding under a new transportation bill. 2014b. http://www.cmap.illinois.gov/documents/10180/245594/2014-02-27-Major-Metros-Freight-Principles-FINAL.pdf/a5f068b8-e4e3-488f-823f-7bc56994bd11. Accessed 8 Oct 2017.

Chicago Metropolitan Agency for Planning (CMAP). Regional mobility, recommendation 12 create a more efficient freight network. 2014c. p. 308–322. http://www.cmap.illinois.gov/documents/10180/21431/Freight_chapter.pdf/6804d3a9-cd94-4f49-b23b-e1d70f9fb8aa. Accessed 9 Oct 2017

Chicago Metropolitan Agency for Planning (CMAP). Emerging priorities for ON TO 2050; public comment draft report. 2016 June 29. http://www.cmap.illinois.gov/onto2050. Accessed 9 Oct 2017.

CMAP About GO TO 2040. 2017. http://www.cmap.illinois.gov/about/2040. Accessed 9 Oct 2017.

Cornell Law School, Legal Information Institute. 43 U.S. Code Chapter 35—Federal lands policy and management. n.d.-a. https://www.law.cornell.edu/uscode/text/43/chapter-35. Accessed 24 Jul 2017

Cornell Law School, Legal Information Institute. Environmental law: an overview. n.d.-b. https://www.law.cornell.edu/wex/environmental_law. Accessed 24 Jul 2017.

Cornell Law School, Legal Information Institute Land use: an overview. n.d.-c. https://www.law.cornell.edu/wex/Land_use. Accessed 24 Jul 2017.

Cornell Law School, Legal Information Institute Natural resources-state statues. n.d.-d. https://www.law.cornell.edu/wex/table_natural_resources. Accessed 28 Sep 2017.

Fischel WA. 2200 Zoning and land use regulation. In: Couckaert B, et al., Editors. Encyclopedia of law & economics. 1998. p. 403–42. http://reference.findlaw.com/lawandeconomics/2200-zoning-and-land-use-regulation.pdf. Accessed 8 Oct 2017.

Gates PW. An overview of American land policy. Agr Hist. 1976;50(1):13–229. http://www.jstor.org/stable/3741919

Global Footprint Network. Ecological wealth of nations. 2017. http://www.footprintnetwork.org/content/documents/ecological_footprint_nations/. Accessed 21 Sep 2017.

Gould S, Rudolph L. Challenges and opportunities for advancing work on climate change and public health. Int J Environ Res Public Health. 2015;12:15649–72. https://doi.org/10.3390/ijerph121215010.

Hancock T et al. One planet regions: planetary health at the local level. The Lancet Planetary Health. 2017;1:e92–e93.

Hultman N. Trump's executive order on energy independence. [PlanetPolicy]. 2017, March 28. https://www.brookings.edu/blog/planetpolicy/2017/03/28/trumps-executive-order-on-energy-independence/. Accessed 23 Oct 2017.
International Organization of Supreme Audit Institutions (INTOSAI) Working Group on Environmental Auditing (WGEA). Land use and land management practices in environmental perspective. 2013. http://www.environmental-auditing.org/LinkClick.aspx?fileticket=NiwOS8 9K5Jk%3D&tabid=128&mid=568. Accessed 24 Jul 2017.
Jowell A, et al. The impact of megacities on health: preparing for a resilient future. Lancet Planet Health. 2017;1:e176–8.
Killenbeck MR, editor. The tenth amendment and state sovereignty: constitutional history and contemporary issues. Lanham: Rowman & Littlefield; 2002.
National Youth Advisory Board. Land use and environmental protection: an overview for addressing environmental problems resulting from land use practices in the United States : report to the Environmental Protection Agency. 1974. Washington, DC, U.S. Government Printing Office.
Nelson L et al. Estimating the proportion of childhood cancer cases and costs attributable to the environment in California. Am J Public Health [Online]. 2017. http://ajph.aphapublications.org/doi/ref/10.2105/AJPH.2017.303690.
Nolon JR. The national land use policy act. 13 Pace. Envtl L Rev, 519-523. 1996. http://digitalcommons.pace.edu/lawfaculty/182/. Accessed 24 Jul 2017.
Nolon JR. Historical overview of the American land use system: a diagnostic approach to evaluating governmental land use control. 2008. http://lawweb.pace.edu/files/landuse/Land_Use_System.pdf. Accessed 24 Jul 2017.
Organization for Economic Cooperation and Development (OECD). United States. In: Land-use planning systems in the OECD: country fact sheets. Paris: OECD; 2017. p. 220–5. https://doi.org/10.1787/9789264268579-35-en
Perdue WC, et al. The built environment and its relationship to the public's health: the legal framework. Am J Public Health. 2003;93(9):1390–4.
Pub Law 94-579 Land Management Act. https://www.gpo.gov/fdsys/pkg/STATUTE-90/pdf/STATUTE-90-Pg2743.pdf. 94th Congress Oct 21, 1976.
Salamon LM. The tools of government. New York: Oxford University Press; 2002.
Santos MJ, et al. The push and pull of land use policy: reconstructing 150 years of development and conservation land acquisition. PLoS ONE. 2014;9(7):e103489. https://doi.org/10.1371/journal.pone.0103489.
Schrag P. Paradise lost, California's experience, America's future. Berkeley: University of California Press; 1998.
Security & Sustainability Forum, National League of Cities (NLC). Webinar, cities on the leading edge of resilience, July 13. 2017. http://securityandsustainabilityforum.org/mc-events/webinar-cities-on-the-leading-edge-of-resilience. Accessed 24 Jul 2017.
United Nations. World development indicators: urbanization. 2017. http://wdi.worldbank.org/table/3.12. Accessed 4 Oct 2017.
United Nations Framework Convention on Climate Change (UNFCCC) Kyoto protocol. 2014. https://unfccc.int/kyoto_protocol/items/1678.php. Accessed 16 Jul 2017.
United States Department of Agriculture (USDA) Economic Research Service. Major land uses. 2016. https://www.ers.usda.gov/topics/farm-economy/land use-land-value-tenure/major-land uses/. Accessed 24 Jul 2017.
United States Department of Health and Human Services (HHS). Agency for toxic substances & disease registry, fiscal year 2017, justification of estimates for appropriation committees. 2017. https://www.cdc.gov/budget/documents/fy2017/fy-2017-atsdr.pdf Accessed 18 Aug 2017.
United States Department of the Interior, Bureau of Land Management. Natural resources: supporting healthy lands. n.d. https://www.blm.gov/programs/natural-resources. Accessed 24 Jul 2017.

United States Department of the Interior, Bureau of Land Management and Office of the Solicitor, editor. The federal land policy and management act, as amended. Washington, DC: U.S. Department of the Interior, Bureau of Land Management Office of Public Affairs; 2001. 69 pp.

United States Department of Transportation, Federal Highway Administration. The nation served by freight. 2017. https://ops.fhwa.dot.gov/freight/freight_analysis/nat_freight_stats/docs/12factsfigures/c1intro.htm. Accessed 8 Oct 2017.

United States Department of Transportation, Federal Highway Administration: Freight Management and Operations. Freight facts and figures. 2012. http://www.ops.fhwa.dot.gov/freight/freight_analysis/nat_freight_stats/docs/12factsfigures/. Accessed 8 Oct 2017.

United States Environmental Protection Agency (EPA). Electric utility generating units: repealing the Clean Power Plan. 2017. https://www.epa.gov/stationary-sources-air-pollution/electric-utility-generating-units-repealing-clean-power-plan. Accessed 23 Oct 2017.

United States Government Accountability Office (GAO). High-risk series: progress on many high-risk areas, while substantial efforts needed on others. Statement of Gene L. Dodaro Comptroller General of the United States before the Committee on Homeland Security and Governmental Affairs, U.S. Senate, GAO-17-407T. Washington, DC: U.S. Government Printing Office; 2017.

Vincent CH, Hanson LA, Argueta CN. Federal land ownership: overview and data. Congressional Research Service. 2017, Mar 3. https://fas.org/sgp/crs/misc/R42346.pdf. Accessed 24 Jul 2017.

World Bank. CO_2 emissions (metric tons per capita). [Data Carbon Dioxide Information Analysis Center, Environmental Sciences Division, Oak Ridge National Laboratory, Tennessee, United States]. 2017a. https://data.worldbank.org/indicator/EN.ATM.CO2E.PC?view=map. Accessed 4 Sep 2017.

World Bank. Urban development. http://www.worldbank.org/en/topic/urbandevelopment. 2017b. Accessed 8 Oct 2017.

Further Reading

Amirtahmasebi R et al Regenerating urban land: a practitioner's guide to leveraging private investment. Urban Development Series. Washington, DC: World Bank. 2016. doi: https://doi.org/10.1596/978-1-4648-0473-1. License: Creative Commons Attribution CC BY 3.0 IGO.

Columbia Law School, Sabin Center for Climate Change Laws. Key environmental issues in U.S. EPA region 2 Conference, 2014 May 29. http://columbiaclimatelaw.com/news-events/events/2014-2/key-environmental-issues-in-u-s-epa-region-2-conference/. Accessed 24 Jul 2017.

Food and Agricultural Organization (FAO) of the United Nations. The state of the world's land and water resources for food and agriculture. Rome: FAO; 2011. http://www.fao.org/docrep/015/i1688e/i1688e00.pdf. Accessed 27 Aug 2017.

Grossman M, Bryner GC. U.S. land and natural resources policy: history, debates, state data, primary documents. 2nd ed. Amenia: Grey House; 2012.

Humboldt State University. Environmental science research guide. 2017. http://libguides.humboldt.edu/c.php? g=303888&p=2029862. Accessed 23 Sep 2017.

James A, Aadland D. The curse of natural resources: an empirical investigation of U.S. counties. 2010. http://www.uwyo.edu/aadland/research/resourcecurse.pdf. Accessed 28 Sep 2017.

Lynn K, et al. Social vulnerability and climate change: synthesis of literature. Gen. Tech. Rep. PNW-GTR-838. Portland: U.S. Department of Agriculture, Forest Service, Pacific Northwest Research Station; 2011, 70 p.

National League of Cities (NLC). Cities strong together. 2017. http://www.nlc.org/. Accessed 24 Jul 2017.

OpenLandContracts.Org. An online repository of open land contracts. n.d. http://openlandcontracts.org/. Accessed 27 Aug 2017.

Our Documents Initiative. 100 milestone documents. n.d. www.ourdocuments.gov. Accessed 30 Aug 2017.

Sacramento County Planning and Environmental Review. Land use planning regulation documents. 2017. http://www.per.saccounty.net/LandUseRegulationDocuments/Pages/default.aspx. Accessed 24 Jul 2017.

United States Department of Agriculture, Natural Agricultural Statistics Services. CropScape: cropland data layer. [Data source: Center for Spatial Information Science and Systems]. 2016. https://nassgeodata.gmu.edu/CropScape/. Accessed 30 Sep 2017.

Chapter 7
Foundations of Community Health: Planning Access to Public Facilities

Kirsten Cook and Beth Ann Fiedler

Abstract While shared use agreement strategies help provide community access to public facilities, the application of this strategy is often an afterthought to community planning and thus, community health. Alternatively, an emerging trend in community health sets an appropriate stage to address community needs by establishing a framework in which various stakeholders build a shared use policy strategy in land use from the onset of development. The application of collaborative community planning as a fundamental component of community health is demonstrated in four case examples from Australia, Canada, and the United States. The qualitative comparative results in the case studies suggest that the partnership framework offers an opportunity to achieve improved community health outcomes. Cumulatively, analysis of a limited number of available shared use performance indicators demonstrates an important need for the development of measurable metrics, reporting, and tracking in which data sharing becomes a necessary element of policy.

7.1 Introduction

The challenge of providing community social services in the United States during and after periods of economic instability is problematic for municipal leaders and across multiple levels of government. Finding innovative methods to optimize existing infrastructure, and develop services, and funding sources to better serve the general health population needs within local communities is important to resolving conditions that decrease quality of life for families experiencing unemployment, obesity, and other environmental conditions that thwart health and optimum lifestyle conditions. Trends, such as the emergence of shared use agreements between parties representing public and private spaces, indicate that educational institutions

K. Cook (✉)
Planner, Partnership for Southern Equity, Atlanta, GA, USA

B. A. Fiedler
Independent Research Analyst, Jacksonville, FL, USA

B. A. Fiedler (ed.), *Translating National Policy to Improve Environmental Conditions Impacting Public Health Through Community Planning*,
https://doi.org/10.1007/978-3-319-75361-4_7

represent viable community assets to promote social and physical activity. While literature suggests that adjusting current policy by promoting the shared use of space between educational leadership and municipal planning can reduce health disparities and provide a venue for physical activity and social interaction for the entire family towards achieving improvements in community health, quantifying shared use activities for effectiveness poses a difficult problem.

A historical overview and case analysis indicate that shared use strategies have been considered as an afterthought leading to the retroactive approach that is necessary in the instances of existing infrastructure and when no plans for new development have been put into place. The review of this approach sheds light on the general scope and obstacles of shared use for two main reasons: first, the way that community and municipal planning has evolved over the last few decades and, second, the disconnect that exists between municipal and educational leadership. Such strategies, however, fail to realize the full potential that exists within a framework of shared use built into policy by various stakeholders from the onset of development.

The National Clearinghouse for Educational Facilities has promoted the concept of collaborative community development since the turn of the millennium. Their concept of schools as an efficient, innovative, and community-driven solution to the demand for new and renovated school buildings (Bingler et al. 2003) provides common facilities and envelopes shared use in the planning stages to optimize facility usage. In practice, this solution has not received the attention it is due, perhaps because of the lack of quantitative research associated with the practice.

The absence of quantifiable analysis and limited quasi-experimental analysis of social public health interventions in school systems (Bonnell et al. 2013) has made the impact of shared use and other measures (e.g., race, distance to parks, socioeconomic status, chronic conditions) on the reduction of obesity—one facet of poor public health—difficult but not impossible to measure. However, funding resources and/or reallocation could be realized by quantifying the physical and cost benefits in coordinated efforts from shared use as with any proposed change to existing policy or attempt to formulate new policy. Thus, consideration for formal shared use policy in the United States could focus on the quantifiable benefit of reducing the long-term costs of poor public health by using a collaborative process prior to community development that maximizes efficiency, reflects the needs of all stakeholders, and collectively benefits the community.

This chapter highlights the Schools as Centers of Community concept as one that sets the foundation for proactive, rather than retroactive, shared use, delving into the approach as a solution not only to infrastructure needs but also to public health challenges. We focus on the impact of deteriorating infrastructure on public health in the U.S. and the existing barriers to shared use agreement policy, demonstrate how communities in Australia, Canada, and the U.S. embed shared use agreements into local policy, and review how localities can influence greater collaboration, particularly through data sharing. Ultimately, we introduce the need for a framework of agreement in which shared use sites are cooperatively managed from the onset to realize the full advantages of shared use to public health.

7.2 Poor Infrastructure, Poor Health in America?

In 2017, America was given a D+ for infrastructure to represent "significant deterioration" and "serious concern with strong risk of failure" (ASCE 2017, *para* 6) in terms of capacity, condition, funding, operation and maintenance, resilience, and innovation. The assessment, released in an *Infrastructure Report Card* given by the American Society of Civil Engineers (ASCE) every four years, indicates that the current U.S. condition and organization of physical structures such as bridges, roads, public parks, schools, railways, and other infrastructure are unable to satisfy the daily operational needs of the American society. Although the report cards do not focus on the impact to public health, one can easily infer the deleterious influence that a national infrastructure of such inferior quality has on the public. An official reporting system of infrastructure relating to the nation's physical activity offerings does not exist, but the available reports, in conjunction with data on public health trends, suggest that the current access to infrastructure is insufficient for promoting a positive quality of life and good public health.

The obesity epidemic is a strong indicator of public health outcomes related to a lack of recreational facilities and safe and accessible spaces for physical activity. Obesity is now widely recognized in the U.S. after years of increasing attention and efforts to curb its' detrimental effects, but the problem is not unique. Between 1980 and 2014, the worldwide prevalence of obesity increased more than twofold. The World Health Organization (WHO) reveals that most of the global population lives in countries where being overweight or obese is linked with more deaths than being underweight (WHO 2016). Obesity impacts 34% of adults and 17% of children and adolescents in the United States, 28% of adults in Australia, and 27% of adults in Canada (NCHS 2016, p.26; WHO 2014) and contributes to the escalating long-term cost of healthcare.

The societal cost of the obesity epidemic is estimated at $315.8 billion per year in the U.S., in 2010 ($983 per capita) (Cawley 2015, p.255). Concurrently, the annual medical expenses for an obese American are on average $2826 higher (in 2005 dollars) than for an American who is not obese (Cawley and Meyerhoefer 2012, p.22). By comparison, other nations have less cost associated with obesity, but the problem is clear. The annual problem of obesity costs Canadians $6 billion or about $171 per capita (Canadian Obesity Network 2017), while Australians pay out $125 billion or $526 per capita (Wade 2016).

Other diseases and health risks associated with lack of quality locations to promote physical activity include diabetes, high blood pressure, and some forms of cancer. Moreover, mental and emotional health stands to benefit greatly from the availability of recreational facilities and access to spaces for physical activity (HHS 2008). Some of these conditions are included in the healthcare costs related to obesity, considering the interdependent nature of many of them. However, some conditions and the medical attention they require, such as depression and other mental health conditions, represent costs that are additional to that already included in the statistics. In sum, all members of society can benefit from increasing access to recreational facilities and other spaces for physical activity that is associated with improved health.

The hardest hit communities exhibiting direct environmental conditions (e.g., unemployment, underemployment, obesity) display immediately recognizable demographics such as low income, which further prohibits access to healthy food due to lack of local business development, land use, and other governed conditions. The difficulty in reaching sustainable solutions that embrace communities and multiple levels of leadership requires an influx of methods that elicit the collaboration of various professionals (e.g., clinicians, municipal leaders, state Department of Health, and US Surgeon General) to promote healthy, sustainable community solutions to this international problem. Developing solutions can begin with (1) understanding the seemingly straightforward but often complex nature of existing environmental conditions, (2) historical policy development, and (3) limited coordinated efforts between multilevel government agencies that often seek independent solutions that are incomplete.

One way in which municipal leaders and school board leaders are seeking to address these environmental problems is evidenced by the National Association of State Boards of Education (NASBE) (2013) in the United States. The NASBE lists states that recognize the value of developing shared use agreements so that private community members can gain legal access to gymnasiums, pools, meeting rooms, and similar facilities in public institutions to engage in physical, social, and educational activity that can lead to improvements in health outcomes. Such actions have paved the way for these local community leaders to combine forces to address the high morbidity and mortality costs of obesity, consequent diabetes, and a myriad of other health hazards brought forth by lack of physical activity for children and adults alike.

This strategy has proven successful in communities across the world and is supported by literature and promoted by global leaders. For example, the World Health Organization supports the establishment of partnerships to share existing recreation and sporting facilities between schools and community partners (WHO 2008-School Policy Framework). In the 2016 Report of the Commission on Ending Childhood Obesity, WHO recommends a whole-of-society approach to combating obesity that involves all actors. The report states, "without joint ownership and shared responsibility, well-meaning and cost-effective interventions have limited reach and impact" (WHO 2016, p.26).

Although no solution is absolute, shared use is an effective strategy that can easily be tailored to communities across the globe. Past efforts have demonstrated, however, that shared use that begins at the operations stage will not successfully meet the imminent infrastructural and health needs of the public. A truly effective framework is one that not only relies on shared uses but also shared ownership, responsibility, planning, operations, and management. Historical review and an examination of four case studies in three countries further demonstrate the need for such a framework.

7.3 Historical Perspective of Shared Use Agreements

Public health and planning professionals vocalized their concern at the turn of the twenty-first century to expand their historical roles to combat the spread of infectious diseases in congested cities, citing that "urban planners, engineers, and architects must begin to see that they have a critical role in public health. Similarly, public health professionals need to appreciate that the built environment influences public health as much as vaccines or water quality" (Jackson and Kochtitzky 2002, p.15). An article linking urban sprawl for the first time to physical activity, obesity, and chronic disease (Ewing et al. 2003) opened the door for the resurgence of shared use agreements as a response to the challenge of public health problems rising in communities resulting from a lack of existing infrastructure and limited methods of collaboration in municipal governance strategies. Further, qualitative evidence continues to support that the built environment influences public health in the inherent potential to either encourage or inhibit physical activity (Ewing et al. 2014). Therefore, developing methods to increase collaboration across professional and governance boundaries becomes the new impetus for shared use. Concurrently, the historical beginnings of shared use provide an informative foundation from which to increase awareness, alter current paths, and generate baselines to take corrective action on existing structures as well as a framework for new infrastructure development.

7.3.1 Increasing Shared Use

Increasing shared use—the relationship between schools and planning—is among one of many policies and design tools that have been suggested in literature since the 1920s to combat the negative ills of urban form. Thus, open-use policies demonstrate the normative interaction between U.S. schools and communities in the early twentieth century. Efficiency was achieved when communities placed schools in the center of neighborhoods to (1) optimize utilization of publicly funded facilities, and 2) maximize social interaction and physical activity for all ages (Cook 2015; Lawhon 2009). Legislation in Victoria, Australia supporting shared use dates back even further. Victoria's Education Act, 1872 included the power to use public school facilities for activities outside of formal schooling. This vision was carried out in subsequent acts—Education Act, 1910 and Education Act, 1928 (McShane et al. 2013).

Subsequent decades of land use decisions favoring urban sprawl and greenfield development, however, generally complicated the community use of schools and made such informal agreements difficult to maintain, particularly in the face of liability and safety concerns. Although some communities pioneered the adoption of formal shared use agreements as early as the 1950s, the tools to make them normative have been a much more recent development, emerging well after the turn of the twenty-first century (SRTS National Partnership 2017). Now, communities across the globe increasingly rely upon shared use policies to address many of the major public health issues they face today.

7.3.2 Shared Use in the United States

Currently, 36 U.S. states (and Washington, D.C.) have laws supporting shared use of school facilities outside of school hours for community recreational use (SRTS National Partnership 2016). A 2016 research brief on shared use found that communities had a higher tendency to address shared use agreements conceptually in plans than through implementation via formal agreements. Furthermore, not all communities specifically addressed shared use via policy with organizations most likely to promote physical activity, such as park districts and recreation leagues. Some partnered instead with community groups that provided benefits besides physical activity, such as libraries and arts organizations.

In 2016, 59% of school districts in the United States had a formal written joint use agreement according to the CDC School Health Policies and Practice Study (2017, p.68). Yet only 48% of districts had a formal written joint use agreement that applies to community use of indoor recreation or sports facilities, 44% had one that applies to outdoor recreation or sports facilities, and less than 14% specified utilization for healthcare services (CDC 2017, p.68). While activity in shared use is growing, the application to physical activity and envelopment of community healthcare continues to lag. Moreover, an important point to note on these study findings is that the percentages only represent district-level policies and practices. While finer than state-level, they may not truly reflect the policies and practices of all individual schools in each district and therefore present the possibility of overestimating the true proliferation of shared use in American schools.

Although the benefits of shared use have thus far proven promising anecdotally in the communities that use it, some impediments still exist to realizing the full potential of shared use to address public health concerns. More broadly, coordinated efforts are needed across the board in decisions relating to schools and land use. Much of the existing state law, however, puts local schools outside the jurisdiction of local land use planning, and local governments rarely collaborate with school districts to determine school siting, building, and renovation that benefits the entire community. Consequently, "a growing chorus of critical voices suggests that current school siting decision-making is inconsistent with efforts to reduce sprawl, encourage compact growth, and increase the sustainability of our built and natural environments" (Miles 2011, p.3). While shared use agreements are certainly a step in the right direction, the crux of the problem goes beyond merely sharing spaces. These problems include the (1) siloed nature of schools and local planning, (2) disconnect between school spaces and community spaces, and (3) lack of holistic involvement in infrastructural planning.

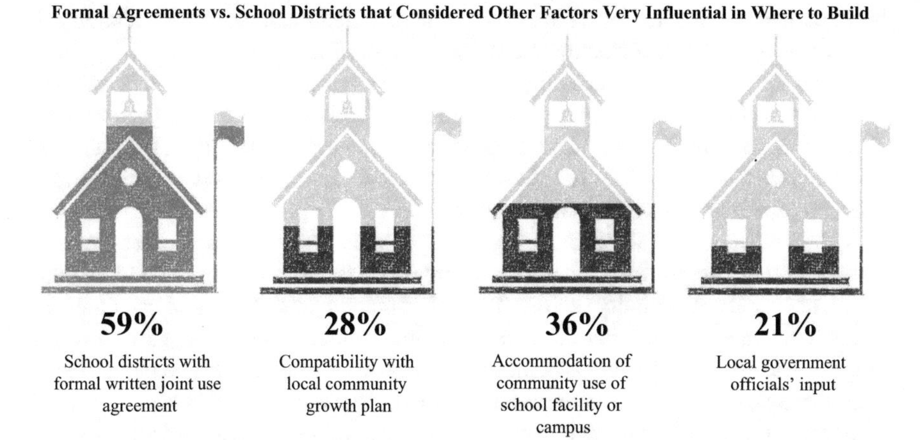

Fig. 7.1 Comparing the existence of formal shared use agreements in the United States and the perception of influential factors when deciding where to build a new school facility demonstrates the need for more coordinated efforts in infrastructural planning (Fiedler and Cook 2017)

Thus, solutions that rely entirely on shared use to overcome poor public health will not likely achieve improvement unless reforms are set in place to address the foundational problems noted here. The 2016 School Health Policies and Practices Study found that only 42% of school districts in the United States considered the desire to accommodate community use of the school facility or campus as a very influential factor in deciding to build a new facility rather than renovate an existing one, and only 36% of districts considered this factor as very influential in deciding where to build a new facility (CDC 2017, p.66). Additionally, when deciding where to build a new school facility, 41% of districts did not take into consideration compatibility with the local community growth plan related to future residential development to be a factor (CDC 2017, p.67). Predictably, consultation or input from local government land use or community planning officials is only required in 47% of school districts when determining whether to construct a new school and 45% of districts when determining where to construct a new school (CDC 2017, p.67). Even among school districts with this requirement in place, fewer still considered input from local government officials to be very influential (only 21%) (CDC 2017, p.67) . The disconnects shown here suggest that local land use and community planning input is viewed as more of a formality in some school districts than a useful part of the process (Fig. 7.1).

The initial need for more coordinated efforts across the board in all decision-making around school facilities is founded in recent studies in Canada and Australia. These studies support a proposition that long-term public health gains can be achieved in the establishment of a community framework of shared use agreement in which shared use sites are cooperatively planned and managed from the onset. For example, a Canadian Active After School Partnership survey that garnered 364 responses from municipal and school sectors determined that lack of communication between partners is cited by 52% as the greatest impediment to creating shared use agreements (Leisure Information Network 2012, p.38).

When the sharing of spaces only begins at the operations stage, good communication is less likely to occur, and miscommunication is more likely to present divisive challenges. On the other hand, a model of shared use that begins at the planning stage increases opportunities for good communication, simultaneously empowering stakeholders to have a voice and to become allies in the process.

The Government of Western Australia Department of Sport and Recreation represents similar support for a collaborative approach prior to development of an education or similar community facility. The department's guide to shared use facilities states "evidence suggests that where preplanning occurs, the ownership by a broader range of stakeholders, partners and user groups is better understood and maintained" (Department of Sport and Recreation n.d., p.10). Preplanning and partnerships tend to ensure a greater sense of ownership across a wide range of stakeholders and users leading to more appropriate design and management as well as long-term success. Partnerships established within this community-school planning framework "will become embedded in a supportive network of relationships that link agencies at many levels of government and the community and that share overlapping reform objectives related to school funding, governance, educational programs, and facilities" (Shoshkes 2011, p.232).

7.4 Shared Use in Action: International Case Studies

The emerging concept of shared use policy development has taken shape in numerous communities across the globe encompassing the unique assets and challenges of each locale. The following four case studies from Canada, Australia, and the U.S. offer some notable differences in shared use implementation, timing in partnerships, policy, and relevant activities undertaken. Cumulatively these cases represent the components necessary for an effective shared use framework.

7.4.1 City of Edmonton, Capital of the Province of Alberta, Canada

Edmonton provides an excellent model of a community maximizing the full potential of shared use because collaboration is evident in policy at the city level in conjunction with the provincial level supporting the integrated planning of school sites (Gunderson et al. 2016). The Edmonton Joint Use Agreement: Land, effective since 2009, clearly lays out the responsibilities of all parties in the various stages of shared use planning and implementation by embedding collaborative principles highlighting components of "Cooperative Planning, Efficiency and Planning, and Transparency and Openness" (City of Edmonton 2009). The agreement maps the planning process, development, and maintenance of land while specifying standard procedure for use of surplus non-reserve school sites and providing a schedule for school properties, among other important features.

The Edmonton Joint Use Agreement was a natural extension of established partnerships between the City, the public-school board, the Catholic school district, the regional French language school board, and Joint Use partners that has benefitted the public since the late 1950s. Representatives from each of these groups communicate with one another regularly to share information and updates about developments, ongoing projects, and opportunities. In Edmonton, shared use collaboration does not begin at the operation stage. Rather, collaboration from the onset enables shared use sites to be planned in such a way that reflects the needs and desires of everyone involved. The partners are founded on a *Joint Use: Land Agreement*, which "guides the planning, assembly, design, development and maintenance of [shared use] sites for school, recreation and park purposes, and provides the framework for decision-making related to surplus reserve and non-reserve sites" (City of Edmonton 2016, p.6).

The 2015/2016 Steering Committee, made up of ten members representing the partners, met six times over the year to carry out many functions critical to the successful implementation of shared use in the City. Among the many tasks, the committee reviewed problems and opportunities common to other cities across the globe such as the status of vacant surplus school sites, land allocation needs and new construction of school park sites, and refinements to improve upon the facilities agreement. Collaboration among the partners also guarantees that the shared use sites are monitored and evaluated on a regular basis to carry out the principles of efficiency, planning, transparency, and openness. An important aspect of the Edmonton Land Use Agreement is the enactment and authority granted to the Land Management Committee to track Edmonton school site status by categorizing a school in one of several categories: (1) operating, (2) ready for school, (3) under assembly, (4) unassembled, (5) surplus, or (6) closed. By following these general guidelines, the Land Management Committee replaced one school; and four new schools were completed and opened to students in 2016, while another 16 schools are anticipated to open in 2017.

The number of hours the community has spent using the school facilities also provides evidence of success in Edmonton. In 2015/2016, the community booked 56,612 hours of school gymnasium use and 99,864 hours of sport field use. These numbers have increased every year since 2012. The agreement benefits the schools too, which booked 17,070 hours of community pool time and 3,131 hours at the community tennis courts (City of Edmonton 2016, p.16), making additional revenue available for other educational uses through reduced costs incurred.

7.4.2 City of Melbourne, State Capital of Victoria, Australia

The development of successful alliances in two communities outside Melbourne, Australia provide another example of the advantages of collaborative and coordinated shared use strategies commonly utilized in southeast Australia. Under development since the late 1990s, the state of Victoria brought forth the *2006 Education and Training Reform Act,* emphasizing policy that focuses on increasing coordination between community and educational services. The Act includes specific powers to support shared use facilities and dedicates eight sections to outlining how school councils might carry out shared use and manage their facilities for public purposes (McShane et al. 2013; Victoria State Government 2006).

The Victorian Competition and Efficiency Commission (VCEC) found that up to two-thirds of government schools in Victoria share facilities or make them available for non-school purposes (McShane and Wilson 2014). The Victoria Department of Planning and Community Development compiled a Guide to Governing Shared Community Facilities that includes noteworthy strategies related to public participation, governance, and operations. The guide also defines a profile for facility vision, size, type, and maintenance and outlines principles of good governance for partners in shared facilities, largely centering on the need for participation, input, leadership, and consensus from all partners and stakeholders (State Government Victoria 2010).

The Department of Planning and Community Development established the Schools and Community Partnerships project in 2007 to meet the need for services and infrastructure in Melbourne's growing suburbs of Caroline Springs and Laurimar. Each suburb also established an alliance made up of a wide range of local partners, both with the objectives of delivering better school and community infrastructure that contributes to stronger, more sustainable communities and exhibiting the advantages and effectiveness of conducting government processes using a different, collaborative approach (Pope 2010).

Because of the partnerships and the resulting efficiencies of shared facilities planning and management, both alliances saved a significant amount of money estimated at over $800,000 in just two years (Pope 2010, pp.18–19), not including the unquantified savings that were redirected either to other related projects or to enhancing the quality of facilities. Moreover, the partnerships delivered infrastructure earlier than expected and ensured that the design of buildings enhanced the overall community feel. The indoor Leisure Center created by the Caroline Springs Alliance is a high-quality facility, reflecting a standard only possible through the partnership model. Further, the center averaged 1,400 visits a week in the first year of operation and continues to serve the community in a variety of ways by providing facilities for strength training, futsal teams (a variant of soccer played on a hard court), hockey, and family-focused social events.

The infrastructure was developed when each partnership made a small investment (0.6% of the overall expenditure) into a broker facilitator, ensuring success of the alliance. All partners agreed that the cost of this position was worth the expense given the generation of significant community outcomes and the ability of most partners to recuperate initial costs through efficiencies and advantages of each alliance (Pope 2010). Developing deliberate investment strategy plays an important role in collaborative shared use.

7.4.3 City of New York, State of New York, United States

New York is an example of a state that authorizes but does not require or even expressly encourage shared use. Rather, New York State Education Law Article 9 §414 grants the trustees or board of education the ability to permit the use of the school and grounds for community purposes, either during or outside of school hours (NY Educ L §414 2015). However, policies developed at the local, school-, or district-level play a leading role in maximizing the extent to which communities rely on shared use by encouraging schools to allow community use of facilities to the greatest extent possible (DASH-NY 2015).

The capacity to maximize resources through shared use to help eliminate disparities in access to recreational facilities was recognized by New York City leaders as the impetus for local policy development. This path led to 132 initiatives, including Schoolyards to Playgrounds, launched in 2007 by then-Mayor Bloomberg as part of the city's PlaNYC 2030 to address the disparity in access to services. The goal of the Schoolyards to Playgrounds program is to put more New Yorkers in closer proximity to parks and playgrounds (specifically, enabling 85% of the population to walk to a park within ten minutes from home). The core strategy of Schoolyards to Playgrounds relies on the collaborative public–private partnership between the Parks Department, the Department of Education, and the Trust for Public Land (DASH-NY 2015) that facilitates a participatory design process with youth input as well as some private funding.

The participatory design process enables students, teachers, and staff to determine the design of spaces that meet the needs of the community. Schoolyards to Playgrounds is an example of shared use in which collaboration permeates every stage of the process—from design to implementation, transforming schoolyards into open public playgrounds and community parks accessible daily from dawn until dusk when school is not in session. As of August 2016, 257 public schoolyards were open to the public, up from the 69 that kicked off the program in 2007 (Chapman and Colangelo 2016).

7.4.4 *Hamilton, County in the State of Tennessee, United States*

The types of disparities seen in Hamilton County exist in communities across the country that often impact populations of similar demographics. These demographics include high minority population and low socioeconomic status. However, Tennessee Code 11–21-108 plays a role in combating some of the inequalities that are evident in the state. The Code requires that the departments of environment and conservation and education provide technical advice, cooperatively with the Tennessee School Boards Association and the Tennessee Parks and Recreation Association, to ensure collaboration between the entities that make school facilities available for recreation (NASBE 2013).

With such a supportive Code in place, Hamilton County was perfectly positioned to receive a grant from the Robert Wood Johnson Foundation. The grant led the Chattanooga-Hamilton County Health Department in 2013 to partner with local organizations and residents in the County to enter a preliminary and important stage of shared use—identification and location of health inequalities and access to recreational spaces. They found that the lack of park space was most prominent in zip codes dominated by minorities and that the health problems the area faces are worst in these same zip codes when compared with the city overall. As one way to combat these inequalities, the County Health Department added an effort through the Step ONE (Optimize with Nutrition and Exercise) initiative, focused on the implementation of shared use as a solution to these inequities (ChangeLab Solutions 2017a). One of the primary Step ONE goals is "to establish a strong organizational network of community partners which includes key leadership from government, area businesses, schools, and community based organizations" supporting the overall mission "to create a culture of health in Hamilton County where residents choose to eat healthy and be physically active" (Step One 2017, *para* 1).

The case of Hamilton County presents an example of a locale that involved residents from the start. The development of two advisory councils, working alongside public health advocates and the county education department, illustrates the cooperative commitment resulting in an open use policy for public access to school playgrounds on all elementary schools successfully passing into district policy in February 2014.

Hamilton County represents the important aspect of data collection and community needs assessment in the development of shared used. Thus, the County established critical areas and is addressing them, beginning with the areas of greatest concern. Moreover, through resident surveys, community engagement efforts, and including residents' involvement in the advisory council, Hamilton County effectively targeted the locations, facilities, and programs that residents requested (Lewis 2016).

7.5 Discussion: Necessary Components of Effective Shared Use

The diversity in the shared use strategies found in Edmonton, Melbourne, New York City, and Hamilton County reflects the diversity of needs, assets, and creativity in each locale. Various elements are consistently evident in all of them. This framework combines both the similarities and differences to reveal the necessary components involved in ensuring cooperative design, management, and implementation of shared use sites that starts at the onset to realize the full advantages of shared use to public health. The establishment or refinement of shared use policy, planning and design participation, alliances and partnerships, facilitation, needs assessments, review of inventory, data tracking and public availability are elements of cooperative shared use that enable greater levels of success.

7.5.1 Guided by Policy

In each of the four case studies, the jurisdiction and its respective school system are guided by policy. The policies vary among the different locales, but they share a likeness in their robustness and affirmation of shared use. New York state's policy merely authorizes shared use; however, more localized policy at the level of schools and districts has stepped in to provide further necessary guidance and support (DASH-NY 2015). Thoughtful, place-based, and commending policy at all levels of government and authority will best serve the effectual implementation of shared use. When such policy is accompanied by guides for application, the potential for success is only magnified. Victoria, Australia's state guide on governing shared community facilities, dependent on a large project team and strong consultation process, is a rare but replicable example for other states providing place-based principles, tools, and checklists (State Government Victoria 2010).

7.5.2 Planning and Design Participation

Planning from the onset is one of the inherent factors in this framework for shared use, and each of the four case studies shows evidence of this element. New York City's participatory process in the case of the Schoolyards to Playgrounds program specifically illustrates how communities should be given opportunity to play an early and significant role in the design process to increase potential for enhanced shared use outcomes benefitting constituents. The program empowers students, teachers, and staff to give ideas and input that shape the design of playgrounds and recreational spaces so that the result reflects the voices of end users of the facilities.

7.5.3 Alliances and Partnerships

Each of the cases also highlights the importance of alliances and partnerships but with notable variation according to the population characteristics. These took different forms in each community, including volunteer steering committees from various sectors, public–private partnerships assembled by local government, and organizational networks of stakeholders. A collective assessment of all four locales demonstrates that the form of collaboration can vary and still prove successful if the composition reflects the needs, desires, and make-up of the unique community.

7.5.4 Facilitation

A reasonable assumption that effective partnership facilitation played a positive influence can be garnered from successful outcomes demonstrated in each case. The only locale that attests to formal facilitation among its partners, however, is Melbourne. The broker facilitator in the two suburbs documented here was responsible for building and mediating relationships, coordinating meetings and working groups between the partners, and building capacity to make the partnerships eventually less dependent on his support. All agreed that the broker played a primary role in the partnership's success and warranted the additional funds supporting this addition. Whether or not the facilitation component is assigned to a specific person or takes on a formal role, facilitation in some capacity is essential to drive the focus of the partnership and manage potential conflict.

7.5.5 Needs Assessment

Hamilton County presents the best example of conducting a needs assessment for creating an effective and needs-based strategy. The partnership with the Health Department particularly ensured that the needs assessment focused on health-based inequalities. Notable is that although shared use can prove effective regardless of location, the specific focus on a prior assessment makes communities aware of the areas of greatest need and prompts them to tackle challenges where they are most deeply felt. Some of the methods for conducting a needs assessment include mapping, resident surveys and focus group interviews, and data collection and analysis.

7.5.6 *Review of Inventory*

A review of inventory, focused specifically on the availability of assets, was conducted in Edmonton. The evaluation is like a needs assessment in that the process requires foresight and advances effective planning. However, in Edmonton the shared use partners conduct reviews on vacant surplus school sites and maintain tracking on school site status to better plan and develop sites for shared use. Awareness of infrastructural stock makes planning for future use easier and strategic.

7.5.7 *Data Tracking and Public Availability*

Perhaps one of the most necessary factors in ensuring the wide promotion and spread of shared use from one community to another is the documentation and reporting of data, both quantitative and qualitative. Those involved in all four case studies documented their stories and made them publicly available. Some took reporting to the next step in terms of providing tangible numbers reflecting their success and challenges. The open and public availability of Edmonton's annual reports on shared use affords other communities the ability to learn what works well (and what doesn't) and how to emulate that success. Furthermore, a clearinghouse for the collection and dissemination of all local data would prove very useful in the future to study and show how best to serve communities and their public health needs through efficient shared municipal and school district planning and facility use.

7.6 Overcoming National, State, and Local Policy Barriers to Shared Use Agreements

Despite the numerous advantages of shared use and the resources available for successful execution, both real and perceived challenges threaten implementation. None of these challenges, however, are significant enough to preclude communities from usage, particularly considering the many benefits that shared use affords. A U.S. national survey of school principals identified the primary rationales behind restricting access to public use of recreational facilities. These included liability concerns, insurance, cost of running activities and programs, staffing for maintenance and security, safety concerns, and maintenance costs and responsibilities (Spengler 2012). Although understandable, the liability and insurance concerns stem from false perceptions of legal and systematic constraints. A survey of state law in all 50 states finds that no state can hold a public school to a legal duty beyond the standard of ordinary, reasonable care. Despite the presence of real liability risks, such risks do not pose threats substantial enough to deny public use of recreational facilities (Baker and Masud 2010).

Certainly, the logistical factors of maintenance, costs, and programming can also present real and significant challenges. Because school districts have for decades designed their buildings and infrastructure solely for the use of the single school rather than to accommodate community use, hesitation to share facilities is rooted in the idea that doing so will compromise the ability to fully service the students. However, the refusal to engage in shared use, although possibly founded upon good intentions, denies holistic use of valuable resources not only to the community but also to the very students whose rights the administration is seeking to protect. These challenges support not the dismissal of shared use strategies but rather the immediate need for a mindset shift in the design and planning of schools. The longer schools and communities fail to engage in the shared use framework discussed here, the longer these difficulties will be proliferated.

The challenges of shared use necessitate a threefold solution. At the state level, policy will prove most effective by extending the "permission" to implement shared use to include support and information repositories to promote and encourage ubiquitous expansion. Beyond the nominal mention of shared use in state code, states can also provide the guiding resources to help school districts and communities navigate the complicated, yet unrestrictive, legal and systematic hurdles. At the local level, the public availability and dissemination of data, resources, and success stories will inspire other communities to engage in the same strategies and activities. A variety of websites and clearinghouses currently exist to make these resources available, but communities will need to play a role in adding to the depth and comprehensiveness for other locales to replicate similar strategies and for future studies to effectively measure their success. Finally, local communities will also need to consider shifting to the framework of shared use presented here to fully circumvent the legal and logistical challenges posed against shared use as played out over the last several years. A holistic approach of shared ownership, planning, and implementation assumes that partnership will ensure that all liability, design, and logistical responsibilities and problems will have a mechanism to continuously address and resolve problems from the onset. Ultimately, the shift towards collaborative shared use proffers the avoidance of all the oft-cited concerns and challenges.

7.7 Recommendations and Discussion

Shared use in any form—proactively or retroactively applied to infrastructure—offers benefits to the community. In many cases, a retroactive application of shared use to existing facilities is perhaps the only option. The ideal model of shared use, however, is one that is built upon collaboration from the onset. True effectiveness lies in collaboration that involves all stakeholders and capitalizes on participation from the municipality, the community, and the school throughout every stage of shared use—design, planning, facility construction, and operations. Moreover, the application of recommended collaborative shared use components—the establishment or refinement of shared use policy, planning and design participation, alliances and partnerships, facilitation, needs assessments, review of inventory, data tracking and public availability, provides a basis for improvement even when these stages have already taken place and the facilities are not slated for future redevelopment. Through application of this framework at any stage of facility development, municipalities and school leadership may only see significant improvements in public health from shared use when they shift the entire mindset about planning, designing, operating, and managing recreational facilities. For instance, school districts and municipal leaders always have a continuous opportunity to improve partnerships, seek greater facilitation, conduct needs assessments, and review inventory. However, meaningful and effective partnership entails representation from all stakeholders and user groups having the opportunity to participate in the process that ultimately determines the spaces they will use.

To proliferate the advantages of the framework, local application of shared use must then be promulgated through a system of data sharing within and across communities. Minimal state-to-state and multilevel government communication has historically limited the efficiencies and effectiveness of strategies that seek to improve public health (Fiedler 2015). However, a mechanism based on an extension of protocols already in place by the CDC for reporting health data can formulate a subset of relevant data related to shared use (Fiedler 2014, 2015). Modifications to data collection, the type of questions being asked, and linking data to patient conditions standardized through the International Classification of Diseases can bring forth the methods to quantifiably model data and assess efficiency and effectiveness of policy (Fiedler and Ortiz-Baerga 2017) (Fig. 7.2).

Further, sharing data and cases across jurisdictions will be most helpful in quantifying and illustrating stories of the impact that shared use can have on public health efforts, specifically conveying which strategies work best under various circumstances. States can support and promote this objective by initiating a centralized outlet for information and data sharing as part of their holistic efforts to not only permit shared use but also expand the concept. Each locale can then follow through by providing the information and data that relates to its own application of shared use within this framework.

This paper has reviewed the insufficiencies in recreational and infrastructural offerings and the related public health challenges to demonstrate the need for a new framework of shared use agreements that begins with municipal-school district partnerships and carries through to all stages of facility planning and management. Available findings indicate that such a framework has the potential to incite real change in how community voices impact the availability of recreational spaces and in public health outcomes. On this foundation, shared use policy serves to improve communication methods between and among multilevel governments to generate awareness, provide revenue sharing opportunities, and offer multiple venues to indirectly achieve the goal of improved health as an important mechanism for change.

Much work can be done to further examine this framework of shared use and its' relationship with public health. Preliminary quantitative analysis of variables in

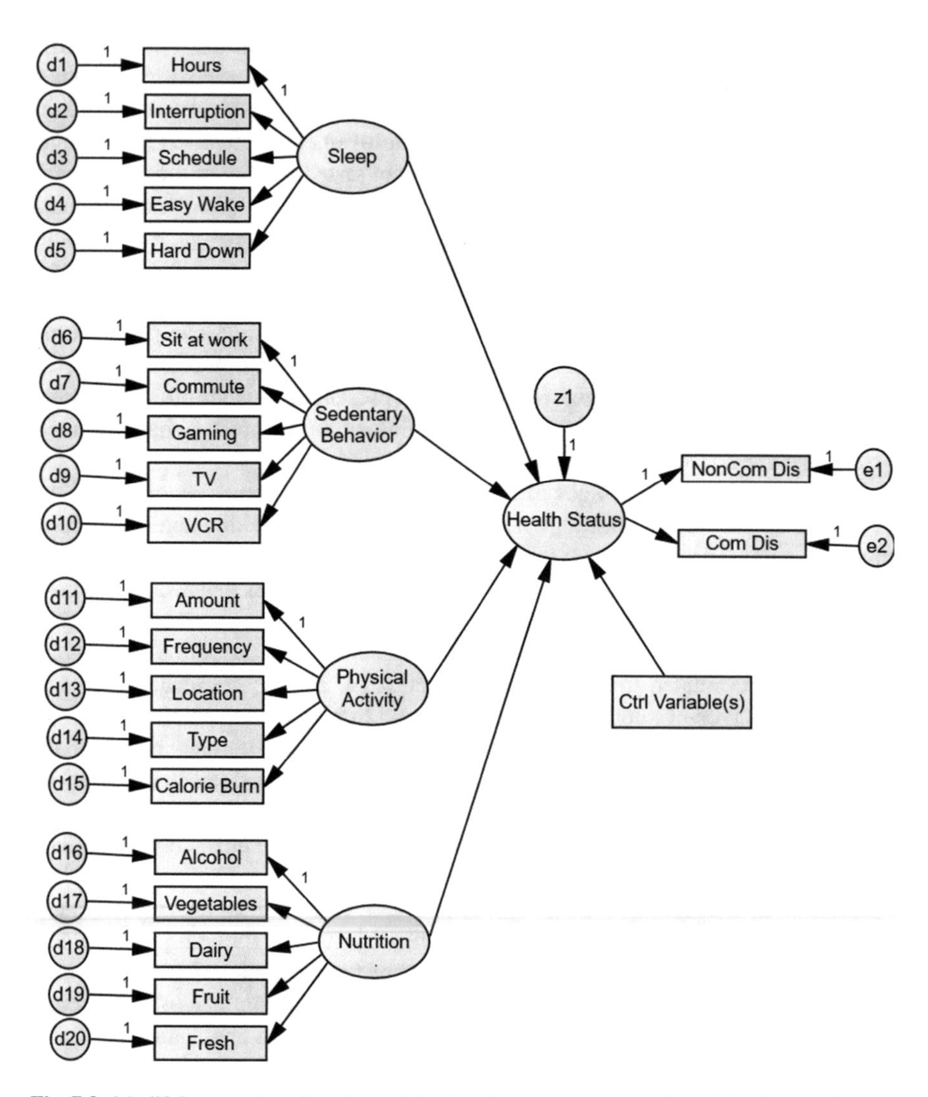

Fig. 7.2 Modifying questions in existing behavioral survey strategies of the United States Centers for Disease Control and Prevention to ordinal questions with a Likert scale represent an opportunity to use these predictive behaviors in relation to existing conditions reported in the International Classification of Diseases to form a structural equation model permitting the capture of overall population health or segments of data (e.g., sedentary behavior, physical activity) such as shared use (Fiedler and Ortiz-Baerga 2017)

available databases listed in additional recommended materials underwent experimental regression analysis without definitive results based on a lack of consistency with variable types and other considerations. Limitations on the available metrics in the United States related to shared use and associated problems linked to inadequate provisions for physical activity were apparent in four factors. These included the variability in local policies, the demographic and environmental characteristics within each state, the short amount of time that shared use policies have been in place, and finally the lack of proliferation of shared use in most jurisdictions at a finer level than the state. Cumulatively these factors are problematic in the analysis, quantification, and correlation between shared use policies and improved public health.

However, case study analysis reveals future strategies that may lead to quantifiable analysis that is dependent on local jurisdictions collecting and reporting information indicating local implementation of shared use and the community use that has taken place as a result. Such self-reported data need not require extensive time or effort on the part of each locale, but a central clearinghouse with this information would greatly enhance data analysis regarding shared use and public health outcomes.

Further, the ability to utilize social capital and networking strategies from the onset of shared use reflected in successful ventures in the case studies illustrates the potential to garner quantitative data on the effectiveness of contributions from multiple stakeholders through the theoretical premise of Social Capital. Social Capital Theory is founded on fundamental predictive variables such as trust, network diversity, network size and demographic diversity that test outcomes such as emotional support, social benefits, and performance (Granovetter 1973; Tsai and Ghoshal 1998) with direct application to international education settings (Bonnell et al. 2013). The relevance of this proposed theoretical approach is based on three facets of the model: (1) structural, (2) relational and (3) cognitive anchors (Tsai and Ghoshal 1998). Applying these anchors in the promotion of shared use policy starts with social interactions that begin to formulate the structure. Eventually, these interactions begin to build relational trust more likely leading to the formation of a shared vision. Finally, the combination of three facets should lead to resource exchange that creates value and produces viable application of proposed policy and thus, an advantageous product or development (Granovetter 1973; Tsai and Ghoshal 1998).

Measuring effectiveness, efficiency, and equity in relation to community services is one way to measure performance (Fig. 7.3). Tracking the number of funding sources, group members, diversity of membership, or measures of trust and cooperation (e.g., the proposed inclusion of school boards in land use and development decisions) can be valid predictive measures in the effectiveness of shared use propositions. Performance can also be measured from the social benefits of community inclusion that has been demonstrated to positively impact health and aid in the reduction of risk behaviors known to contribute to poor public health outcomes (Lin 2001).

> There is nondefinitive evidence for the feasibility and effectiveness of school environment interventions involving community/relationship building, empowering student participation in modifying schools' food/physical activity environments, and playground improvements … This evidence lends broad support to theories of social development, social capital, and human functioning and school organization (Bonnell et al. 2013, p.vi).

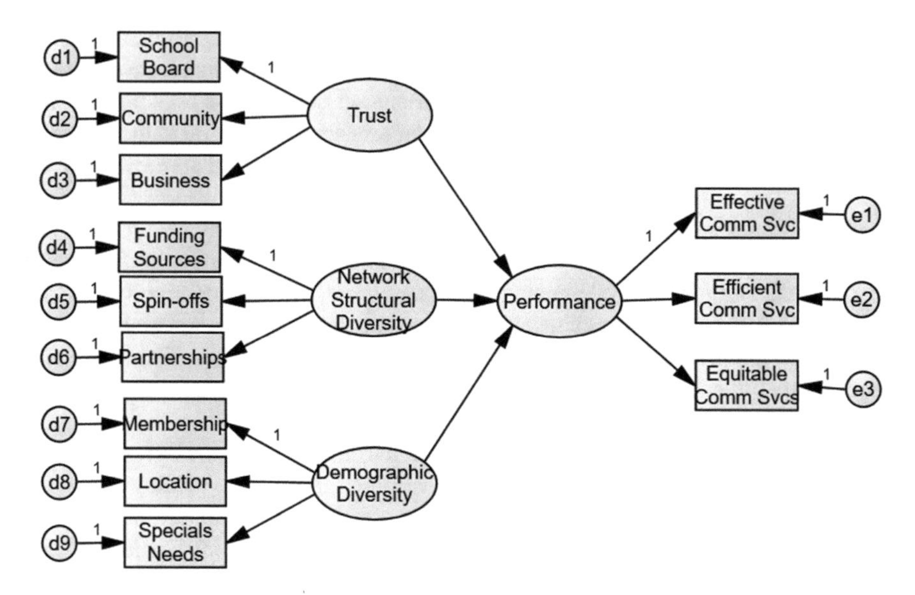

Fig. 7.3 Advanced statistical analysis could be conducted using a method of structural equation modeling (a graphical depiction of data) using information from community members, employees, and contributors as predictive measures to gauge performance measured by outcome scales associated with effective, efficient and equitable community services (Fiedler and Cook 2017)

Ultimately, the value derived from shared use and how communities can advance their health and social status can be demonstrated through constructs embedded in Social Capital Theory providing a foundation for baseline metrics to enhance data sharing. The approach capitalizes on the aspect of personal information, measuring both predictors and outcomes, to better understand organizational performance and population health. Thus, defining organizational performance metrics in measurable terms based on Social Capital, or using the premise to advance data exchange, will permit the universal collection and analysis of data that could quantitatively demonstrate the effectiveness and efficiency of shared use and other programs.

7.8 Summary

This chapter began with an emphasis on the historical application of shared use and the relationship between poor infrastructure and poor health. Four case studies from three countries (Canada, Australia, and the United States) formed the basis of a framework for embedding shared use agreements into the municipal planning process. Several important aspects of application of shared use include the conduct of a community needs assessment, an inventory of assets that could be shared, partnerships, and the important nature of data strategies to enhance performance metrics and increase decision-making.

Glossary

Community A group of people living in a common location or sharing a certain set of attributes; used in this context to refer to the citizens who share a stake in the subject area.

Facilitation The act of easing communication and collaboration among various groups and/or individuals.

Greenfield development Construction on previously undeveloped land that has never been used, often outside the boundaries of existing urban infrastructure and buildings.

International Classification of Diseases (ICD) An international standard for coding and terminology for medically diagnosed diseases or injuries (e.g., 250.00 Diabetes Mellitus, Type II, without complication); in Fig. 7.2, diabetes would be an example of a noncommunicable, chronic disease.

Likert scale Measures a level of agreement or disagreement with a given statement; normally incremental in 3, 5 or 7 depending on the method of statistical analysis (agree, neither agree or disagree, or disagree is an example of a 3-point Likert scale).

Ordinal A categorical data type used in survey research to rank variables; response scales can be Yes/No (dichotomous) or have multiple values such as in a Likert scale.

Quality of life The general well-being of a society and its members, largely dependent on physical, social, economic, and other indicators that either positively or negatively affect one's satisfaction with life.

Recreational facilities A physical building or space that provides opportunities for physical activity and leisure, such as a walking path, swimming pool, running track, or sports field; used most often in this context about publicly available spaces.

Shared use or joint use An agreement, either formal or informal, between two or more entities that enables the collective use of a facility or property by different groups; most commonly referenced in this context to describe an agreement between a school district and its respective municipal leaders that allows community use of a school building or property.

Structural equation modeling (SEM) Data elements are portrayed graphically; advanced method of statistical analysis where survey responses to exogenous (independent, predictor, X) variables can be measured for statistical significance against endogenous (dependent, outcomes, Y); the fundamental algebraic relationship between exogenous and endogenous variables in Fig. 7.2 is that Health Status = f (Sleep + Sedentary Behavior + Physical Activity + Nutrition) or $y = f(x_n)$ + measurement error.

Urban sprawl Unconstrained spread of development and human populations outside of a centralized urban core, which often results in suburbanized, low-density, and car-dependent populations.

References

American Society of Civil Engineers (ASCE). What makes a grade? 2017 infrastructure report card. 2017. http://www.infrastructurereportcard.org/making-the-grade/what-makes-a-grade/. Accessed 18 Sep 2017.

Baker T, Masud H. Liability risks for after-hours use of public school property to reduce obesity: a 50-state survey. J Sch Health. 2010;80:508–13. https://doi.org/10.1111/j.1746-1561.2010.00535.x.

Bingler S, et al. Schools as centers of community: a citizen's guide for planning and design. 2nd ed. Washington, DC: National Clearinghouse for Educational Facilities; 2003.

Bonnell C, et al. Systematic review of the effects of schools and school environment interventions on health: evidence mapping and synthesis. Public Health Res. 2013;1(1)

Canadian Obesity Network. Obesity in Canada. 2017. http://www.obesitynetwork.ca/obesity-in-canada. Accessed 18 Sep 2017.

Cawley J. An economy of scales: a selective review of obesity's economic causes, consequences, and solutions. J Health Econ. 2015;43:244–68.

Cawley J, Meyerhoefer C. The medical care costs of obesity: an instrumental variables approach. J Health Econ. 2012;31(1):219–30.

ChangeLab Solutions. Hamilton county, Tennessee. 2017a. http://www.changelabsolutions.org/shared-use-hamiliton-tn. Accessed 24 Feb 2017.

Chapman B, Colangelo L. Mayor de Blasio will open 22 school playgrounds for public use under plan to provide more parkland to New Yorkers. New York Daily News. 2016, August 2. http://www.nydailynews.com/new-york/nyc-schools-widen-playground-access-public-article-1.2736051. Accessed 18 Sep 2017.

City of Edmonton. Edmonton joint use agreement: land. 2009. https://www.edmonton.ca/programs_services/documents/PDF/JUALand2.pdf. Accessed 18 Sep 2017.

City of Edmonton. Edmonton's joint use agreements: annual report 2015/2016. 2016. https://www.edmonton.ca/programs_services/documents/PDF/COE_JointUse_AnnualReport_2016.pdf. Accessed 18 Sep 2017.

Cook K. Planning through the shared use of resources: a case study of DeKalb County (Thesis). Georgia: Georgia Institute of Technology, School of City & Regional Planning; 2015.

DASH-NY. New York shared use agreement policy implementation guide: a guide to expanding healthy living through shared use agreements. NY Acad Med:1–30. 2015. http://www.dashny.org/wp-content/uploads/2015/10/SharedUseGuide-Final-09082015-A.pdf. Accessed 18 Sep 2017.

Department of Health and Human Services. Physical activity guidelines advisory committee report. Washington, DC. 2008. https://health.gov/paguidelines/pdf/paguide.pdf. Accessed 18 Sep 2017.

Department of Sport and Recreation. Guide to shared use facilities in the sport and recreation community. Government of Western Australia. n.d. https://www.dsr.wa.gov.au/support-and-advice/facility-management/managing-facilities/guide-to-shared-use-facilities. Accessed 18 Sep 2017.

Ewing R, et al. Relationship between urban sprawl and physical activity, obesity, and morbidity. Am J Health Promot. 2003;18:1.

Ewing R, et al. Relationship between urban sprawl and physical activity, obesity, and morbidity—update and refinement. Health Place. 2014;26:118–26.

Fiedler BA. Constructing legal authority to facilitate multi-level interagency health data sharing in the United States. Paper presented at American Society of Public Administration Conference (ASPA), Washington, DC, 14-18 March 2014.

Fiedler BA. Constructing legal authority to facilitate multi-level interagency health data sharing in the United States. Int J Pharm Healthc Mark. 2015;9(2):175–94.

Fiedler BA, Cook K. Foundations of community health: planning access to public facilities. Paper presented at Southeastern Conference of Public Administration (SECoPA) on education, health, and social welfare policy, Hollywood, FL, October 4-7 2017.

Fiedler BA, Ortiz-Baerga J. Extending public health surveillance reporting through digital data collection of behavior patterns and existing conditions. United States Centers for Disease Control and Prevention, CDC Data Challenge, Phase I, August 4 2017.
Granovetter MS. The strength of weak ties. Am J Sociol. 1973;78(6):1360–80.
Gunderson T et al Joint use agreements and school site planning. Edmonton: Alberta School Boards Association. 2016. http://www.asba.ab.ca/wp-content/uploads/2014/07/sgm16_joint_use.pdf. Accessed 18 Sep 2017.
Jackson R, Kochtitzky C. Creating a healthy environment: the impact of the built environment on public health. Sprawl Watch Clearinghouse Monograph News. 2002. http://www.sprawlwatch.org/health.pdf. Accessed 17 Sep 2017.
Lawhon L. The neighborhood unit: physical design or physical determinism? J Plan Hist. 2009;8(2):111–32. http://jph.sagepub.com/content/8/2/111. Accessed 20 Sep 2017
Leisure Information Network. National report on joint use agreements survey 2012. Canadian Active After School Partnership. 2012. http://lin.ca/shared-use. Accessed 18 Sep 2017.
Lewis H. Fair play: advancing health equity through shared use. Community Commons. 2016. https://www.communitycommons.org/tag/shared-use/. Accessed 17 Sep 2017.
Lin N. Building a network theory of social capital. In: Lin N, et al., editors. Social capital: theory and research. New York: Aldine de Gruyter; 2001. p. 3–29.
McShane I et al Opportunity spaces: community engagement in the planning, use and governance of shared school facilities. Australian Research Council Linkage Project. 2013.
McShane I, Wilson C (2014) .Making better use of school facilities—what are the issues? https://oppspaces.files.wordpress.com/2014/05/making-better-use-of-school-facilities.pdf. Accessed 18 Sep 2017.
Miles R. Introduction and problem context. In: Miles R, Adelaja A, Wyckoff M, editors. School siting and healthy communities. Michigan: Michigan State University Press; 2011. p. 3–12.
National Association of State Boards of Education (NASBE). State school health policy database. 2013. http://www.nasbe.org/healthy_schools/hs/bytopics.php?topicid=3181&catExpand=acdnbtm_catC. Accessed 18 Sep 2017.
National Center for Health Statistics. Health, United States, 2015: with special features on racial and economic disparities. 2016. https://www.cdc.gov/nchs/data/hus/hus15.pdf. Accessed 18 Sep 2017.
Pope J. Strengthening local communities: a partnership approach to delivering school and community infrastructure in Melbourne's growth areas of Laurimar and Caroline Springs. Melbourne: Strategic Policy, Research and Forecasting Department of Planning and Community Development; 2010. http://www.futurecommunities.net/files/images/melbourne_strengthening_local_coms.pdf. Accessed 17 Sep 2017.
Spengler J. Promoting physical activity through the shared use of school and community recreational resources. Active Living Research Brief, Robert Wood Johnson Foundation. 2012. http://activelivingresearch.org/promoting-physical-activity-through-shared-use-school-and-community-recreational-resources. Accessed 17 Sep 2017.
Safe Routes to School (SRTS) National Partnership. Making strides: 2016 state report cards. 2016. http://www.saferoutespartnership.org/sites/default/files/resource_files/072616_sr2s_statereport_2016_final.pdf. Accessed 19 Jan 2017.
Safe Routes to School (SRTS) National Partnership. Shared use of school and community facilities. 2017. http://www.saferoutespartnership.org/state/bestpractices/shareduse. Accessed 17 Sep 2017.
Shoshkes E. Engaging the public in comprehensive planning and design for healthy schools. In: Miles R, Adelaja A, Wyckoff M, editors. School siting and healthy communities. Michigan: Michigan State University Press; 2011. p. 221–35.
State Government Victoria. Guide to governing shared community facilities. Department of Planning and Community Development. 2010. http://www.localgovernment.vic.gov.au/__data/assets/pdf_file/0025/48625/Guide-to-Governing-Shared-Community-Facilities.pdf. Accessed 18 Sep 2017.

Step One. Our mission. 2017. http://www.hcstep1.org/Mission.aspx. Accessed 17 Sep 2017.
Tsai W, Ghoshal S. Social capital and value creation: the role of intrafirm networks. Acad Manag J. 1998;41(4):464–76.
United States Centers for Disease Control and Prevention (CDC). Results from the School Health Policies and Practices Study 2016. 2017. https://www.cdc.gov/healthyyouth/data/shpps/pdf/shpps-results_2016.pdf. Accessed 25 Sep 2017.
Victoria State Government. Education and training reform act. 2006. http://www.legislation.vic.gov.au/Domino/Web_Notes/LDMS/PubStatbook.nsf/f932b66241ecf1b7ca256e92000e23be/575C47EA02890DA4CA25717000217213/$FILE/06-024a.pdf. Accessed 17 Sep 2017.
Wade E. The four factors that drag Australians down. The Sydney Morning Herald. 2016, June 8. http://www.smh.com.au/comment/the-four-things-that-drag-australia-down-20160607-gpdfrg.html. Accessed 17 Sep 2017.
World Health Organization (WHO). Interactive charts: prevalence of obesity. 2014. http://gamapserver.who.int/gho/interactive_charts/ncd/risk_factors/obesity/atlas.html. Accessed 17 Sep 2017.
World Health Organization (WHO). Fact sheet: Obesity and overweight. 2016. http://www.who.int/mediacentre/factsheets/fs311/en/. Accessed 17 Sep 2017.

Further Reading

Active Living Research. Resources for schools. 2017. http://activelivingresearch.org/taxonomy/schools. Accessed 12 Apr 2017.
ChangeLab Solutions. What is a joint use agreement? 2017. http://www.changelabsolutions.org/publications/what-is-JUA. Accessed 12 Apr 2017.
City of Ann Arbor, MI. FY2018–2023 Capital improvements plan. 2017. https://www.a2gov.org/departments/systems-planning/programs/Documents/Composite_CIP_%20Jan-17-2016%20Public%20Hearing%20Documents.pdf. Accessed 17 Sep 2017.
Community Commons. Animated Obesity rate map 1985–2008. [Animation: Nevit Dilmen]. [Data source: United States Centers for Disease Control and Prevention (CDC)]. n.d. https://www.communitycommons.org/2013/04/animated-obesity-rate-map/. Accessed 20 Sep 2017.
Kaiser Family Foundation. Health care expenditures per capita by state of residence. 2009. http://kff.org/other/state-indicator/health-spending-per-capita/?currentTimeframe=0&sortModel=%7B%22colId%22:%22Location%22,%22sort%22:%22asc%22%7D. Accessed 10 Feb 2017.
National Assn of County and City Health Officials (NACCHO). Healthy community design toolkit. 2017. http://archived.naccho.org/topics/environmental/landuseplanning/index.cfm. Accessed 12 Apr 2017.
Thrun E et al Disparities in shared use agreements, policies, and plans. Bridging the Gap program. 2016. http://www.bridgingthegapresearch.org/_asset/zqqge6/BTG_SUA_disparities_brief_Feb2016.pdf. Accessed 17 Sep 2017.
United States Census Bureau. American FactFinder: Community facts. American community survey 5-year estimates. 2015. https://factfinder.census.gov/faces/nav/jsf/pages/community_facts.xhtml. Accessed 30 Jan 2017.
United States Centers for Disease Control and Prevention. Chronic disease and health promotion data & indicators. 2017. https://chronicdata.cdc.gov/health-area/heart-disease-stroke-prevention?limit=25&view_type=rich. Accessed 18 Sep 2017.
University of California, Berkley. Center for cities and schools. 2017. http://citiesandschools.berkeley.edu/. Accessed 12 Apr 2017.

Chapter 8
Food Reservations at the Reservation?

Rebecca Webster

Abstract The growing problem of Americans facing chronic health conditions—Type 2 diabetes, heart disease, and obesity—is exacerbated within the Native American population who live on reservations. Their rate of these chronic conditions exceeds those for all other races bringing forth a greater need for methods to improve health through the development of local food security. Fortunately, the indigenous food sovereignty movement has brought attention to their struggle for access to healthy and culturally appropriate foods that are grown and harvested in accordance with tribal agricultural practices. The Oneida Indian Reservation in Wisconsin provides a case study demonstrating how tribal government farm operations, backyard gardening, and agricultural cooperatives combine to reintegrate Iroquois white corn into diets to improve health outcomes. Collaboration between the Oneida Nation's Tsyunhehkwa (life sustenance), Cannery, and Oneida Market and the Sustainable Agriculture Research and Education Program financially support the commitment to farming and food preservation that contribute to the development of informal agricultural cooperatives. Oneida families developed their own backyard gardens and formed Ohe•láku (among the cornstalks). This chapter provides a historical overview of the external forces contributing to the current Native American health crisis, illustrates the growing strength of tribal governance and how the people have reconnected with the land to produce healthy crops and restore lost culture. Their resilience and spiritual revival demonstrates several methods that can be translated to other Indian reservations and communities to aid in the resolution of national health and food security problems throughout the United States.

8.1 Introduction

Indicators of poor health expressed in the development of chronic diseases are prevalent in the general population in the United States. However, one sector of the population demonstrates higher rates of chronic disease than all others—the

R. Webster (✉)
University of Minnesota, Duluth, MN, USA
e-mail: rwebster@d.umn.edu

B. A. Fiedler (ed.), *Translating National Policy to Improve Environmental Conditions Impacting Public Health Through Community Planning*,
https://doi.org/10.1007/978-3-319-75361-4_8

Native American population representing 567 federally recognized tribes (National Congress of American Indians n.d., *para* 2), 5.4 million people, and 2% of the US population (United States Census Bureau 2016, *para* 2). The Native American incidence of chronic disease such as type 2 diabetes, heart disease, and obesity surpass rates for all other races (Dion-Buffalo and Mohawk 1999; Kuhnlein and Receveur 1996; Milburn 2004). For example, Native Americans are twice as likely to develop type 2 diabetes than the rest of the population (CDC 2016). Two factors emerge as causal indicators in prior literature including (1) persistent colonial assimilation policies, and (2) reliance on nonindigenous foods that are replete of nutrients due to over processing. The consequent loss of knowledge from these historical indicators is also the impetus to compel Tribal Governance to action to restore a system of tribal agriculture practices in which healthy and culturally appropriate foods are grown and harvested in accordance with tradition. European colonization to the United States provides a starting point to understanding the path leading to this persistent health crisis in the Native American population.

The health crisis is one of a string of detrimental impacts of colonization and forced assimilation initiated by European contact in the late 1400s (Parker 1910) that persist in Native American culture and identity (Loew 2001). Indigenous people across the world have strikingly parallel stories in which the loss of language and culture are common outcomes of external contact. But recent scholarly attention is focusing on the health impact of forced dietary changes on the health of Native American people (Grey and Patel 2015) as well as among indigenous population throughout the world (Haman et al. 2010).

"Part of the history of colonization of Native American peoples was to take away both native lands and the native foods which flourished upon these lands" (Walter 2012, p.586) resulting in the generational health crisis apparent today. The problem became pervasive during the boarding school era in the late 1800s and early 1900s when children were taken away from their homes and forced to eat foods foreign to them to assimilate them into mainstream society (Loew 2001). Similarly, pursuant to the Indian Relocation Act of 1956, the federal government encouraged the relocation of Native American people from their reservations into larger metropolitan areas by paying for trade schools and offering to help with relocation expenses while simultaneously decreasing subsidies to Native Americans continuing to reside on reservations. Removal from tribal lands and culture meant that participants were also separated from tribal agricultural practices and traditional foods. Thus, attempts by colonists to assimilate Native Americans is a factor contributing to the present problem as knowledge was lost spawning "numerous trans-generational health consequences for Indigenous populations," (Bodirsky and Johnson 2008, p.1). "These diseases are enduring legacies of land dispossession, de-culturalisation through boarding schools, and the concomitant loss of cultural, agricultural, spiritual and ancestral knowledge," (Walter 2012, p.586).

Genetics may explain some of the high prevalence of these diseases among indigenous populations when compared to Caucasians, but it is certainly not the

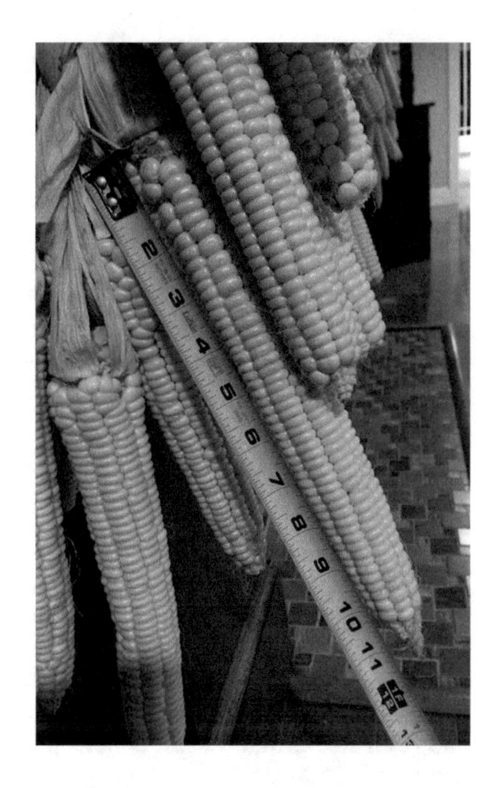

Fig. 8.1 Cob of Iroquois white corn

sole factor. Reliance on nonindigenous and highly processed foods can, at minimum, partially account for higher rates of chronic conditions than any other ethnic groups in the United States (Coté 2016; Walter 2012). Thankfully, collaborations with organizations such as the North Central Region—Sustainable Agriculture Research and Education Program (NCR-SARE) (http://www.northcentralsare.org/) in conjunction with the United States Department of Agriculture (USDA) (https://www.usda.gov/wps/portal/usda/usdahome) represent opportunities to restore traditional food staples into the Native American diet.

This brief, historical overview provides the basic context of the old policy versus new federal efforts informing the balance of this chapter that unfolds the chronic health condition of Native Americans, identifies the problems of food security and food sovereignty on reservations, and presents the Oneida Nation case study. Then, the chapter will view the rule of tribal governance to address the debilitating nature of the environmental and behavioral conditions that impact this sector of population health. Next, efforts of the Oneida tribe in collaboration with new agencies demonstrate how their activities can help to improve the health status of Native Americans. Finally, the reintroduction of Iroquois white corn is discussed as one solution to promote health improvements (Fig. 8.1).

8.2 Native American Tribal Response to Health, Food Security, and Sovereignty

The adoption of Western diets has proven critical on the health outcomes for Native Americans requiring a tribal governments' response to food problems that they are facing. Nonindigenous diets have brought forth the need to (1) examine Native American health conditions, (2) incorporate food security within reservations, (3) integrate food sovereignty within reservations, and (4) unify the tribal governments' response to food issues facing Native Americans. Cumulatively, these items play a significant role in the return of traditional crop growth using tribal agricultural practices.

8.2.1 Native American Chronic Health Conditions

Rapid change in diet among a population can impact cultural knowledge and lead to drastic health consequences, especially with indigenous populations that are genetically unable to process western foods in the same manner as those of European ancestry (Haman et al. 2010). Two factors that influence food selection over the last century are (1) policies that moved education outside of the reservation (e.g., mission schools, boarding schools) acting as a barrier to transfer cultural knowledge and (2) media-driven federal policy applying population health standards of the dominant culture to indigenous people without sensitivity to divergent cultural and nutritional benefits of traditional food.

The introduction of each new item to the Native American food chain (e.g., sugar, refined grain flour and bread, sweetened tea, and alcohol) slowly eroded indigenous traditions, cultures, languages, as well as tribal political and economic systems (Coté 2016; Kuhnlein and Receveur 1996). These foods in the modern Western diet are high in fat, calorie-dense, and nutrient-poor (Milburn 2004). Many epidemiologists claim that the shift from wild and near-wild foods to super-domesticated crops and highly refined foods are to blame for the high rates of type 2 diabetes, heart disease, and obesity in the Native American population (Dion-Buffalo and Mohawk 1999; Kuhnlein and Receveur 1996; Milburn 2004).

The epidemiologist claims are consistent with the Centers for Disease Control and Prevention (CDC) reports that Native Americans are twice as likely to develop type 2 diabetes as other races (CDC 2016). Heart disease was the number one cause of death among Native Americans and the death rate from heart disease was 20% higher for Native Americans than the national average. While the CDC does not track obesity rates for Native American populations nationwide, in one study spanning 14 states, the CDC found that 40.1% of Native Americans were obese as compared to 26.5% of African Americans, 26.6% of Hispanic Americans, and 2.7% of Asian Americans (CDC 2003) .

Some scholars have called into question the integrity of the United States Department of Agriculture's (USDA) food and nutrition policies based on an inherent conflict in their responsibility to advocate for both agribusiness and public health (Milburn 2004). The USDA developed the four-food group approach consisting of milk, meat, fruit, and vegetables in the 1950s. However, this food grouping reflected not only the dominant Western diet but also the power of the meat and dairy industries. When the USDA attempted to revise the food groupings in the 1980s, the meat and dairy industries challenged their attempts. In 1991, the USDA adopted the food pyramid to stress the importance of consuming more fruits, vegetables, and whole grains and less meat, milk, sugar, and fats. Despite a number of successful lawsuits filed by the Physicians Committee for Responsible Medicine (PCRM), most notably *PCRM v. Glickman*, in the United States District Court for the District of Columbia arguing that the USDA failed to disclose conflicts of interest with the dairy, meat, and egg industries (Physicians Comm. for Responsible Med. v. Glickman 2000), the USDA continues to recommend diets that include products from these industries in amounts that are not based on science, but more likely are influenced by economic pressure from these industries (PCRM 2016).

An example of an element to be considered in a culturally and economically driven food policy is the continued inclusion of milk products in recommended daily food consumption when studies indicate that many ethnic populations are unable to properly digest these foodstuffs (Milburn 2004). An enzyme called lactase, found in the people of northern European descent and in some African groups, is required for a person to digest milk sugar lactose but many ethnic groups lack this ability. For example, studies have shown that 74% of Native Americans are lactose intolerant (Milburn 2004). For certain populations, the public health benefits from the USDA's classification of milk and dairy as an essential food group is difficult to envision when considering that a large portion of the American public is physically unable to digest milk products. Therefore, inclusion of alternative items to dairy products would be universally beneficial and embrace the needs of this population sector.

In addition to the USDA's continued classification of milk and dairy as an essential food group, the agency fails to account for different dietary needs of ethnic populations. Instead, the USDA attempts to establish food guidelines that apply to all Americans.

> These [g]uidelines…embody the idea that a healthy eating pattern is not a rigid prescription, but rather, an adaptable framework in which individuals can enjoy foods that meet their personal, cultural, and traditional preferences and fit within their budget. [There are] [s]everal examples of healthy eating patterns that translate and integrate the recommendations in overall healthy ways to eat. (USDA 2015)

Current recommended food groups include fruits, vegetables, protein, dairy, grains, and oils. The only variations on these recommendations are for vegetarians and Mediterranean diets; there are no variations that address the dietary needs of Native Americans. While the United States Department of Health and Human Services, Indian Health Service (IHS 2012) does have dietary recommendations for Native Americans called "My Native Plate," they are essentially the same as the standard USDA recommended guidelines with some additions, such as wild rice and wild game, while retaining dairy as well as breads and cereals made from highly processed grains. "These government models [for Native American dietary guidelines] would fall into the camp of not making much difference in the end," (Milburn 2004 p.429).

8.2.2 *Food Security on Reservations*

Statistical evidence suggests that there is a strong correlation between food insecurity and health problems such as Type 2 diabetes, heart disease, and obesity (Jernigan et al. 2011). The problem of food security on Reservations is twofold in nature. First, food security requires that people have access to food that is "nutritionally adequate, culturally acceptable, and safe" (Bauer et al. 2012) and second, people must also have access to locally grown produce (Jarosz 2014). Thus, several factors that lead to food insecurity also describe inhabitants of Reservations such as low socioeconomic status, receipt of low quality food assistance, residence in a rural area, a lack of a healthy food supply including locally grown produce, and limited, if any, access to public transportation. The dependence on government food assistance because of low economic status (Gundersen 2008) with nutritional contents that are inconsistent with the Native American diet, and the cost and availability of food influencing dietary choices (O'Connell et al. 2011) combine to build the walls limiting access to fresh produce. People of lower socioeconomic status often choose to maximize their spending power by choosing less expensive, lower quality, and therefore less nutritious, foods.

With the increase in globalization, more of our daily food comes from distant sources (Kuhnlein and Receveur 1996). This may serve as a benefit to many people living in urban areas that can afford the variety and supply of fresh produce. However, lack of available public transportation in rural areas where many Indian reservations are located can limit access to higher quality foods (Baek 2016). Often referred to as a "food desert," many families end up purchasing food from fast food restaurants and small grocery or convenience stores (Bauer et al. 2012). These establishments typically have a limited supply of high quality produce and low-fat foods. To compound the problem, many Native Americans living on reservations receive food assistance from the United States Department of Agriculture Food Distribution Program (Jernigan et al. 2011). These foods are typically canned or packaged, highly processed, and high in fat, sugar, and salt. The combination of these factors serves as further evidence that the colonial impacts on food extend beyond the decreased growth of traditional foods and spread well into the preparation, storage, consumption, and exchange of food today (Grey and Patel 2015).

When compared to the general population, Native Americans have the lowest health and economic rates and the highest rates of food insecurity (Mullany et al. 2013). This assessment is supported by data revealing Native Americans' per capita income is calculated at 40 percent less than the general population (Gundersen 2008). Further, in a study relying on data collected between 2001 and 2004, Gunderson reported that 28% of Native American households with children were food insecure and 16.3% of Native American households without children were food insecure (Gundersen 2008, p.201). Comparatively, 15.7% of non-Native American households with children were food insecure and 7.8% of non-Native American households without children were food insecure (Gundersen 2008, p.201). However, Native Americans did not always wrestle with the problem of food insecurity. Tribal members produced nearly all of their own food locally until the early 1900's. Unfortunately, today, less than 20 percent of the food tribal members consume is grown locally (LaDuke et al. 2010, p.19).

Despite the bleakness of current condition of Native Americans' food security, many tribes have the potential to address this problem by making better use of land held by tribes and tribal members, estimated to be over 54 million acres (LaDuke et al. 2010), where growing indigenous food can serve as a revitalization of cultural identity (Slocum 2006). Approximately 47 million acres of this land is cropland and rangeland. However, tribes and tribal members lease 70% of the cropland and 20% of the rangeland to non-Indians, leaving tribal communities with less control over their food systems (LaDuke et al. 2010, p.19). Only a handful of the 8000 Native American farmers that operate on reservations produce food for local tribal members. Tribes' prioritization of tribal members' agricultural needs when designating land uses is critical to improving food security within reservations and would simultaneously promote increased indigenous food sovereignty.

8.2.3 Indigenous Food Sovereignty

One definition classifies indigenous food sovereignty as "right of [p]eoples to define their own policies and strategies for the sustainable production, distribution, and consumption of food, with respect for their own cultures and their own systems of man aging natural resources and rural areas, and is considered to be a precondition for [f]ood [s]ecurity" (Consultation 2015, p.2). In the past few decades, the indigenous food sovereignty movement has gained momentum (Grey and Patel 2015). While the triggering event sparking the food sovereignty movement is unknown, some argue that the food sovereignty movement began over the fishing controversies of the 1970s where Native Americans fought for and secured their rights to harvest fish (Adamson 2011). "The food sovereignty movement has deep roots in indigenous campaigns to force states to abide by treaty obligations including the right to 'first foods' like salmon, elk, deer, camas, geoduck, and huckleberry," (Adamson 2011, p.215).

The use of the term "food sovereignty movement," often criticized for being vague and lacking a concise definition, is defined herein to encompass three main goals for indigenous populations. First, indigenous people should have access to healthy and culturally appropriate food. Second, indigenous people should be able to engage in sustainable food production. Third, indigenous people should be able to safeguard their agricultural practices including planting, harvesting, and preservation. While these goals may also promote food security, the main difference between a focus on food sovereignty and food security is that food sovereignty necessitates that Native American people be able to accomplish these goals for themselves, without external interference.

Food sovereignty can serve as a "means to discuss the marginalization of Native Americans as both producers and consumers within the existing food system and to envision how their situation could be improved," (Fairbairn 2012, p.225). Further, regaining control of the food system can be a means for Native Americans to address some of the long-term effects of colonization (Coté 2016). For example, the First Nations Development Initiative (2014) produced the First Nations' Food Sovereignty Assessment Tool to assist Native American communities to reclaim their local food systems. The program provides a toolkit to assist communities to "measure and assess food access, land use and food policy in their communities" with the goal of reclaiming those food systems (First Nations Development Initiative 2014, p.6).

8.2.4 Tribal Government Response

Tribal governments are tackling health problems, food security and food sovereignty with a wide range of external and internal responses. They include utilizing the court system to protect against nonnative attempts to appropriate indigenous foods for a profit, taking greater interest in implementing tribal governance, and promotional campaigns inviting Native Americans to become more physically active.

Tribes across the nation are undertaking measures to regain control of their traditional food systems and to make traditional foods more available to their communities (Ahtone 2016) to address the problems of food security and sovereignty. One example includes the food sovereignty summits hosted by tribes in all areas of the country. For example, in September 2016, Red Lake in Minnesota hosted a food summit that addressed organic certifications, strengthening fisheries, maple syrup tapping, soil health, and seed keeping (Intertribal Agriculture Council 2016).

Tribes may also battle such appropriation by developing their own agricultural laws. For example, to prevent cross-pollination with the wild rice, one Anishnaabeg tribe—White Earth, passed a law prohibiting genetically modified seeds within their reservation boundaries. Other tribes that have developed food and agriculture codes have received assistance from the University of Arkansas, School of Law, Indigenous Food and Agriculture Initiative (University of Arkansas n.d.).

Many tribes are implementing the "Just Move It" campaign to promote physical activity for their members and to improve the overall health of their members (Just Move It n.d.). Several organizations have also been implemented with the goal of getting tribes together to address specific health issues. For example, the National Indian Health Board formed a Tribal Leaders Diabetes Committee to explore ways to address diabetes and other chronic health conditions (NIHB n.d.).

These varying tribal responses to Native American health, food security and food sovereignty speak to the complexity of the matter as the responses span from community exercise programs, internal land use assessment, intertribal research, discussion and communication, and legislative and potential litigious actions.

8.3 Case Studies: Iroquois White Corn History, Culture, and Health

Iroquois white corn has the power to address the population health, food security and food sovereignty problems facing Native American people today. The history of white corn, historical relevance to Native American culture and diet, and the scope of Native Americans who are reclaiming white corn as one of their traditional foods, including the Oneida Nation and community members in Wisconsin, provides a basis for understanding the important nature of these concepts in relation to the potential for improved health outcomes by working diligently to get more white corn into their diets.

8.3.1 Historical Significance of Iroquois White Corn

Tribes formed sophisticated government structures and established trade routes that spanned North and South America prior to European contact (Beauchamp 1898). Scholars agree that agriculture, specifically corn crops, led to the rise of civilization throughout the New World. "Ubiquitous throughout the New World at the time of European contact, maize is heralded as a plant full of possibilities, serving as the backbone for the rise of complex societies in the Americas" (Briggs 2015, p.113).

One formal group came to be known as the Iroquois Confederacy. Referring to themselves as Haudenosaunee (people of the longhouse), the confederacy consisted of the Mohawk, Oneida, Onondaga, Cayuga, Seneca and Tuscarora nations. This group was primarily located in what is now known as the State of New York. In addition to hunting, fishing, and gathering, the Haudenosaunee were well known for farming varieties of corn, beans, and squash (Harrington 1908).

Written accounts of Haudenosaunee farming practices date back to 1535 (Mt. Pleasant 2011) and consist of discussion on the varieties of corn, the lack of farm animals to plow the fields, and the predominance of women as laborers in the fields. Of the many different varieties of corn—white corn, also referred to as flint corn or Tuscarora corn, was and continues to be the most common variety (Perrotto 2015) (Fig. 8.2).

Unfortunately, many Indian tribes lost millions of acres of land through illegal land transactions and invalid treaties in the early 1800's (Webster 2015). Pressure for tribes to move westward pushed relocation in that direction away from their original territories. A group of Oneida people migrated to what is now the State of Wisconsin at that time and later entered a treaty with the United States in 1838 establishing their reservation boundaries there. The Oneida people continued their agricultural practices until the late 1800s when Congress' General Allotment Act resulted in the dispossession of roughly 95% of their land (Webster 2016). Agricultural practices throughout the United States faced a similar decline in the1930's (Mt. Pleasant 2011).

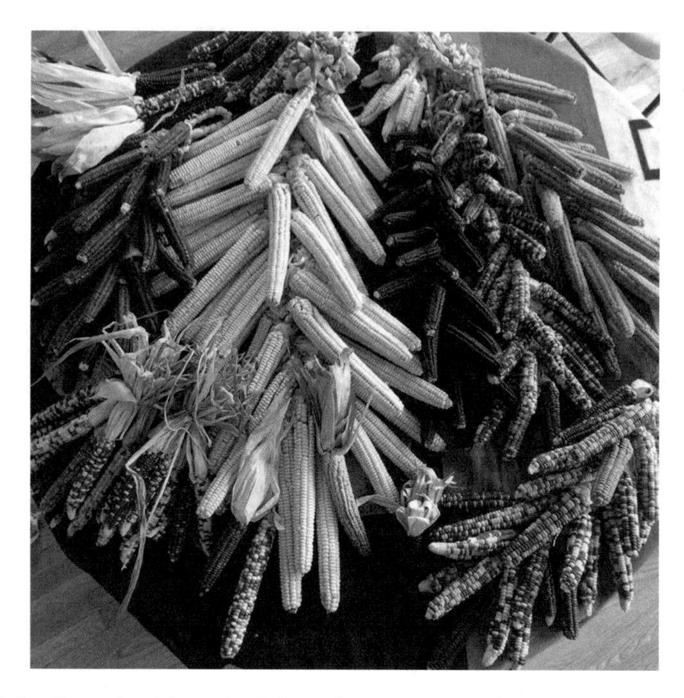

Fig. 8.2 A Small sample of the variety of corn from North and South America including Iroquois white corn

8.3.2 Iroquois White Corn: Place in Culture and Diet

Arthur C. Parker, a Seneca descendant and well-known archaeologist in the early 1900s, wrote extensively about Haudenosaunee culture and agricultural practices. "The mythology of the Iroquois is full of allusions to corn, its cultivation and uses" (Parker 1910, p.37). Along similar lines, Dr. Carol Cornelius, an Oneida tribal member and retired Area Manager of the Oneida Cultural Heritage Department, encouraged the use of Iroquois corn as a culture-based curriculum in K-12 classrooms. His proclamation that, "Corn is integral to all aspects of the Haudenosaunee way of life" (Cornelius 1999, p.91) was evident as corn served as a symbol of hospitality and played roles in wedding customs and traditional ceremonies (Fenton 1962).

Haudenosaunee stories make numerous references to white corn including the creation story, stories about the formation of the Iroquois Confederacy before contact (the Great Law) as well as the revival of the Confederacy in the 1700s (Handsome Lake). Jeff Metoxen, Manager of the Tsyunhehkwa (life sustenance), which is the Oneida Nation department responsible for growing white corn, relays a brief portion of the creation story relative to white corn.

> The beginning of our Mother Earth occurred when Sky Woman fell from a hole near the Tree of Life. When she was falling from her world, she grabbed at the sides of the ground near the tree and took with her seeds of various plant life. A number of birds saw her fall from the sky and came together to help her descend safely and placed her on the back of a

> large turtle. Life at that time was mostly birds and water animals, with no land in sight. They understood she needed more to survive in their world, so some of the animals dove deep into the water to bring clay up from the bottom. The clay was placed on the back of the turtle, which began to expand to form Turtle Island, and become part of Mother Earth. The seeds that Sky Woman had brought with her began to grow into the plants and herbal life needed for survival. Plants grown from those first seeds included Corn, Beans, and Squash, and became the Three Sisters for our people. They are the main providers for our sustenance. It is our tradition and responsibility to honor our sustainers. (Metoxen 2005, p.1–2)

Haudenosaunee people held ceremonies and planted their fields in accordance with the natural cycles around them filled with colorful illustrations from nature. “Planting usually took place when leaves on the oak trees were as big as a red squirrel’s foot, or when the Juneberry blossomed” (Cornelius 1999, p.107). Part of the preparation for planting includes the process of the Haudenosaunee people soaking the corn in a tea made from plants to prevent birds from digging up the seeds (Parker 1910). Any unfortunate bird that chose to eat the seed “becomes dizzy and flutters about the field in a way which frightens the others,” (Parker 1910, p.26).

Planting corn, beans, and squash together was a common practice among many Native American people dating back to 1200 B.C. (Kuhnlein and Receveur 1996). Referred to as the “three sisters,” these plants create a symbiotic relationship with the corn serving as a support for the beans to climb and the bean roots supporting nitrogen-fixing bacteria colonies as the squash leaves covered the ground to keep down weeds and retain moisture in the soil (Cornelius 1999). The three sisters were planted together with fish, localizing the concentration of fertilizer and preventing soil erosion, on permanent hills spaced about three feet apart in rows the same distance apart. Modern agronomists agree that their method of elevating mounds provide a better climate for certain crops such as corn (Mt. Pleasant 2006). The Haudenosaunee people were knowledgeable and skilled agriculturalists as the planting and harvesting for each plant was different (Fig. 8.3).

Fields were planted, cared for, and harvested communally (Parker 1910). While individuals could cultivate their own fields, they could not claim a share of the communal harvest if they did not help in the communal fields. In one of his accounts, Parker describes the corn harvest gathering and food preparation for storage. “Husking time was another time for a long season of merry industrial gatherings. Work was play in those days when mutual helpfulness made money unnecessary” (Parker 1910, p.31).

Parker (1910, p.32) further explains:

> The [corn husking] “bees” were often conducted out of doors under the white moonlight. A roaring fire of sumac bush or logs tempered the crisp air of the night but left it sufficiently invigorating to keep up spirit and keep the workers active. There was nothing unhealthful in these night carnivals where the smell of the corn plant, the breath of the pines blown by the autumn wind, the smoke of the fragrant burning wood and the pure merriment of the workers and the knowledge of good work furnished the sole exhilaration.

During these husking bees, the people would harvest the corn, pull the husks back, trim the stem and all but two or three of the husks, then braid the corn cobs together (Cornelius 1999). Next, they hung the braids of corn from the rafters of the

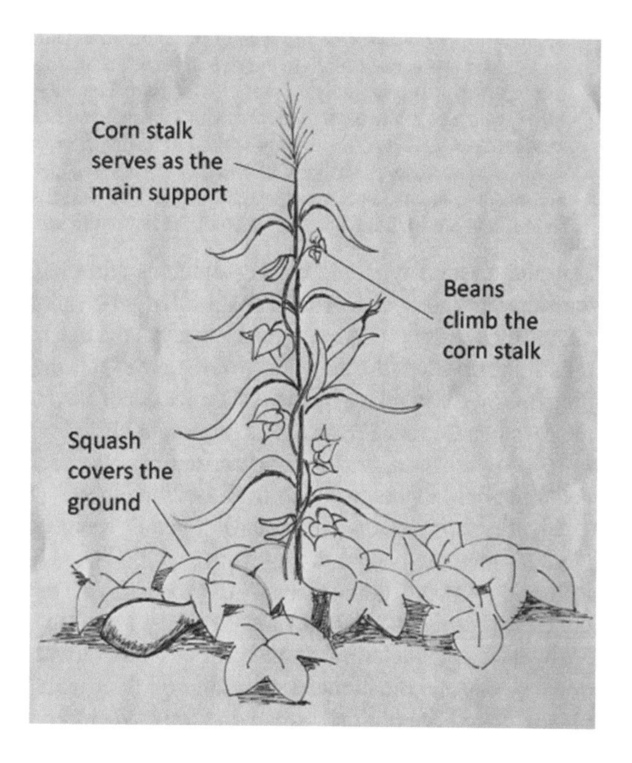

Fig. 8.3 "Three sisters" growing in a traditional garden (Drawing by Rebecca Webster, Used by Permission)

longhouse to dry. The cooking fire smoke helped to dry the corn and keep pests away. The husks of the corn were eventually used to make corn husk dolls, floor mats, footwear, baskets, and ceremonial masks (Fig. 8.4).

After the corn dried out, the Haudenosaunee people would shell the corn, taking the kernels off the cobs, setting aside seeds from the best cobs for replanting (Cornelius 1999) followed by a sifting process removing debris from the dried corn (Parker 1910). They stored the dried and shelled corn, beans, and squash in bark containers or underground corncribs lined with long grass or hemlock boughs. Some historical accounts claim that the Haudenosaunee stored three to four years' worth of corn and often used stored corn for trading and to help neighboring Haudenosaunee people in the event of a shortage.

The Haudenosaunee prepared the corn for cooking using a two-step process that began with pre-boiling (Cornelius 1999) followed by a method to remove the hard, outer hull of the corn (Fenton 1962). The ground white corn, resembling wheat flour (Enfield 1866), was often a main ingredient for breads or cornmeal-type of dish called mush often garnished with fresh items such as berries or nuts (Harrington 1908). Partially ripened corn, available several weeks before the fall harvest (Perrotto 2015) could be boiled and eaten off the cob like sweet corn or baked in the ashes of a fire (Fig. 8.5).

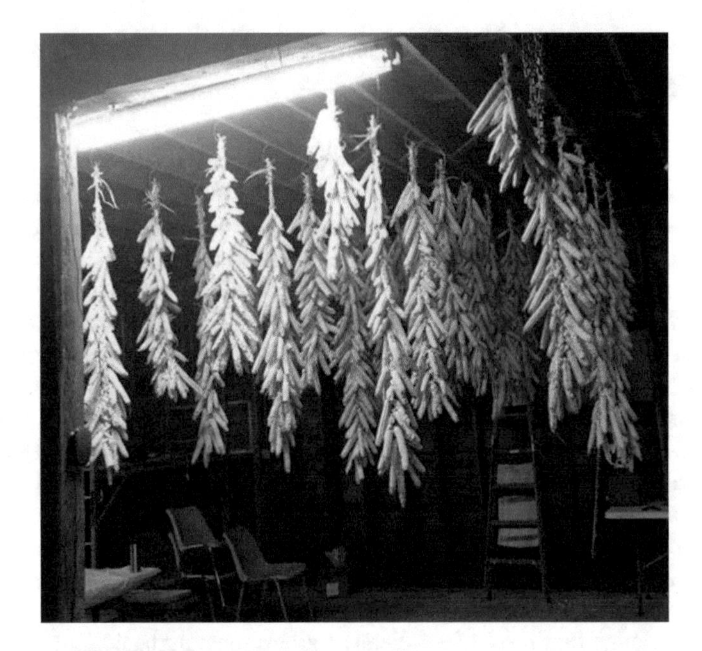

Fig. 8.4 Corn braids hanging in a barn to dry

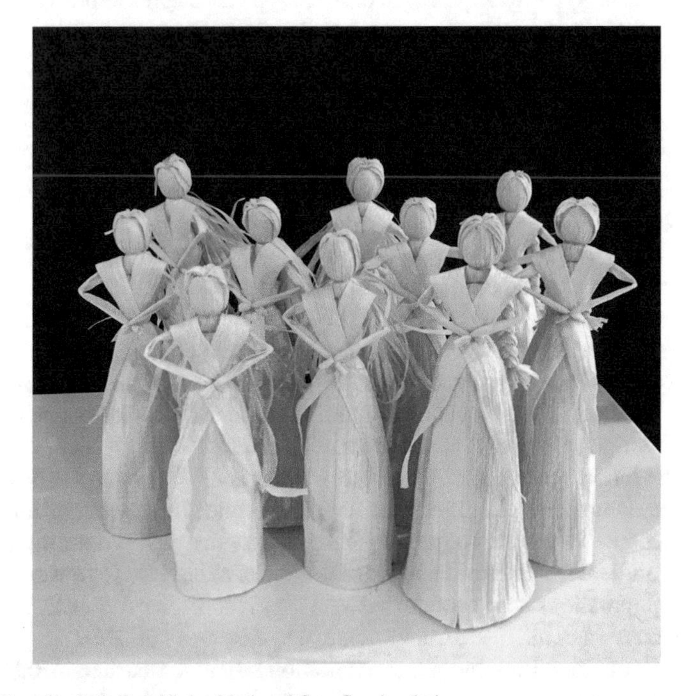

Fig. 8.5 Corn husk dolls with braided and free-flowing hair

8.3.3 Indigenous White Corn Foods and Impact on Overall Health

Indigenous food systems are comprised of items from the local and natural environment that are also considered culturally acceptable (Kuhnlein and Receveur 1996) and healthier containing many health benefits for indigenous people including traditional foods such as corn, beans, and squash. Nutritional factors that are beneficial to indigenous food systems include the higher protein content of white corn when compared to commercial varieties (Metoxen 2005) and the addition of nitrogen-rich beans (Mt. Pleasant 2006). Eaten together, corn and beans provide a complex protein and a complete array of amino acids (Hart 2008). Squash contributes significant calories, protein and oil, as well as vitamins and minerals not found in either corn or beans (Mt. Pleasant 2006). "Supplementing agricultural foods with wild game, fish, berries, wild greens, nuts, roots, and maple sugar more than met the nutritional principle of food diversity" (Milburn 2004, p.423).

Evidence suggests that traditional diets combined with an active lifestyle protect indigenous populations from chronic disease when reliant upon indigenous foods. Indigenous nutrition is defined as "culturally and bioregionally [sic] specific food-related knowledge that results in a dietary pattern meeting basic nutritional needs while avoiding Western diseases" (Milburn 2004, p.421).

While there is no medically proven cure for type 2 diabetes at present, the medical community is in general agreement that proper diet can control the disease and prevent complications such as limb amputation, kidney failure, and blindness (Kowalski et al. 2016; Steven et al. 2016). A two-month study of aboriginal people in Australia revealed that reincorporating indigenous foods back into their diet resulted in improved insulin metabolism, decreased blood sugar levels, decreased blood pressure, improved levels of cholesterol and triglyceride, and weight loss (Milburn 2004).

Dietary changes have also reversed heart disease in recent studies when participants ate indigenous foods (Björck et al. 2016; Lacroix et al. 2017) and returned after participants resumed their western diets (Massera et al. 2016). Similarly, in a five-year study, participants from the general population that were exposed to diets like the Haudenosaunee which consisted primarily of corn, beans, and squash could reduce the atherosclerotic blockage of their arteries while heart disease in the control group continued to progress and worsen (Milburn 2004).

While the linkage between diet and obesity may seem like common sense, recent studies have demonstrated that earlier research did not fully account for the wide array of complex issues in body weight regulation that involve multiple genetic, epigenetic, and environmental factors (Zarrinpar et al. 2016). However, studies of indigenous populations demonstrate that a return to traditional diets can help reverse obesity (Broussard et al. 1995; Liaw et al. 2011; Rowley et al. 2001).

Despite the colonial attempts at assimilation discussed earlier in this chapter, traditional diets remain a significant aspect of the contemporary lifestyles of indigenous people (Bodirsky and Johnson 2008), especially evident as cultural knowledge of traditional food systems is experiencing a resurgence. Mt. Pleasant described the persistence of growing corn in Haudenosaunee communities throughout the 1900's as follows.

> But despite the persistent decline in agriculture in Iroquois communities, even in the 1950s and 1960s individuals and families continued to grow traditional varieties of corn in home gardens and on small acreages, supplying their communities with corn for ceremonies and traditional corn-based foods. Beginning in the 1970s, Iroquois communities began to reassert their political and cultural sovereignty, reclaiming many of the traditions that had been damaged and marginalized by centuries of colonization. As these communities pushed to control their own school, healthcare, political, judicial, and economic systems, there was also resurgence in preserving and learning traditional languages and revitalization of traditional agricultural crops and foods. (Mt. Pleasant 2011, p.14–15)

Fostering this resurgence is not only "necessary in healing the trauma emerging from colonialism" (Bodirsky and Johnson 2008, p.1), but also necessary in improving the overall health of indigenous populations.

8.3.4 Oneida Nation Collaborative Strategies to Reintroduce White Corn

The Oneida Nation has three main tribal departments that work with white corn (Metoxen 2005). Tsyunhehkwa (life sustenance) plants, grows, and harvests the corn. The Oneida Cannery processes the corn into many food products. Oneida Retail, in the Oneida Market, sells the food products. To help with white corn operations, these three departments work with elders in the area as well as several different tribal areas such as the Cultural Heritage Department, Oneida Museum, Conservation Department, and Environmental Health & Safety Division. This section will discuss how the three main tribal departments work together to protect, grow, and share white corn.

While a handful of community members in Oneida continued to grow white corn on family plots, the seed for the corn currently grown at Tsyunhehkwa came during a visit to New York in 1992 when Jeff Metoxen, Tsyunhehkwa manager, traveled there to learn more about other Haudenosaunee people's planting, growing, and harvesting practices (Metoxen 2005). Tsyunhehkwa soon began to expand their white corn operations by incorporating modern equipment and tractors but all harvesting is still done by hand and dried through traditional methods. The hand harvesting, husking, and braiding is a labor-intensive task and requires help from the community so members of the Tsyunhehkwa regularly invite everyone from the community to come help with the husking bee. Teachers from nearby schools also incorporate a visit to the event as part of their annual student field trip schedule.

Tsyunhehkwa is located on an 86-acre farm (Metoxen 2016) where they also raise chickens, cattle, and a variety of vegetables. Planting white corn on a rotating basis remains their focus to keep up with community demand for the product. Limited planting (10 acres in 2016) and high demand often leads to shortages of the locally grown commodity (Cornelius and Betters 2016), requiring the Oneida Nation to import white corn from other Haudenosaunee communities. Tsyunhehkwa has plans to work with other tribal departments, such as the Eco Services Project, to improve better yields in future planting seasons (Johnson 2016).

Tsyunhehkwa also teaches community members important skills of organic farming practices beginning with how to secure seed, providing 150 families with seed and plants in 2016, and prepare gardens for planting, tilling the gardens of about 50 families (Metoxen 2016). The shared identity of growing, preparing, and eating traditional foods begins with this foundation to connect community members with these needed resources.

The Oneida Cannery was established using grant funds in the 1970s to establish a food preservation program (Metoxen 2005). The Cannery now provides tools for community members to grow and preserve their own food (Cornelius and Betters 2016). They offer on-site tours, classes, and presentations on proper food preservation techniques as well as on preserving and passing on knowledge about how to prepare white corn.

In 2016, the Cannery processed 6878 pounds of white corn into 3146 pounds dehydrated white corn, 1399 quarts of fresh hull corn, 222 pounds of corn mush flour, 1721 large loaves of corn bread, and 300 mini corn breads (Cornelius and Betters 2016). Cannery classes in 2016 helped families make a variety of products ranging from apple pie filling to maple syrup and spaghetti sauce. Cannery staff help ensure the processing is done correctly so that food is properly preserved. In addition to helping prepare the food, Jamie Betters, a Cannery Worker, organized a community garden where she helped 20 families grow individual 40'x 40′ plots of white corn on a piece of tribal land (Cornelius and Betters 2016; Metoxen 2016).

Oneida Retail sells products from Tsyunhehkwa and the Cannery at a store called the Oneida Market. The Oneida Market is located on the Oneida Reservation and is accessible to both Oneida tribal members as well as the public. Various jams, apple butter, and green salsa are produced in addition to the wide variety of corn product ingredients and finished goods (Cornelius and Betters 2016), beef products from the Oneida Farms and Tsyunhehkwa (Metoxen 2005), and other food (e.g., coffee, wild rice, and free-range chicken eggs) and nonfood items such as essential oils, homeopathic remedies, and natural cleaning supplies. Together, Tsyunhehkwa, the Cannery, and the Oneida Market do their best to help get more indigenous foods and other environmentally safe products to community members.

8.3.5 Backyard Gardening

Individual families that choose to grow white corn in their own gardens have autonomy over all aspects of planting, harvesting, and food preparation. A handful of families have been growing white corn for generations throughout the Oneida community. However, as Tsyunhehkwa recognized, many community members lack the technical

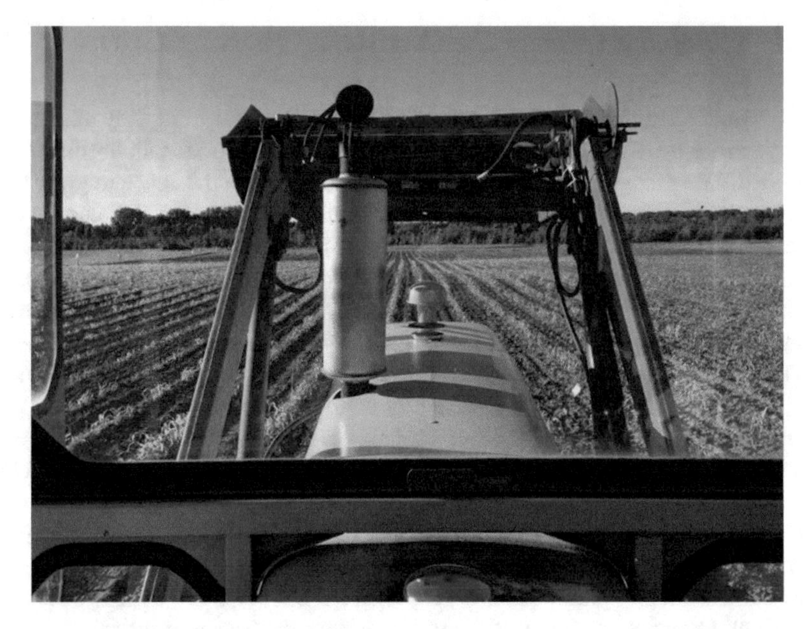

Fig. 8.6 Using modern equipment in the agriculture process to spray fish emulsion on a field of young, white corn stalks

expertise to secure seeds, prepare the garden site, properly fertilize, adequately maintain the garden, and to properly harvest and prepare the corn for storage.

In early 2015 two Oneida women, Laura Manthe and her daughter, Lea Zeise set out to complement the services Tsyunhehkwa already provided, and to tap into the existing knowledge base of those families that have grown corn for generations. These two women assembled a loose knit group of eight Oneida families interested in forming a network to learn more about how to successfully grow white corn in their backyards. Based on their own less than successful attempts at growing white corn themselves, the two women secured funding through the North Central Region—Sustainable Agriculture Research and Education Program (NCR-SARE). This grant, dubbed the "beginning farmer rancher grant," provided technical expertise and funds to improve the success rate of backyard white corn gardens. Grant funds were used to purchase fish emulsion, a compromise from the traditional use of fish in gardening as well as a more cost-effective way to get the nutrients from the fish distributed evenly throughout the field (Fig. 8.6).

The NCR SARE grant also covered the expenses for the participating families to travel to New York in the spring of 2017 to learn more about growing white corn from other Haudenosaunee farmers. Together, these eight families of backyard gardeners incorporated language and culture into their gardening practices, shared stories and recipes, and served as a network for learning more about growing white corn.

8.3.6 Ohe·Láku (Among the Cornstalks) Farming Co-Op

While Manthe and Zeise were assembling the backyard gardeners, they realized that many families were interested in growing white corn, but three main obstacles were persistent. The first obstacle was that families did not have the space to grow white corn in their own yards; the second, was that families' yards were too close to commercial corn fields that used seeds that were genetically modified organisms (GMO) where Iroquois white corn was at risk for contamination that destroyed the option for seed yield; and the third obstacle, was that several families were interested in pooling their resources to explore large-scale white corn farming operations.

The two women set out to interview Tsyunhehkwa employees, community members, as well as Haudenosaunee community members from New York to learn more about large-scale white corn farming. They recognized that growing heirloom white corn would not yield as much as growing commercial GMO sweet corn or GMO field corn, but aside from that they were unsure what to expect from large scale white corn farming. The pair, armed with some basic knowledge, other farmers and encouragement from a handful of backyard gardeners sought to assemble more families and apply earned funding grants in 2015 (e.g., Mifflin Street Co-op, Global Greengrant Funds, and Intertribal Agriculture Council) to move the project forward.

In early 2016, Manthe and Zeise obtained permission to use a 3.5-acre site from a local 4-H group for the co-op to plant their corn. With a group assembled and a site for planting, they considered which type of corn seed to purchase. The group considered their limited funds, the quickly approaching planting season, uncertainly about group dynamics, and the risk associated with the surrounding GMO corn pollen that could impact their own corn plants. Based on these factors, the co-op's planting was a lesser quality soup grade seed, which means that the seed they obtained was good enough to eat, but not of a high enough quality to be considered for planting. With the white corn seed purchase from the Onondaga Tribe and a secure site, the co-op named themselves Ohe•láku (among the cornstalks). Then they established roles and responsibilities and made a commitment to work in the field. The balance of their needs was met through the financial assistance from grants and Ohe•láku pooled resources leading to access to a nearby water source, someone to plow the field, a sprayer for fish emulsion and compost tea, a corn planter, and a barn to store their corn harvest. Recognizing grant funds were limited, Ohe•láku improvised. For example, instead of paying someone money to rent a barn to hang the corn harvest, Manthe found an Oneida family with a barn that was willing to trade use of their barn for traditional beadwork that led the women in Ohe•láku to make a beaded collars and cuffs. Before planting the corn, the Ohe•láku prepared the soil by removing rocks and fertilizing. After the corn was planted, scarecrows were placed, and a border of squash planted around the field of corn to help keep critters away. Weeding the field and modifications to the barn to accommodate the white corn harvest kept the families busy.

Securing funding (e.g., Oneida Nation in Wisconsin, the Manzanita Fund, Cultural Conservancy, South Central Farmers Health and Education Fund, and Wise

Women Gathering Place) was a top priority for Manthe and Zeise for an event during harvest time in the fall after a full summer of assisting with farm operations. They partnered with Braiding the Sacred, which is a network of Native American farmers, faith keepers, seed keepers, and allies maintaining seed diversity. With their help, Ohe•láku and Braiding the Sacred hosted approximately 50 people from the Midwest and New York to educate them about growing different varieties of traditional heirloom corn in their communities and the tradition of the husking bee while participants were introduced to practical skills in the field such as harvesting, barn husking, and braiding the corn. The financial assistance enabled the groups to host the conference, pay for travel for the participants, and to produce a video about growing corn.

The persistence of the pair in seeking grants continued to pay off in 2016 when they secured another grant from the Great Lakes Commission and then worked with the Oneida Nation's Environmental Health and Safety Department to obtain funding to help keep phosphorus runoff out of the waterways. The reduction of environmental strain on the land will help to promote sustainable agriculture as the planting area grows from land use of tribal property for additional fields granted by the Oneida Nation's Land Commission. Ohe•láku planted this field in the spring of 2017 using alternative farming methods that included leaving the cover crop on the ground and planting the seeds under existing vegetation that will act as a natural fertilizer while decomposing during the summer months. These activities, one of the many learned skills of the group, will help prevent water from running off the field and into nearby waterways.

8.4 Summary of Recommendations/Conclusion

Health and food security are problems that many Americans face daily but are experienced in disproportionate rates by Native Americans. One potential solution to help alleviate these concerns is a return to indigenous diets. This chapter examined the health and social benefits of returning to tribal agricultural indigenous practices to enrich diets using Iroquois white corn as an example. Through education and advocacy, federal health policy can become more responsive to the benefits of indigenous diets. Tribes can continue to enact legislation to protect their resources, regain control of their existing resources, and consider ways to encourage more tribal members to pursue agriculture. Individual tribal members can also find ways to connect with the resources to grow, harvest, and prepare their indigenous foods. However, these solutions are not unique to tribes and Native Americans. States, local governments, and everyday citizens could place locally grown produce as a priority. They can encourage community members to grow, harvest, prepare local produce, and develop ways to get these foods to the community members whose health requires access to fresh produce. The benefits of such a change in lifestyle are also not unique to Native Americans as replacing highly processed, imported foods with local, fresh produce in daily diets can improve overall health in any community.

Glossary

Boarding school A school where the students live away from family adult members for all or part of the year.

Colonization The act of settling among and establishing control over indigenous people in an area.

Food security People have access to food that is nutritionally adequate, culturally acceptable, and safe and that people have access to locally grown produce.

Food sovereignty A collective right based on rights to our lands, territories, and natural resources, the practice of our cultures, languages, and traditions, and is essential to our identity as Peoples.

Food system Activities involved in growing, harvesting, processing, and distributing food.

Haudenosaunee A group of Native American Tribes consisting of the Mohawk, Oneida, Onondaga, Cayuga, Seneca, and Tuscarora tribes. Haudenosaunee means "people of the longhouse" referring to the type of dwellings they built. Another term commonly used to refer to the Haudenosaunee is Iroquois.

Heart disease A general term used to describe a disease of the heart or blood vessels.

Husking bee A gathering of community members to husk corn.

Indian Reservation The legal designation for an area of land occupied by an Indian tribe.

Indigenous The original inhabitants of an area.

Native American People indigenous to the United States.

Native American tribe A separate and distinct community of Native American people.

Obesity The condition of having an excess of body fat.

Three sisters Native American practice of planting corn, beans, and squash together in their fields.

Type 2 diabetes Chronic health condition that impacts the way a person's body metabolizes sugar.

White corn A variety of corn historically grown by the Haudenosaunee and served as the primary staple for their diets. It is also referred to as flint corn or Tuscarora corn.

References

Adamson J. Medicine food: critical environmental justice studies, native North American literature, and the movement for food sovereignty. Environ Justice. 2011;4(4):213–9.

Ahtone T. Tribes create their own food laws to stop USDA from killing native food economies. Yes! Magazine. 2016, May 24. http://www.yesmagazine.org/people-power/tribes-create-their-own-food-laws-to-stop-usda-from-killing-native-food-economies-20160524. Accessed 17 Feb 2017.

Baek D. The effect of public transportation accessibility on food insecurity. East Econ J. 2016;42(1):104–34.

Bauer KW, et al. High food insecurity and its correlates among families living on a rural American Indian reservation. Am J Public Health. 2012;102(7):1346–52.
Beauchamp WM. Indian corn stories and customs. J Am Folklore. 1898;11(42):195–202.
Björck L, et al. Changes in dietary fat intake and projections for coronary heart disease mortality in Sweden: a simulation study. PLoS One. 2016;11(8):e0160474.
Bodirsky M, Johnson J. Decolonizing diet: healing by reclaiming traditional Indigenous foodways. J Can Food Cult Cuizine. 2008;1(1):1–10.
Briggs RV. The hominy foodway of the historic native eastern woodlands. Native South. 2015;8(1):112–46.
Broussard BA, et al. Toward comprehensive obesity prevention programs in Native American communities. Obes Res. 1995;3(S2):289s–97s.
Center for Disease Control and Prevention (CDC). Health status of American Indians compared with other racial/ethnic minority populations. 2003. https://www.cdc.gov/mmwr/preview/mmwrhtml/mm5247a3.htm. Accessed 17 Feb 2017.
Centers for Disease Control and Prevention (CDC). American Indian and Alaska Native Heart Disease and Stroke Fact Sheet. 2016. https://www.cdc.gov/dhdsp/data_statistics/fact_sheets/fs_aian.htm. Accessed 17 Feb 2017.
Consultation AG. Declaration of Atitlán, Guatemala. 2015. http://cdn5.iitc.org/wp-content/uploads/2013/07/FINAL_Atitlan-Declaration-Food-Security_Apr25_ENGL.pdf. Accessed 17 Feb 2017.
Cornelius C. Iroquois corn in a culture-based curriculum: a framework for respectfully teaching about cultures. Albany: SUNY Press; 1999.
Cornelius V, Betters J. Oneida Cannery year in review. Kalihwisaks, 2016, December 15, p. 20.
Coté C. "Indigenizing" food sovereignty: revitalizing indigenous food practices and ecological knowledges in Canada and the United States. Humanities. 2016;5(3):57.
Dion-Buffalo D, Mohawk J. Daybreak farm and food project seeks revitalization of white corn usage. In: Cajete G, editor. A people's ecology: explorations in sustainable living. Santa Fe: Book Marketing Group; 1999.
Enfield E. Indian corn: its value, culture, and uses. New York: D. Appleton; 1866.
Fairbairn M. Framing transformation: the counter-hegemonic potential of food sovereignty in the US context. Agr Hum Values. 2012;29(2):217–30.
Fenton WN. This island, the world on the turtle's back. J Am Folk. 1962;75(298):283–300.
First Nations Development Initiative. First Nations' food sovereignty assessment tool, 2nd ed. 2014. http://www.firstnations.org/knowledge-center/foods-health/FSAT-2nd-Ed. Accessed 17 Feb 2017.
Grey S, Patel R. Food sovereignty as decolonization: some contributions from Indigenous movements to food system and development politics. Agr Hum Values. 2015;32(3):431–44.
Gundersen C. Measuring the extent, depth, and severity of food insecurity: an application to American Indians in the USA. J Popul. 2008;21(1):191–215.
Haman F, et al. Obesity and type 2 diabetes in Northern Canada's remote First Nations communities: the dietary dilemma. Int J Obes. 2010;34:S24–31.
Harrington MR. Some Seneca corn-foods and their preparation. Am Anthropol. 1908;10(4):575–90.
Hart JP. Evolving the three sisters: the changing histories of maize, bean, and squash in New York and the greater Northeast. Current Northeast Paleoethnobotany II. NY State Mus Bull. 2008;512:87–99.
Indian Health Service (IHS). My native plate. 2012. https://www.ihs.gov/MedicalPrograms/Diabetes/HomeDocs/Resources/InstantDownloads/MyNativePlate2_508c.pdf. Accessed 17 Feb 2017.
Intertribal Agriculture Council. Event Summary—Red Lake Food Summit. 2016. https://iacgreatlakes.com/2016/09/29/event-summary-red-lake-food-summit/. Accessed 17 Feb 2017.
Jarosz L. Comparing food security and food sovereignty discourses. Dialogues in Hum Geo. 2014;4(2):168–81.
Jernigan VBB, et al. Addressing food insecurity in a Native American reservation using community-based participatory research. Health Educ Res. 2011;cyr089:168–81.

Johnson W. Partnerships for white corn. Kalihwisaks, 2016, November 17, p. 7.
Just Move It. Welcome to just move it. n.d. https://wwwjustmoveitorg/jmi/ Accessed 13 Jul 2017.
Kowalski GM, et al. Reversing diet-induced metabolic dysregulation by diet switching leads to altered hepatic de novo lipogenesis and glycerolipid synthesis. Sci Rep. 2016;6:1–10.
Kuhnlein HV, Receveur O. Dietary change and traditional food systems of indigenous peoples. Annu Rev Nutr. 1996;16(1):417–42.
Lacroix S, et al. Contemporary issues regarding nutrition in cardiovascular rehabilitation. Ann Phys Rehabil Med. 2017;60(1):36–42. (In press)
LaDuke W, et al. Sustainable tribal economies: a guide to restoring energy and food to Native America. Minneapolis: Honor the Earth; 2010.
Liaw ST, et al. Successful chronic disease care for Aboriginal Australians requires cultural competence. Aust N Z J Public Health. 2011;35(3):238–48.
Loew P. Indian nations of Wisconsin: histories of endurance and renewal. Madison: Wisconsin Historical Society Press; 2001.
Massera D, et al. Angina rapidly improved with a plant-based diet and returned after resuming a Western diet. J Geriatr Cardiol. 2016;13(4):364.
Metoxen J. Tsyunhehkw^. Toward a sustainable agriculture: module II. Center for Integrated Agricultural Systems, University of Wisconsin: Madison. 2005. http://www.cias.wisc.edu/curriculum/modII/secb/Tsyunhehkwa2.pdf. Accessed 17 Feb 2017.
Metoxen J. Tsyunhehkwa ag updates 2016. Kalihwisaks, 2016, June 2, p. 12.
Milburn MP. Indigenous nutrition: using traditional food knowledge to solve contemporary health problems. Am Indian Q. 2004;28(3):411–34.
Mt. Pleasant J (2006) The science behind the 'three sisters' mound system: an agronomic assessment of an indigenous agricultural system in the northeast. In Staller J et al (eds) Histories of maize: multidisciplinary approaches to the prehistory, linguistics, biogeography, domestication, and evolution of maize. Academic Press, Burlington, p 529–538.
Mt. Pleasant J. Traditional Iroquois corn: its history, cultivation, and use. Plant and Life Science, Ithaca; 2011.
Mullany B, et al. Food insecurity and household eating patterns among vulnerable American-Indian families: associations with caregiver and food consumption characteristics. Public Health Nutr. 2013;16(04):752–60.
National Congress of American Indians. About tribes. n.d. http://wwwncaiorg/about-tribes. Accessed 4 Apr 2017.
National Indian Health Board (NIHB). Tribal leaders diabetes committee. n.d. http://www.nihb.org/tribal_resources/tldc.php. Accessed 13 Jul 2017.
O'Connell M, et al. Food access and cost in American Indian communities in Washington State. J Am Diet Assoc. 2011;111(9):1375–9.
Parker AC. Iroquois uses of maize and other food plants, vol. 144. New York: University of the State of New York; 1910.
Perrotto D. The agency of Iroquois women through corn production. J Student Res. 2015;4(2):44–8.
Physicians Comm. for Responsible Med. v. Glickman, 117 F.Supp.2d 1 (D.C. Cir. 2000. http://law.justia.com/cases/federal/district-courts/FSupp2/117/1/2450079/. Accessed 12 Jul 2017.
Physicians Committee for Responsible Medicine (PCRM). The physicians committee praises new dietary guidelines for strengthening cholesterol warnings, but demands investigation into cholesterol money trail. 2016. http://wwwpcrmorg/USDA. Accessed 17 Feb 2017.
Rowley KG, et al. Improvements in circulating cholesterol, antioxidants, and homocysteine after dietary intervention in an Australian aboriginal community. Am J Clin Nutr. 2001;74(4):442–8.
Slocum R. Anti-racist practice and the work of community food organizations. Antipode. 2006;38(2):327–49.
Steven S, et al. Very low-calorie diet and 6 months of weight stability in type 2 diabetes: pathophysiological changes in responders and nonresponders. Diabetes Care. 2016;39(5):808–15.
United States Census Bureau. Population. 2016. https://www.census.gov/newsroom/facts-for-features/2015/cb15-ff22.html. Accessed 4 Apr 2017.

United States Department of Agriculture (USDA). Dietary guidelines 2015-2020. 2015. https://wwwcnppusdagov/dietary-guidelines. Accessed 17 Feb 2017.
University of Arkansas, School of Law. Indigenous food and agriculture initiative. n.d. http://indigenousfoodandag.com/model-food-code-project/. Accessed 13 Jul 2017.
Walter P. Educational alternatives in food production, knowledge and consumption: the public pedagogies of growing power and Tsyunhehkw^. Aust J Adult Learn. 2012;52(3):573.
Webster RM. Service agreements: exploring payment formulas for tribal trust lands on the Oneida Reservation. Am Indian Q. 2015;39(4):347–63.
Webster RM. This land can sustain us: cooperative land use planning on the Oneida Reservation. Plan Theory Prac. 2016;17(1):9–34.
Zarrinpar et al. Daily eating patterns and their impact on health and disease. Trends Endocrin Met. 2016;27(2):69–83.

Further Reading

Braiding the Sacred. A gathering of corn and people. 2017. https://wwwyoutubecom/watch?v=EScfVBAxAow&feature=youtube. Accessed 23 Feb 2017.
Decolonizing Diet. Center for Native American Studies at Northern Michigan University Blog. 2017. http://decolonizingdietproject.blogspot.com. Accessed 23 Feb 2017.
Iroquois White Corn Project. Iroquois white corn. 2017. http://wwwiroquoiswhitecornorg/ Accessed 23 Feb 2017.
Well for Culture. Tribal food sovereignty. 2017. http://wwwwellforculturecom/tribal-food-sovereignty/ Accessed 23 Feb 2017.
WLUK-TV Fox 11. Corn harvest and husking bee. 2014, October 6. https://wwwyoutubecom/watch?v=zP5SCH6P3G0. Accessed 23 Feb 2017.

Chapter 9
The Buzz About Restoring Mother Nature at the Urban Core

Beth Ann Fiedler

Abstract The environmental justice approach to restoring the urban core envelopes the needs of minorities, including Native American Indians and indigenous peoples, and low-income populations with these and other problematic socioeconomic conditions that impact public health. This chapter provides an overview of existing environmental regulation in the United States indicating two primary objectives: (1) to protect environmental and population health and (2) to identify and remediate the adverse effects of various enacted legislation and programs on minority and low-income populations. This chapter suggests best practices identified in transitioning urban ecosystems in the metropolitan District of Columbia encompassing the area surrounding the United States national capitol. Further recommendations suggest that including the provisions of the Clinton Administration Executive Order 12898 stipulating federal actions to address environmental justice in minority and low-income populations in all policy as intended can improve upon current health and income disparities.

9.1 Introduction

There is much more to the story of the birds and the bees than you may once have been told. Honey bees have been buzzing about the roof of the Paris opera house for nearly 35 years now and they are not alone. In 2015, more than 700 colonies graced the roof tops of local restaurants and landmark buildings in the city of Paris as bees thrive on flora there with significantly less dangerous pesticides than rural areas where they are endangered (Malsang and Uwimana 2017). While bees gather nectar to eventually form honey, they also participate in ecosystem services by pollinating plants—plant proliferation is a significant component of nutrient recycling that helps to purify air (Fig. 9.1). Pollination and air purification (Mace et al. 2012) are two ecosystem services directly and indirectly conducted by bees in the natural environment.

B. A. Fiedler (✉)
Independent Research Analyst, Jacksonville, FL, USA

B. A. Fiedler (ed.), *Translating National Policy to Improve Environmental Conditions Impacting Public Health Through Community Planning*,
https://doi.org/10.1007/978-3-319-75361-4_9

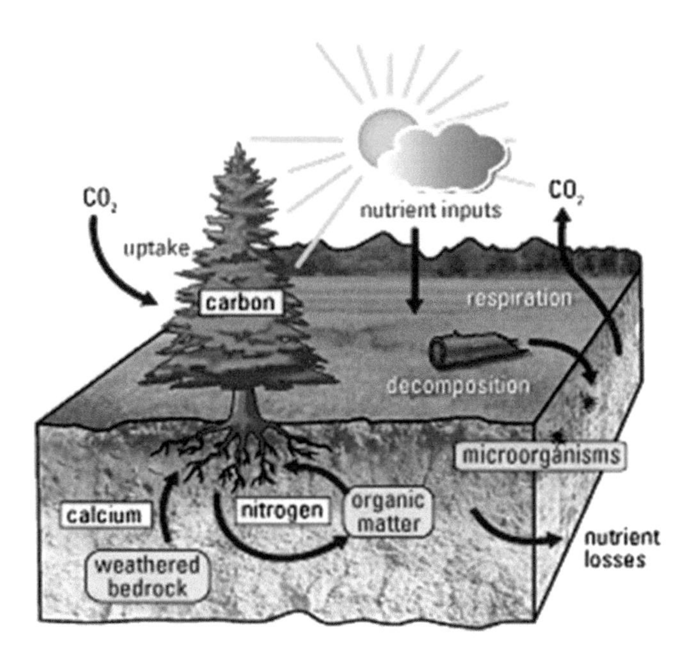

Fig. 9.1 Ecosystem processes, such as the nutrient cycle shown here, depicts how essential elements (e.g., Carbon, Calcium, and Nitrogen) are recycled through biological, chemical, and geological processes in the environment to sustain life (Beldin and Perakis 2009, used by general permission under public domain)

Other ecosystem services include microclimate regulation, water infiltration, noise reduction, cultural services, recreation, and education (Grêt-Regamey et al. 2016; Mace et al. 2012). Restoring a balance in the built environment with the natural environment has been a topic of global importance. For example, the role of ecological restoration through conservation planning and regenerative design is often channeled to efforts in a variety of global urban restoration (Ahern 2016; Boada and Maneja 2016; Conniff 2014; Gobster 2010; Ingram 2008; Niemelä et al. 2010; Ravetz 2016; Ravetz 2015). In the U.S., urban restoration is also equated with addressing environmental urban health disparities under the formidable umbrella of environmental justice (NIEHS 2016). Urban health disparities, commonly known as the social determinants of health, include urban environmental factors such as "the complex relationships between genes and the environment, individual behaviors, access to health services, socioeconomic status, literacy levels, and legislative policies" (NIEHS 2015, *para* 1) influencing the occurrence of and the potential to abate disease.

The National Institute of Environmental Health Sciences (NIEHS) in the United States envelopes two primary goals: (1) reduction of health disparities due to environmental conditions, and (2) educating the population on the ethos of environmental justice (NIEHS 2015). Environmental justice, adopted from an individual movement and brought forth by the U.S. Environmental Protection Agency (EPA), is defined as "the fair treatment and meaningful involvement of all people regardless of race, color, national origin, or income with respect to the development, implementation, and enforcement of environmental laws, regulations, and policies" (EPA 2009; NIEHS 2016).

This chapter discusses the current legislative policies that address the urban ecosystem following the environmental justice approach to restoring Mother Nature at the urban core where a large minority population and those with low socioeconomic status reside. Details of the social determinants of health in the urban ecosystem follow emphasizing health and income disparities. Then, the chapter turns to the brief overview of the metropolitan District of Columbia as an example of the restoration of an urban ecosystem that promotes healthy and sustainable living. Finally, the case analysis brings forth general best practices followed by recommendations to fill gaps in the prominent legislative policy of Executive Order 12898 (1994).

9.2 Current Legislative Policies in the Urban Ecosystem

While U.S. federal environmental and health regulation, such as National Environmental Policy Act (NEPA) of 1969 (Public Law 91-190) and the Clean Water Act of 1972, provide standards to protect natural resources against contamination leading to public harm, other legislation stipulates protection for specific population sectors. In 1994, President William J. Clinton signed Executive Order 12898 (1994) stipulating federal actions to address environmental justice in minority and low-income populations, access to human health and environmental planning public information through the Freedom of Information and the Emergency Planning and Community Right-to-Know Acts, and the establishment of agencies to ensure all federal agencies incorporate environmental justice.

The EO established two agencies: (1) an Interagency Working Group (IWG), and (2) the Office of Environmental Justice (OEJ). The IWG is comprised of representatives from the White House and multiple agencies including the EPA Administrator who is tasked as the chair (EPA 1994b). The OEJ "works to protect human health and the environment in communities overburdened by environmental pollution by integrating environmental justice into all EPA programs, policies and activities" (EPA 2017, *para* 1).

Inherently, EO 12898 is linked to Title VI of the Civil Rights Act of 1964 summarily stipulating that any agency or program relating to public or environmental health in receipt of federal funds must comply with nondiscriminatory conditions (e.g., race, color, national origin) or else jeopardize funding (EPA 1994a). Though all agencies receiving federal support are called upon to address disproportionate suffering, "with the exception of the Environmental Protection Agency, very little federal regulatory activity included references to EO 12898" (Geltman et al. 2016, p.143). Funding through the U.S. EPA Superfund has also been under scrutiny for the lack of minorities and low-income populations able to benefit from the program. Recent evaluation of funding allocation and distribution indicate that, "increases in minority populations, families in poverty, or people without high school diplomas all lower the chances of a Superfund listing" (O'Neil 2007, p.1090). Low participation by the target population is an example of problems with effectiveness of the policy towards meeting the equitable intent of the policy.

While ecosystem services can improve environmental and public health in urban areas and legislation can abate environmental and public harm, the impact of urbanization on ecosystems (e.g., poor air quality, traffic) and thus, urban dwellers, is the other side of the coin. Reputable U.S. agencies, such as the National Institute of Health (NIH), the National Quality Forum (NQF), and others address the unequal problem of health and income disparities in urban ecosystems. Understanding these prominent inequalities in minority and low-income populations is important to addressing the needs of these sectors.

9.2.1 Health Disparities in Urban Ecosystems

"Health disparities … are differences in the incidence, prevalence, mortality, and burden of diseases and other adverse health conditions that exist among specific population groups" (National Institute of Minority Health and Health Disparities n.d., p.6). In response to mounting health disparities (AHRQ 2017; NIH 2013), the NQF Roadmap for Promoting Health Equity and Eliminating Disparities targets some specific health conditions experienced in disproportionate levels against the general population. They hope to alleviate these inequalities through the development of performance measures linked to policy such as monitoring, accountability and data-driven performance (2017).

The NQF roadmap targets health conditions, such as heart disease, in which those with low income and lower levels of education have a higher prevalence and "African Americans are more likely to die prematurely" (NQF 2017, p.2). The perinatal period, where "infants born to black women are 1.5–3 times more likely to die than infants born to women of other races/ethnicities (CDC 2011, p.1), was another important area of health. Other prominent areas of disease include cancer, abnormal kidney function, and mental illness compounded by various social risk factors associated with higher incidence of these diseases. These social risk factors include "socioeconomic position, race/ethnicity, gender, social relationships, and residential/community context" (NQF 2017, p.8).

Key findings of the Agency for Healthcare Research and Quality (AHRQ) indicate that racial disparities persist in the Black and Hispanic communities and that households with low socioeconomic status (e.g., poor, low income) confirm worse care than affluent families (2017, p.1). Overall, the report demonstrates that greater than half of 250 assessment measures within several topical indicators (e.g., access to care, preventive care, women's health, affordable care) are not improving.

9.2.2 *Income and Other Compounding Disparities in Urban Ecosystems*

"Income can influence health by its direct effect on living standards (e.g., access to better quality food and housing, leisure-time activities, and health-care services)" (Beckles and Truman 2011, p.13). Thus, income inequality is a major factor in health status. In 2016, the black population had 22% of their people in poverty with Hispanics at 19.1% compared to white people in poverty at 11% (Semega et al. 2017, p.13). Those of minority status comprise more than 40% of people impacted by poverty or about 16.7 million of the 40.6 million people in 2016 that were classified as in poverty; the U.S. poverty rate hovered at 12.7% during the same time (Semega et al. 2017, p.12). Jarosz and Mather graphically depict the level of poverty in the U.S. from 1989 to 2014 indicating that "high levels of poverty and inequality are more prevalent across all types of counties [more than 2/5th of all counties] today than two decades ago" (2016, *para* 4). The sheer number impacted by income inequality also has implications in the capacity for the urban ecosystem, where many low income and minorities reside, to incorporate sustainability goals.

The impact of urban income disparity, one of many fractured human characteristics of urban ecosystems, has been studied recently in relation to the capacity of neighborhoods to achieve social and environmental sustainability. Other factors also reveal how mass urbanization in the existing infrastructure must be overcome to introduce and sustain ecosystem services into the built environment. They include the "compounded deprivation, racial cleavages, civic engagement, institutional cynicism, and segregated patterns of urban mobility and organizational ties that differentially connect neighborhood resources" (Sampson 2017, p.8957). The study of three U.S. cities (e.g., Boston, Chicago, and Los Angeles) demonstrates that the future of "smart cities" is dependent on the capacity to address neighborhood diversity and the social welfare needs of specific population sections therein (Sampson 2017).

Thus, "global urbanization creates opportunities and challenges for human well-being and transition towards sustainability" (Leuderitz et al. 2015, p. 98). Recognizing the impact of social determinants, such as income inequality, is just the beginning. Addressing the long-term population growth in urban areas and the impact of climate change there (e.g., wastewater contribution to flooding, microclimatic heat effects of heat islands due to increased city temperatures derived from built infrastructure, air pollution from traffic congestion) is important. Sampson's (2017) premise also supports the urgency of supporting the minority population because of the cumulative benefits to all urban residents towards sustainability. Therefore, addressing inequalities that impact the social and environmental fabric of urban populations must become a high priority.

Notable is that each city or urban designation has a unique history, cultural attributes, and built environment vested within the natural surroundings requiring special attention by residents, politicians, and skilled urban planners. We demonstrate how urban planners and various stakeholders adjust to the local environmental conditions and population needs in the U.S. capital of Washington, DC.

9.3 Case Study: Metropolitan Washington, DC

The changing dynamics of industrialization, globalization, urbanization, immigration, and others has left many locations strained of natural resources and sometimes abandoned to population sectors unable to relocate. Faced with urban blight and decline, three methods are prominent in reclaiming deteriorating urban landscapes. First, urban regenerative design—a restorative process introducing indigenous species and natural diversity into a built environment to promote self-sufficient nutrient cycling; second, ecological restoration—process of removing harmful contaminants; and conservation planning—a comprehensive natural resource plan spanning one of many components from grazing to wildlife preservation. Faced with declining natural resources, we look at the metropolitan area of the U.S. national capital of Washington, DC to demonstrate how an infusion of ecosystem services through these methods can reclaim resources with a positive impact on public health.

9.3.1 Anacostia River

Sometimes the buzz is about America's national past time—baseball. But what does baseball have to do with restoring Mother Nature at the urban core? A lot! The playing field of the Washington Nationals, a Major League Baseball™ franchise in the National League Eastern Division, is a brownfield development and a green ballpark (MLB 2017). A brownfield development is repurposed land likely fraught with soil contaminants, pollution, or sometimes early restoration efforts gone wrong. But the ball park, completed in 2005, is one of the many improvements along the more than 8-mile portion of the Anacostia River (Fig. 9.2) that flows from Maryland to Washington, DC where it meets the Potomac River. Both rivers feed the Chesapeake Bay so work upstream is vital to the recovery of the ecosystem there.

After industrial pollutants, sewage, and harmful sediments from agricultural runoff accumulated in the waterway by 1972, the Anacostia River underwent dredging operations leading to changes that transformed the area into a recreational area in the 1980s. However, three centuries of exploitation were a difficult obstacle to overcome as the area ecosystem was further damaged by this early attempt to revitalize the area. In 1989, area conservationists formed the Anacostia Watershed Society and began plans to restore the original freshwater tidal marsh that once served Anacostan Native Americans with a variety of wildlife and vegetation (Anacostia Watershed Society 2017). With assistance from the United States Geological Survey (USGS) and a consortium of organizations (e.g., Baltimore District of the Army Corps of Engineers, District of Columbia Department of Environmental Health, The Patuxent Wildlife Research Center and the University of Maryland) (USGS 2008), the long journey to restore the marsh and wetland areas was underway (Anacostia Watershed Society n.d., 2017). The conservation of a variety of natural habitats for indigenous species such as fowl and fish, as well as abatement for invasive species,

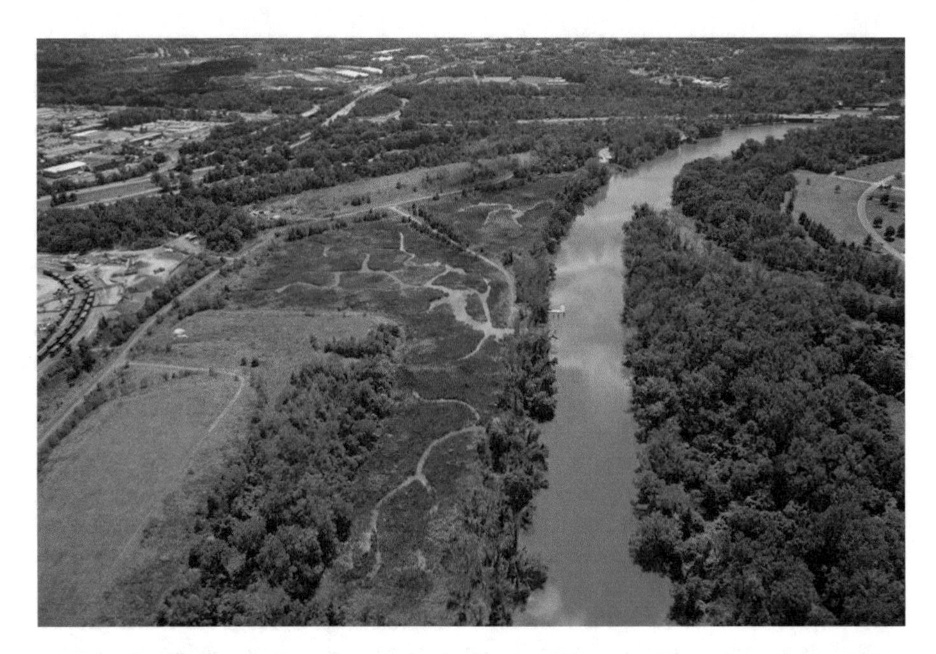

Fig. 9.2 The Bladensburg Wetlands was a landfill known as "ANA 11" until the Maryland State Highway Wetland Mitigation Project transformed the area into this natural water filter and wildlife habitat in 2008 (Photo courtesy of the Anacostia Watershed Society, used by permission)

continues in their long-term vision of a national park conservatory and environmentally responsible resource for public recreation.

There is still much work to be done toward the advocacy group goal of completion by 2025 to address infrastructure and toxic hotspots to permit full water contact events like swimming and fishing. While funding was primarily gained from negotiated settlements, key work continues to unfold in the interest of public health under the auspices of environmental justice. About 17,000 people annually consume fish caught in the Anacostia River. Research to determine the public health impact on the vast number of minority fisherman that consume fish caught in the river is a major concern due to several remaining contaminated areas (Lambert 2014; Wilson 2014). Wilson recommends that limiting water contact and reducing consumption of fish caught in the river is advisable until contaminated areas are addressed in ongoing and forthcoming projects (2014).

A far cry from the period when the Anacostia River was a haven for disease, the area is a growing example of collaboration between nonprofit, academic, and government agencies addressing multiple public administration services through ecological restoration. Mixed-use development, public transportation access and new housing in "The Yards" (Cooper 2016) together anchor 800,000+ residents who live in the over Anacostia Watershed spanning more than 170 square miles (Cooper 2017).

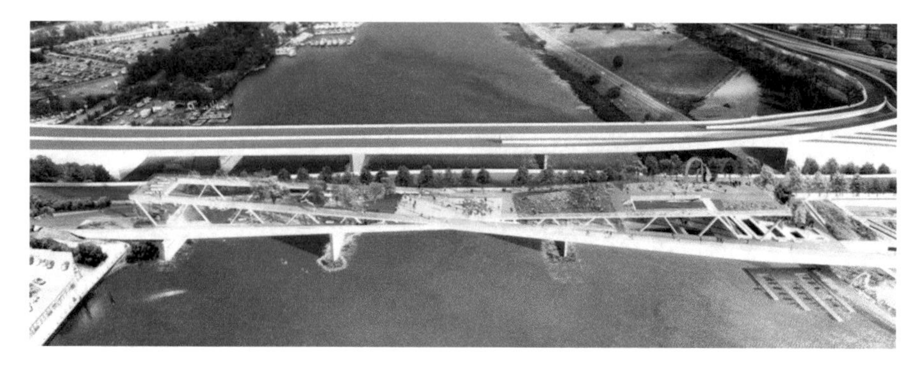

Fig. 9.3 The Anacostia River continues to transform the watershed with pedestrian and education friendly developments, such as the Plans for the 11th Street Bridge Park (Photo Courtesy of OMA+OLIN, used by permission)

Plans to improve the area include the 11th Street Bridge Park (www.bridgepark.org), a project of the Ward 8 nonprofit Building Bridges Across the River, will reutilize existing pylons from the old bridge to create a pedestrian walkway connecting the DC side of the river with Anacostia (Courtney 2017) (Fig. 9.3). The project endeavors to physically and socially connect residents from both sides of the Anacostia River—Washington, DC and Anacostia.

9.3.2 *Chesapeake Bay*

Addressing environmental contaminants in the upstream Anacostia River watershed is important to ongoing Maryland Department of Natural Resources (DNR) projects in conjunction with the Chesapeake Bay Trust (CB Trust 2015) and several organizations. The Chesapeake Bay Trust located in Annapolis, MD offers multiple resources for education, grants, capacity building, and opportunities for civic engagement. "The mission of the Chesapeake Bay Trust is to promote public awareness and participation in the restoration and protection of the water quality and aquatic and land resources of the Chesapeake Bay region and other aquatic and land resources of the State" (CB Trust 2015, *para* 1).

The CB Trust will simultaneously address stormwater runoff by adding green space at MedStar Harbor Hospital, one of 15 newly announced projects, which will also aid in the overall well-being of the patient population (DNR 2017). Combining outdoor patient care with environmental strategies to offset the built environment through green space planning is an example of multipurpose planning that is both effective and efficient.

This green infrastructure project is one of more than a dozen projects funded by various Watershed Assistance programs from 2016-2017 spanning concept design for soil conservation along with restoration of streams and ponds to reduce the problem of stormwater runoff in the area (DNR 2017). Multiple stakeholders from the city of Baltimore; town of Templeville; faith-based organizations such as Peoples' Community Lutheran Church; and federal funding provide an overarching water quality improvement plan for the area serving several counties (DNR 2017).

Many local and federal organizations provide several ways to inform and engage the public. For instance, the CB Trust is one example of a local portal (https://www.youtube.com/user/ChesBayTrust). Other public information opportunities regarding environmental justice can be obtained by subscribing to a EJ Listserv (https://lists.epa.gov/read/all_forums/subscribe?name=epa-ej). Finally, another agency that can provide financial guidance and support is the USDA Natural Conservation Resources Services (https://www.nrcs.usda.gov/wps/portal/nrcs/main/national/programs/financial/). Announcements range from opportunities to volunteer, learn about conservation, and access funding and other support to address environmental conditions that impact health and well-being in your community.

9.4 Discussion and Recommendations

Many agree that EO 12898 was groundbreaking in bringing the problem of environmental conditions that disproportionately impacts minority and low-income populations; but further actions are required to reach the intended goal of environmental justice. This section highlights some best practices in urban ecological restoration and suggests how recognized gaps in EO 12898 can be a platform for improvement.

9.4.1 Best Practices in Urban Regenerative Design

Several overarching lessons can be learned from the urban ecological restoration projects in the brief case study. For example, overcoming decades of contamination is no small task. While advocacy is crucial, securing a funding stream is important to see a project come to fruition. Impacting legislation through advocacy strategic litigation and utilizing existing legislation, such as the EO 12898, are methods that both legitimize and fund urban ecological restoration projects. Both approaches represent opportunity but offer different levels of planning as access to funds are allocated differently. Strategic litigation offers a substantial reward for persistent advocacy that builds legal pathways and long-term funding for multiple infrastructure projects required to incorporate sustainable design and restoration. But time and personnel capable of pursuing this path have recognizable limits. On the other hand, EO 12898 provides an established path but funding is dependent on available portion awarded from the federal budget.

Three key ingredients to the success of the Anacostia Watershed Society are important. First, the organization worked diligently to generate a series of legislation to protect the area and hold industry accountable. "Most major issues facing the river and the parties responsible for them have been identified and held liable to ensure that environmental justice for the river is served" (Anacostia Watershed Society n.d., p.3). Second, strategic litigation was instrumental in securing a funding stream to support the ongoing advocacy efforts and pay for planned changes to infrastructure that include mechanisms to prevent sewerage overflow and manage stormwater (Anacostia Watershed Society n.d.). Third, long-term commitment and persistence are essential ingredients.

Overarching lessons learned in the metro DC case is that (1) urban development can accompany ecological restoration, (2) urban planning is a collaborative project across many stakeholders to concurrently address population, wildlife, vegetation and utilization of natural resources such as waterways, (3) economic development can be sustainable, and (4) small scale projects over time can reinvigorate and reinvent significant areas previously written off. Thus, the big picture of Chesapeake Bay improvements suggests the critical nature of multipurpose strategic solutions in small bites that incorporate the varied interests of multiple stakeholders towards a common goal.

9.4.2 How Addressing Gaps in EO 12898 Can Improve Policy

The groundbreaking intent of EO 12898 is monumental in both recognizing and attempting to address environmental justice for minority and low-income populations that have historically and continue to be disproportionately subjected to the ill health effects of environmental hazards. Undeniably, the EO lacks specific guidance on siting and permitting, two major areas where structured rules with substantive standing would be valuable (Huang 2014). "Instead, the Order directed agencies to adopt an [environmental justice] EJ strategy and then implement it. To date, not every federal agency has fulfilled the Order's EJ mandates" (Huang 2014, *para* 4).

Further, mechanisms to draw attention to available funding in target populations have relied on grass root organizations working with local political representatives to acquire information, a right granted by EO 12898, to access funds. That is why state efforts to identify and address specific populations in harms' way through substantive state legislation (Bonorris 2010) is vital to assessing contaminated sites and housing, establishing public health concerns, and acting as a conduit to funding for population sectors in most need.

Of course, the environmental conditions and population sectors vary widely but the expressed purpose remains the same—meet the needs of "communities across the country [that] continue to be unnecessarily exposed to toxic pollution that threatens their health and quality of life" (Huang 2014, *para* 8). Nevertheless, civic engagement is critical to accessing funding to facilitate cleanup. Be a part of the buzz. That means citizens must apply the process of access to information, utilize standards to establish environmental hazards, and work with various agencies to address health hazards related to environmental conditions.

9.5 Summary

This chapter brings forth awareness of the growing concern for urban population growth and the need to expand development inclusive of ecological restoration and regenerative design of ecosystem services. These are viewed considering disproportionate health and income disparities that exist in minority and low-income populations resulting from hazardous environmental conditions. Existing legislation to provide environmental and public health relief for this population sector in the U.S. through the Clinton Administration Executive Order 12898 (1994) underwent a cursory review for areas of improvement. While urban planning with ecosystem solutions are generally custom solutions for a specific area, a review of the case study on the transformation of the Anacostia River Watershed and Chesapeake Bay leads to several general best practices. They include nonprofit advocacy and strategic litigation as a source of funding for the high costs associated with returning ecosystem services into the urban environment. But also speak to the importance of effective and efficient multipurpose strategic planning that serves multiple interests for population health.

Glossary

Biomass Release of carbon by burning wood and other organic matter as fuel

Brownfield development Repurposed land in the U.S. previously used for industrial/commercial business with poor soil, potentially hazardous soil and other natural resource conditions, and environmental pollutants

Conservation planning The record of decisions and supporting information for treatment of a unit of land meeting planning criteria for one or more identified natural resource concerns because of the planning process; the plan describes the schedule of implementation for practices and activities needed to solve identified natural resource concerns and takes advantage of opportunities (USDA n.d., *para* 1)

Cultural services One of several ecosystem services; often referred to as the nonmaterial or aesthetic benefits derived from surrounding culture, a sense of belonging, or ethereal experience from nature (FAO 2017)

Microclimate regulation One of several ecosystem services; a variance in temperature and humidity experienced locally when compared to surrounding areas such as a city compared to neighboring suburbs

Minorities Smaller sector of a larger group; the smaller portion of Native Americans, Hispanics, and African Americans in the U.S. population compared to Caucasians

Nutrient cycling An ecosystem process in which biological, chemical, and geological activity in the environment help to recycle elements essential to life such as carbon, hydrogen, calcium, phosphorus, and nitrogen

Regenerative design Instead of just restoring damage, this approach focuses on improving environmental conditions to promote nutrient cycling and other ecosystem services that support life

Soil formation Several factors contribute to soil formation including the breakdown of rock (parent material) over time, climatic conditions, various organisms, and area landscape; also known as pedogenesis

Urban ecosystem The interaction of various elements within a densely populated area such as a city or large metropolitan area (https://www.britannica.com/science/urban-ecosystem)

Water infiltration One of several ecosystem services; process where rain or melting snow moves through gaps and other shallow openings in top soil to provide moisture or through sediment to replenish groundwater sources

References

Agency for Healthcare Research and Quality. 2016 National healthcare quality and disparities report, AHRQ Pub. No. 17-0001. Rockville: AHRQ; 2017.

Ahern JF. Novel urban ecosystems: concepts, definitions and a strategy to support urban sustainability and resilience. Landscape Architecture & Regional Planning Faculty Publication Series, 66. Landscape Archit Front. 2016;4(1):10–21. http://scholarworks.umass.edu/larp_faculty_pubs/66

Anacostia Watershed Society. Wetland restoration. 2017. http://www.anacostiaws.org/programs/stewardship/native-plant-restoration/wetland-restoration. Accessed 16 Oct 2017.

Anacostia Watershed Society. A waterway to 2025: a vision for the Anacostia river. n.d.. http://www.anacostiaws.org/userfiles/file/A%20Waterway%20to%202025%20brochure-WEB.pdf. Accessed 17 Oct 2017.

Beckles GL, Truman BI. Education and income—United States, 2005 and 2009, p. 13–17. In: United States Centers for Disease Control and Prevention (CDC) (2011) CDC health disparities and inequalities Report —United States, 2011. MMWR, 60(Suppl):1–114.

Beldin S, Perakis S. Unearthing secrets of the forest, fact sheet 2009-3078. https://pubs.usgs.gov/fs/2009/3078/. 2009. Accessed 23 Oct 2017.

Boada M, Maneja R (2016) Cities are ecosystem: urban green governance increases the quality of life and protects vital services. http://www.unep.org/ourplanet/october-2016/articles/cities-are-ecosystems. Accessed 12 Oct 2017.

Bonorris S (ed) (2010) Environmental justice for all: a fifty state survey of legislation, policies and cases, 4. Center for State and Local Government Law, UC Hastings College of the Law. San Francisco. http://gov.uchastings.edu/public-law/docs/ejreport-fourthedition.pdf. Accessed 14 Oct 2017.

Chesapeake Bay (CB) Trust. Strategic plan 2015-2020. 2015. https://cbtrust.org/strategic-plan/ Accessed 20 Oct 2017.

Conniff R. Rebuilding the natural world: a shift in ecological restoration [Yale Environmental 360]. 2014, March 17. http://e360.yale.edu/features/rebuilding_the_natural_world_a_shift_in_ecological_restoration. Accessed 12 Oct 2017.

Cooper R. Anacostia River (Things to know about the Anacostia Watershed). [TripSavvy]. 2017, August 7. https://www.tripsavvy.com/anacostia-river-info-1040510. Accessed 15 Oct 2017.

Cooper R. Anacostia Waterfront in Washington DC. [TripSavvy]. 2016, March 14. https://www.tripsavvy.com/anacostia-waterfront-guide-1040563. Accessed 15 Oct 2017.

Courtney S. The 11th street bridge park isn't just a vanity project. [Washingtonian]. 2017, April 17. https://www.washingtonian.com/2017/04/14/11th-street-bridge-park-isnt-just-vanity-project/. Accessed 23 Oct 2017.

Executive Order 12898 of Feb. 11. 1994 (59 F.R. 7629, Feb. 16, 1994) Federal actions to address environmental justice in minority populations and low-income populations. http://www.dot.ca.gov/ser/vol1/sec1/ch1fedlaw/EO12898.pdf. Accessed 13 Oct 2017.

Food and Agricultural Organization (FAO) of the United Nations. Ecosystem services & biodiversity (ESB). 2017. http://www.fao.org/ecosystem-services-biodiversity/background/cultural-services/en/. Accessed 17 Oct 2017.

Geltman E, et al. Beyond baby steps: an empirical study of the impact of environmental justice Executive Order 12898. Fam Community Health. 2016;39(3):143–50. https://doi.org/10.1097/FCH.0000000000000113.

Gobster PH. Introduction: urban ecological restoration. Nat Cult. 2010;5(3):227–30. https://doi.org/10.3167/nc.2010.050301.

Grêt-Regamey A et al Urban ecosystem services: planning of landscape and urban systems. 2016. https://www.ethz.ch/content/dam/ethz/special-interest/baug/irl/plus-dam/documents/lehrveranstaltungen/msc/landscape-planning-and-environmental-systems/UrbanES.pdf. Accessed 13 Oct 2017.

Huang A. The 20th anniversary of President Clinton's Executive Order 12898 on environmental justice. [National Resources Defense Council]. 2014, February 10. https://www.nrdc.org/experts/albert-huang/20th-anniversary-president-clintons-executive-order-12898-environmental-justice. Accessed 14 Oct 2017.

Ingram M. Urban ecological restoration. Ecol Restor. 2008;26(3):175–7.

Jarosz B, Mather, M. Poverty and inequality pervasive in two-fifths of U.S. counties. [Population Reference Bureau]. 2016. http://www.prb.org/Publications/Articles/2016/Poverty-and-Inequality-US-Counties.aspx. Accessed 16 Oct 2017.

Lambert K. Commitment to environmental justice leads fish and wildlife service to study Anacostia River Fishing. [EPA Blogs]. 2014, August 14. https://blog.epa.gov/blog/2014/08/commitment-to-environmental-justice-leads-fish-and-wildlife-service-to-study-anacostia-river-fishing/. Accessed 17 Oct 2017.

Leuderitz C, et al. A review of urban ecosystem services: six key challenges for future research. Ecosyst Serv. 2015;14:98–112.

Mace GM, Norris K, Fitter AH. Biodiversity and ecosystem services: a multilayered relationship. Trends Ecol Evol. 2012;27(1):19–26. https://doi.org/10.1016/j.tree.2011.08.006

Major League Baseball, Official Site of Washington Nationals. Green ballpark. 2017. http://washington.nationals.mlb.com/was/ballpark/information/index.jsp?content=green_ballpark. Accessed 15 Oct 2017.

Malsang I, Uwimana S. Paris's urban rooftop hives hope to preserve honeybees. [Phys Org, Science X Network]. 2017, August 4. https://phys.org/news/2017-08-paris-urban-rooftop-hives-honeybees.html. Accessed 13 Oct 2017.

Maryland Department of Natural Resources. Green infrastructure project connects human health and environmental health. 2017, April 4. http://news.maryland.gov/dnr/2017/04/04/green-infrastructure-project-connects-human-health-and-environmental-health/. Accessed 12 Oct 2017.

National Institute of Environmental Health Sciences (NIEHS). Contributions of the National Institute of Environmental Health Sciences Division of Extramural Research and Training to Environmental Justice: 1998-2012. 2015. http://1.usa.gov/1Ag7E9a. Accessed 13 Oct 2017.

National Institute of Environmental Health Sciences (NIEHS). Environmental health disparities and environmental justice. 2016. https://www.niehs.nih.gov/research/supported/translational/justice/index.cfm. Accessed 13 Oct 2017.

National Institute of Health. Health disparities. 2013. https://report.nih.gov/NIHfactsheets/ViewFactSheet.aspx?csid=124. Accessed 14 Oct 2017.

National Institute of Minority Health and Health Disparities. NIH health disparities strategic plan and budget fiscal years 2009-2013, extended to FY2016. n.d.. https://nimhd.nih.gov/docs/2009-2013nih_health_disparities_strategic_plan_and_budget.pdf. Accessed 14 Oct 2017.

National Quality Forum. A roadmap for promoting health equity and eliminating disparities: the four I's for health equity. 2017. http://www.qualityforum.org/Publications/2017/09/A_Roadmap_for_Promoting_Health_Equity_and_Eliminating_Disparities__The_Four_I_s_for_Health_Equity.aspx. Accessed 12 Oct 2017.

O'Neil SG. Superfund: evaluating the impact of Executive Order 12898. Environ Health Perspect. 2007;115(7):1087–93.

Ravetz J. Future of the urban environment & ecosystem services in the UK. London: Government Office of Science; 2015. Report No. Working Paper 15. 2015. https://www.gov.uk/government/publications/future-of-cities-ecosystem-services. Accessed 13 Oct 2017.

Ravetz J. Sustainable urban futures: contested transitions and creative pathways. In: Archer K, Bezdecny K, editors. International Handbook of Cities and the Environment. Cheltenham: Edward Elgar; 2016. p. 119–59.

Sampson RJ. Urban sustainability in an age of enduring inequalities: advancing theory and ecometrics for the 21st-century city. Proc Natl Acad Sci U S A. 2017;114(34):8957–62. www.pnas.org/cgi/doi/10.1073/pnas.1614433114

Semega JL et al Income and poverty in the United States: 2016, P60-259. [Data source: United States Census Bureau]. 2017. https://www.census.gov/library/publications/2017/demo/p60-259.html. Accessed 12 Oct 2017.

United States Centers for Disease Control and Prevention (CDC). CDC health disparities and inequalities Report—United States, 2011. MMWR Suppl. 2011;60:1–114.

United States Department of Agriculture Natural Conservation Service Conservation planning: productive lands, healthy environment. n.d.. https://www.nrcs.usda.gov/wps/portal/nrcs/detail/national/programs/technical/cta/?cid=stelprdb1049425. Accessed 16 Oct 2016.

United States Environmental Protection Agency. About EPA: Office of Environmental Justice. 2017. [Last update August 28, 2017]. https://www.epa.gov/aboutepa/about-office-enforcement-and-compliance-assurance-oeca#oej. 13 Oct 2017

United States Environmental Protection Agency (EPA). Environmental justice homepage. http://www.epa.gov/environmentaljustice/. 2009. Accessed 13 Oct 2017.

United States Environmental Protection Agency (EPA). EPA Insight Policy Paper: Executive Order #12898 on Environmental Justice; Statement from EPA Administrator Carol Browner. 1994a. https://www.epa.gov/fedfac/epa-insight-policy-paper-executive-order-12898-environmental-justice. Accessed 13 Oct 2017.

United States Environmental Protection Agency (EPA). Summary of Executive Order 12898—Federal Actions to Address Environmental Justice in Minority Populations and Low-Income Populations. 1994b. https://www.epa.gov/laws-regulations/summary-executive-order-12898-federal-actions-address-environmental-justice. Accessed 13 Oct 2017.

United States Geological Survey (USGS) Patuxent Wildlife Research Center and the University of Maryland Department of Biological Resources Engineering. Anacostia freshwater tidal reconstructed wetlands. 2008. https://www.pwrc.usgs.gov/resshow/hammerschlag/anacostia.cfm. Accessed 15 Oct 2017.

Wilson S. Community-based assessment of exposure to substances in the Anacostia River Region (CAESARR). 2014. https://www.epa.gov/sites/production/files/2016-03/documents/sacoby_iwg_presentation_sept_2014.pdf. Accessed 17 Oct 2017.

Further Reading

Principles of Environmental Justice. First National People of Color Environmental Leadership Summit held on October 24–27. 1991. http://www.ejnet.org/ej/principles.pdf 13 Oct 2017.
Advancing Science, Serving Society (ASSS). Urban ecosystems. n.d.. http://sciencenetlinks.com/lessons/urban-ecosystems-1/. Accessed 12 Oct 2017.
Breuste J, et al. Urban ecosystem services on the local level: urban green spaces as providers. Ekológia (Bratislava). 2013;32(3):290–304. https://doi.org/10.2478/eko-2013-0026.
Elmqvist T, et al. Benefits of restoring ecosystem services in urban areas. Curr Opin Environ Sustain. 2015;14:101–8.
Gogal D, et al. EPA policy on environmental justice for tribes and indigenous peoples & ej tools, webinar. Washington, DC: Office of Environmental Justice, U.S. Environmental Protection Agency; 2017, October 19.
Health Disparities Calculator, Version 1.2.4. Division of Cancer Control and Population Sciences. National Cancer Institute: Surveillance Research Program and Healthcare Delivery Research Program; 2013, October 29.
National Partnership for Action to End Health Disparities. Compendium of publicly available datasets and other data-related resources. 2016. https://www.minorityhealth.hhs.gov/npa/templates/browse.aspx?lvl=1&lvlid=46. Accessed 12 Oct 2017.
Niemelä J, et al. Using the ecosystem services approach for better planning and conservation of urban green spaces: a Finland case study. Biodivers Conserv. 2010;19(11):3225–43. https://doi.org/10.1007/s10531-010-9888-8

Chapter 10
Green Business: Not Just the Color of Money

Naz Onel and Beth Ann Fiedler

Abstract Sustainable business development has moved into the social fabric of corporations alongside historical parameters of business performance such as profit margins and return on investment. The transition to envelope a mindset beyond profits has been supported by initiatives founded by the United Nations (UN) Millennium Development Goals and more recently the Sustainable Development Goals (SDGs). However, sustainable business development faces challenges in both emerging and developed nations to infuse corporate social responsibility and innovation to address current environmental conditions that endanger public health. The UN suggests that to achieve these measures will require new economic paradigms, behavioral pattern changes in corporate and consumer consumption of natural resources, adaptive policy, and commitments to limit resource use. This chapter defines the evolution of sustainability and presents key components from a business perspective. Next, the impact of business environmental sustainability on public health is discussed using several examples of how corporations address important problems such as e-waste, natural habitat conservation, and employee safety and health. From there, we review management tools to assess sustainability providing insight to corporate business ventures that are best aligned with SDGs. Finally, we summarize key points of the material and present a high-level list of best practices.

10.1 Introduction

Corporate Social Responsibility (CSR), the Triple Bottom Line (TBL), and other sustainable business perspectives are driving the application of environmental sustainability to the core of business principles under equal consideration with traditional business performance measures such as profit margins and returns on

N. Onel (✉)
School of Business, Stockton University, Galloway, NJ, USA
e-mail: naz.onel@stockton.edu

B. A. Fiedler
Independent Research Analyst, Jacksonville, FL, USA

B. A. Fiedler (ed.), *Translating National Policy to Improve Environmental Conditions Impacting Public Health Through Community Planning*,
https://doi.org/10.1007/978-3-319-75361-4_10

investment. The application of sustainability principles is no longer tenuous or an urgent response to remedy bad public relations after hazardous contamination has been uncovered. Instead, they have become important factors in new business development considering the impact to the community, public health, and the planetary ecosystem from the onset.

(PWC Global 2015, p.6):

> Increasingly, companies from all sectors are having to confront and adapt to a range of disruptive forces including globalization, increased urbanization, intense competition for raw materials and natural resources and a revolution in technology that is challenging the business models of many sectors while forcing all companies to be more accountable to, and transparent with, all their stakeholders.

The well-being of all living things is dependent upon understanding the functioning of the Earth's systems and taking actions to eliminate detrimental causes towards the healthy operation of the global ecosystem. With this aim, in 2000, world leaders gathered at the United Nations (UN) Headquarters in New York and developed the first set of Millennium Development Goals (MDGs). Later, at the beginning of 2016, the Sustainable Development Goals (SDGs) came into effect with a leading focus on eradicating poverty and hunger. Other SDGs are specifically important items to this chapter including—Goal 3, "Ensure healthy lives and promote wellbeing for all at all ages"; Goal 8, "Promote sustained, inclusive and sustainable economic growth, full and productive employment and decent work for all"; Goal 9, "Build resilient infrastructure, promote inclusive and sustainable industrialization and foster innovation"; and Goal 12, "Ensure sustainable consumption and production patterns." These highlighted SDGs demonstrate the elegant, interdependent, complex, and interconnected nature of the multiple objectives that prompt strategies to improve the plight of humanity without devouring limited natural resources.

Worldwide actions by proponents of sustainable development, such as the UN MDGs and SDGs, have had remarkable influence towards the incorporation of these goals into the role of business entities. However, the transition from sound, global environmental objectives to local implementation has been fraught with typical policy hurdles—political and economic feasibility. Unlike the MDGs, SDGs are proposed to be universal and therefore apply to all countries. Thus, achieving the SDGs requires worldwide collaboration, such as the partnership of governments, participation of organizations, private sector, civil society, and consumers. Collaboration in this fashion may be the backbone from which the possibility of transferring a healthy and livable planet for future generations can be realized.

Furthermore, UN projections for success recognize the need for new economic paradigms, behavioral pattern changes, policy adaption, and resource commitments. This suggests the emergence of a circular economy—one in which the resource inputs and waste generated by production can be regenerated minimizing resource depletion through a system of multiple strategies for reutilization.

A recent study on SDGs assessment scores display relevant and significant challenges even for the most developed nations (Osborn et al. 2015). The study identifies the most common transformational challenges facing developed countries as the goals of sustainable consumption and production (SDG 12), sustainable energy (SDG 7) and combating climate change (SDG 13) (Osborn et al. 2015).

The greatest transformational challenges for emerging countries are variable but generally face limited opportunity for economic development. Thus, they are entering their own industrial era without the benefit of advanced technologies to abate persistent environmental problems such as pollution or waste management. Additionally, limited infrastructure and regulatory representation represent small but growing areas of opportunity or platforms from which leaders can initiate change.

A brighter future for emerging nations and thus, global health, will incorporate the collaborative visions of C-suite senior corporate executives to positively influence change and achieve competitive advantage by moving from "sustainability attempts" to ingraining the notion into their foundation. In the words of Yoda, Star Wars' (a registered trademark of Lucasfilm, Ltd) Jedi leader, "Try not. Do. Or do not. There is no try" (https://www.youtube.com/watch?v=XZbVLvT7qBU). Moving forward, business leaders, business stakeholders, and impacted communities must grasp that sustainability and responsible business practices outline the new path to business survival, solutions to countless environmental problems, and present an opportunity for green employment.

"As companies navigate this uncertain business landscape, having a cohesive vision of environmental and social sustainability will help them develop new models for growth and opportunities to be product, service and market leaders" (PWC Global 2015, p.6). In turn, these actions should prompt individual citizens to respond and engage through innovative methods that promote sustainable consumption patterns under environmental conditions that support public health.

Therefore, this chapter provides a general overview of the evolution of sustainability in the business world and defines the important constructs of sustainable business perspectives leading to the positive impact of business environmental sustainability actions on societal well-being. Next, the chapter highlights some of the best sustainable business practices in leading corporations and discusses how their actions meet some of the important global sustainability goals. The chapter concludes with a summary highlighting key information and recommendations.

10.2 Evolution of Sustainability in the Business World

The meaning of sustainability and how companies view the concept have changed dramatically over the last few decades. Initially, sustainability was perceived by business entities as "little more than a peripheral 'green' issue—useful for reducing energy and waste disposal costs or supporting some worthy community causes but hardly central to a company's core business" (PWC Global 2015, p.6). Sustainability has been elevated in current application and is defined as "a balance between ecological, social and economic indicators that ensures the maintenance of the environment and society over time" (Boxer 2007, p.87). Prior to this paradigm shift, the main objective of a corporation was to maximize profits to distribute earnings to those who had invested in the company according to the number of stock shares they held. At that time, the word "sustainability" was perceived by business leaders as "to connote a company that had steady growth in its earnings" (Werbach 2013, p.8) before the concept of sustainability was cited in "Our Common Future" of UN World Commission on Environment and Development (Werbach 2013). The meaning of the term in the business world has changed over time because of the shifting perceptions of individuals, such as business leaders and grass root organizations, who began to realize the interdependence of development on environmental systems and social welfare in relation to the community and public health. Furthermore, consumers have pushed companies towards reforms that target business objectives beyond the notion of profits. Together, these factors form and continue to refine the current definition of sustainability.

True sustainability should cover four components with equal importance: (1) social, (2) economic, (3) environmental, and (4) cultural aspects (Werbach 2013). The social aspect focuses on the inclusion of all members of society to promote sustainability from several perspectives—public health, education, labor, and human rights, creating the conditions for improvement. Next, a focus on sustainability does not negate the need for the economic reality of profitable businesses; but achieving financial gain should not undermine social responsibility or the other aspects of sustainability. Environmental well-being is the third component of true sustainability that should be taken into consideration in every action. Protecting and restoring the ecosystem is on equal footing with the important social and economic aspects of sustainability. Cultural aspects are the final component of true sustainability (Werbach 2013) but are often considered a part of the social element or not specified in every sustainability definition. However, cultural diversity is an important merit of different societies. Protecting and valuing this asset is significant to achieving true sustainability as communities are permitted to maintain their unique identities from generation to generation.

Today, most corporations have come to the realization that sustainable business strategies must emphasize each one of Werbach's (2013) components to achieve long-term success. Thus, integration of environmental, social, ethical, and economic issues into all corporate decisions should be at the core of today's business sustainability principles (Mukherjee et al. 2016).

10.3 Sustainable Business Perspectives

Being sensitive and responsive to social and environmental welfare is not a new phenomenon in the business world. Today, corporate leaders and businesses are increasingly aware of the interdependence of environmental systems, social welfare (such as community and public health), and the companies' well-being and growth. They follow this awareness by embedding sustainable business strategies into the core of their business functions. Organizational strategies that build environmental protection, economic development, stakeholder value improvement, and a safe, just, and equitable societal support system (e.g., creating meaningful jobs, minimizing inequalities in quality of life) into their decision-making processes to bring forth best practices. This section covers information about how companies adopt these processes and what they can achieve resulting from these implementations. This section details some of the key aspects of sustainable business practices—Corporate Social Responsibility (CSR) and Triple Bottom Line (TBL)—and the importance of adopting sustainable business strategies.

10.3.1 Corporate Social Responsibility (CSR)

In the early twentieth century, growing concerns about large corporations and their extensive powers steered a new way of thinking, including initiating internal debates about corporate voluntary actions, as well as shaping the ideas of charity, responsible operations, and stewardship. During the 1970s, corporations were moved by social pressures to undergo an objective and systematic review of the impact of business on society (Frederick 1986, 1994). A focus on ethics shaped the relationship between business and society over time creating new social norms and requiring that businesses become involved with a wider span of problems, such as equal employment opportunities, pollution abatement, and poverty alleviation, previously restricted to government purview (Cannon 1992). Corporate leaders and managers began to think beyond improving monetary value for the corporate stockholders or improving statutory obligations to minimally comply with legislation. As a result, organizations increasingly began to take voluntary action to improve the quality of life for employees, their families, the local community, and society at large. Today, this concept is known as *Corporate Social Responsibility* (CSR).

CSR is defined as a concept whereby organizations consider the interests of society by taking responsibility for the impact of their activities on customers, employees, shareholders, communities, and the environment in all aspects of their operations. The term is still widely used "even though competing, complementary and overlapping concepts such as corporate citizenship, business ethics, stakeholder management and sustainability are all vying to become the most accepted and widespread descriptor of the field" (Carroll and Shabana 2010, p.86).

Companies are adopting CSR in different ways to meet their varied perspectives on responsibility to society. Some of the corporations are taking very small steps in practicing CSR because their approach reflects Friedman's controversial point of view. He defines social responsibility as spending "corporate resources for socially beneficial purposes regardless of whether those undertaken expenditures are designed to help achieve the financial ends" (Friedman 1970 p.298). In his article published by the *New York Times Magazine*, Friedman (1970) states that the spending of corporate resources for socially beneficial purposes is wrong and unacceptable. He advocates that "those who support the idea of 'social responsibility' of business executives in addition to maximizing the profits of the company, are incorrect" (Mukherjee et al. 2016, p.201). He argues that the executives' job should be focused on maximizing company profits and if the management spends company financial sources on socially responsible acts, this indicates that they are using money that belongs to the corporate owners, employees, or customers without their consent. First introduced about fifty years ago, the Friedman approach typically undertakes the value maximization of the shareholders (also called stockholders) as the ultimate basis for the corporate decision-making process. This argument, today known as shareholder theory, remains one of the most prominent, argued, as well as controversial approaches against corporate CSR management strategies.

Although some companies and their executives that reflect Friedman's point of view may see CSR as a burden on the companies' bottom line, many others counter the approach of solely maximizing the shareholder value by accepting the challenge of CSR and managing teams to infuse a moral compass into corporate decision-making. If the subject matter is argued within the context of moral terms, "at least some of Friedman's professed adherents appear to offer incoherent moral views" (Schaefer 2008, p.297) and instead choose to remain primarily concerned with their duties towards their shareholders.

Alternatively, there are numerous examples of companies that have embedded the notion of CSR in business management practices that include strategies to make a positive impact on society (Samy et al. 2010). As a part of their CSR activities, large companies are now issuing a CSR report containing their nonfinancial societal activities along with their annual fiscal report. The increased awareness of CSR has also come about because of the UN MDGs, in which a major goal is the increased contribution of assistance from large organizations, especially multinational corporations, to help alleviate poverty and hunger, global health and environmental issues, and for businesses to be more aware of their impact on society. CSR continues to offer a strong foundation from which community-based initiatives and business development can be applied, especially in poverty-stricken countries or communities.

10.3.2 Moving Towards a Sustainable Business Strategy: Triple Bottom Line

"The business community became fascinated with the notion of sustainability, or sustainable development, and this theme became an integral part of all CSR discussions" (Carroll and Shabana 2010, p.88) at the turn of the millennium. Efficient and effective characteristics of sustainability began to emerge including a long-term adopted business strategy, formally recognizing resource limits, protecting natural habitats, transforming current business practices, practicing fairness, and enhancing creativity. In this sustainability model, production and consumption of resources requires careful planning and management in a manner that produces economic gain while contributing to the social and environmental well-being of the community. This approach is also called a triple-bottom-line (TBL) (Elkington 1998) requiring three elements to measure if a business is successful—people, profit, and the planet. The TBL strategy can be built into all aspects of business (e.g., manufacturing, supply chain management, labor practices, transportation, facilities management) to achieve corporate sustainability.

Corporations have devised community-oriented strategies to participate in creating a society that is more just and equitable while operating under the foundation of the TBL approach. New corporate TBL models have advanced from initial one-time community service projects to include broader community activating strategies, such as educational grants for local schools, and the incorporation of a methodological process to reuse materials obtained from foreign suppliers (Laff 2009; Liebowitz 2010). These anti-stockholder theory corporate strategies demonstrate two important factors as opposed to strictly focusing on how they are financially performing within the marketplace. First, corporations are placing an increased emphasis on the image they portray to the greater community by integrating social equity and justice factors into daily operations within the corporate structure. Second, they recognize that their community image reflects their position in the marketplace. This necessitates an emphasis on employee satisfaction, involvement, and participation that ensures that TBL and social equity factors specifically are ingrained in, as opposed to merely appended, to strategic plans after economic and environmental considerations have been considered. Therefore, a greater emphasis is placed on positively impacting the lives of employees and society at large (i.e., all the stakeholders) in ways that benefit not only the corporation, but local and global communities.

10.3.3 Importance of Adopting Sustainable Business Strategies: Company Perspective

The introduction of new strategies to create value and meet different stakeholder expectations in the evolving new business era has opened the door for companies to adopt a variety of sustainable business initiatives. Over twenty years ago renowned Harvard Business School Professor Michael Porter introduced the Porter hypothesis which states that "environmental regulation can benefit companies by nudging them to explore their current production methods and eliminate costly waste that they have been blissfully unaware of" (Kahn 2017, *para* 3; Porter and Van der Linde 1995). While cost reduction is prominent, there are many key benefits for companies that adopt sustainable business strategies including the following:

- **Reduced Costs:** Sustainable practices, such as using less natural resources, eliminating unnecessary processes, or altering supply chain, that can help companies reduce their costs associated with these activities and save money in the long run. Cost savings can be added into the company's bottom-line and applied to other functions of the corporation towards achieving growth and a better position for the company in the marketplace (Mukherjee et al. 2016).
- **Market Opportunity**: Sustainability in the business setting is a new market opportunity for products and processes with fast pace growth that can help

companies to achieve sustainable competitive advantage in the long-term with products that cannot be easily copied by competitors.

- **Source of Differentiation**: Competition drives companies to differentiate themselves as much as possible. Sustainability strategy adoption can provide a source of differentiation for companies to uniquely position themselves in the market.
- **Waste Reduction:** Sustainable business actions can address waste management and elimination to offset one of the costliest business functions.
- **Innovation and Long-Term Growth:** Companies, such as General Electric and their Ecomagination program (http://www.ge.com/about-us/ecomagination), that invest in research, reinvent business processes, and innovate green products to support their sustainable focus can achieve multiple corporate and community benefits. These actions also ensure sustained long-term company growth and profitability (Nidumolu et al. 2009).
- **Competitive Advantage:** A focus on corporate sustainability leads to outperforming the industry average by gaining competitive advantage through new market opportunities. Research shows that those corporation with adopted sustainable business strategies have been consistently outperforming their rivals that neglect the dimensions of sustainable development (Eccles et al. 2014).
- **Environmental Protection:** Widespread sustainable business activities can achieve and maintain a healthy natural environment, prompt corporate longevity, and preserve the ecological balance providing natural resources for future generations. Adopting sustainable business models and practices will optimize utilization of natural resources in the present and in the future.
- **Employee Motivation and Retention:** Companies that are environmentally responsible and value sustainability instills a sense of belonging, connection, and pride in their employees that, in turn, creates a unique corporate culture and team motivation leading to more engaged and productive employees. "At least one recent study found that companies that effectively engage employees on sustainability issues outperform others by wide margins, demonstrating 2.6 times higher earnings-to-share growth rates" (Ceres 2010, p.72).
- **Social Sphere and Cultural Diversity:** Sustainable business practices can contribute towards the operating environment of companies by introducing social and cultural improvements in the business and the community.
- **Added Value:** Companies continuously aim to improve their perceived value by consumers and investors by adding value to their products, services, and internal operations. Sustainable activities can innovate new processes, achieve higher market share with new or existing sustainable products, and improve employee retention and motivation.
- **Increased Corporate Social Responsibility (CSR):** In today's competitive marketplace, practicing CSR is important for corporate survival. Corporate ideology that adopts sustainable strategies can significantly increase the social responsibility performance of companies and project an image of accountability to shareholders, government regulators, and consumers.

- **Increased Consumer Knowledge and Awareness:** The detrimental impact of many environmental problems could be solved by increasing consumer knowledge and awareness (Onel and Mukherjee 2016). Sustainable business actions can provide information about the status of the ecosystem and direct individuals to join in the fight. Moving towards responsible consumption habits could be possible with the help of environmentally responsible companies.
- **Responsiveness:** Consumers who are environmentally sensitive constitute a growing segment of the market. These consumers wish to put their money where their values are, demanding that companies function sustainably while they are producing goods and services that they purchase (Ceres 2010). Companies that promptly respond to consumer demands by incorporating sustainable practices benefit from doing the right thing and capturing this market segment.
- **Corporate Reputation:** Corporate reputation is defined as "a collective representation of a firm's past actions and results that describe a firm's ability to deliver valued outcomes to multiple stakeholders" (Fombrun and Van Riel 1997, p.10). A good reputation can be a way of differentiating the company from competitors (Pollach 2015). Good intention based on eco-sensitivity can establish a good company reputation with the positive benefits of competitive advantage and increased profits resulting from gaining customer trust.
- **Building Consumer Trust and Loyalty:** Moving a step forward by undertaking green initiatives demonstrates the company level of involvement with society and genuine moral obligation to be socially responsible. These are crucial aspects that increase consumer trust and generate loyalty. A long-term loyal customer can be more profitable than a single-transaction customer (Myler 2016). Therefore, maintaining a larger percentage of loyal customers for a longer time can build on a revenue foundation that is more predictable and, eventually, more profitable.
- **Improving Investor Perception and Relations:** Today, investors are increasingly interested in business sustainability initiatives and, therefore, they demand companies to detail and calculate sustainability risks and opportunities in their financial disclosures. As company owners, long-term investors demand solid management, strong governance and long-term thinking about future growth potential. Sustainability indicators are one in which investors evaluate these conditions. Thus, they value those companies that integrate sustainability into their strategic planning (Ceres 2010).
- **Meeting Regulations:** In recent years, there have been a growing number of rules and regulations related to environmental and human health protection. This trend is expected to continue due to global stakeholder pressure as many governmental bodies are working diligently to reduce or eliminate harm caused by unsustainable business practices. Adopting a sustainable roadmap can help companies to meet these laws and regulations in advance without additional costs, such as fines for noncompliance that may be incurred once they become enacted.

10.4 The Impact of Business Environmental Sustainability on Public Health

By adopting advanced business strategies, such as CSR and TBL, companies are increasingly becoming oriented towards environmental sustainability. Among the list of benefits from this new way of thinking are the remarkable positive impacts on societal well-4being. In this section, we unfold the public health implications of business environmental sustainability activities to battle waste (particularly, electronic waste) and harmful emissions, partnering to address specific health crisis, actions to address employee well-being, such as employee safety and health, natural habitat conservation, conflict resources, customer protection and safety, and sustainable fair trade in some multinational conglomerates.

10.4.1 Corporate Action to Reduce Waste and Harmful Emissions

Companies affect the well-being of the planet, humans, and all other living entities through the accumulation of waste by-products of manufacturing, natural resource overconsumption, and pollutants in the air, water, and soil. Today, a growing number of firms are developing "innovative, resource-efficient solutions and effective waste management systems" so that they can capture value in their business settings and contribute to sustainable development (Kurdve et al. 2015, p.304). We will cover two important areas of focus under this category: reduction of electronic waste (e-waste) and harmful emissions.

10.4.1.1 E-waste

Although electronic products satisfy many of our needs including 24/7 global connectivity, these innovations are being rapidly replaced with new products as soon as they are introduced into the marketplace. As consumers are not aware of the ultimate consequences of their purchase and usage behaviors, they easily replace outdated products but often update perfectly viable systems to obtain the latest bells and whistles. This combination of negative behavioral patterns—consumer overconsumption and corporate behavior of rapid turnover innovation, result in massive amounts of electronic products discarded into landfills or shipped overseas to lesser developed nations to handle as recycling materials. This problem, often referred to as e-waste (i.e., variety of discarded electrical or electronic equipment and component parts), pollutes the environment and is becoming the fastest growing waste stream issue in the world (Lundgren 2012). Projections indicate that the global e-waste generated by humans can reach 65.4 million tons in 2017 (Breivik et al. 2014).

The health implications of e-waste are devastating when humans are exposed to hazardous substances decaying in soil, leaching into water supplies, or becoming particulate matter in dust or food supplies (Norman et al. 2013). Whether the exposure is direct or indirect, the health and environmental effects from many of the individual hazardous substances often found in e-waste are well established from existing studies, including studies in children (Grant et al. 2013; Lundgren 2012). Health consequences from e-waste exposure are plausible and may include changes in thyroid function, altered cellular expression and function, adverse neonatal outcomes, cognitive and behavioral changes, and decreased lung function (Grant et al. 2013). Several known developmental neurotoxicants are found in e-waste, such as lead, mercury, cadmium, and brominated flame retardants, which can lead to irreversible cognitive deficits in children and behavioral and motor skill dysfunction across their lifespan (Chen et al. 2011). These inform the public regarding the significant priority that electronic companies must place on their environmental activities: (1) to reduce the amount of harmful materials in their products, and 92) their obligation to implement actions to reduce post-use electronics with appropriate recycling programs. As a result, a growing number of companies, as well as nonprofits and industry associations such as the International Electronics Manufacturing Initiative (http://www.inemi.org/), are working to reduce or eliminate the use of toxic chemicals in electronic products and replace them with safer alternatives. Furthermore, those companies that are in the business of e-waste operations are implementing programs for their workers and surrounding communities by providing a variety of protective and exposure reduction systems.

A good example of corporate responsible action to reduce e-waste comes from Dell Inc. In 2014, the company launched a closed-loop recycling program that provides the company with an opportunity to turn old plastics into new Dell products. Hewlett Packard (HP), another large electronics company along a similar vein, is at work to get poly vinyl chloride (PVC) out of their power cables and to eliminate halogenated substances (SDG 9). Apple Inc., the world's largest information technology company by revenue and total assets, has eliminated their lead usage, reduced brominated flame retardants inclusion and stopped PVC usage in their power cords. The company also has eliminated using dangerous solvents that are harmful to workers during manufacturing processes (Cernansky 2016) addressing SDGs 9 and 12.

Dr. Paul Mazurkiewicz, senior scientist at HP's laboratory in Colorado, states that the company is striving to the point where electronics fit very neatly into the circular economy (SDG 12). He explains that for this reason they are developing the concept of a fully edible computer which they believe can be achieved within a reasonable timeframe (Cernansky 2016; HP 2017).

10.4.1.2 Other Waste and Harmful Emissions

Though an important step, electronic companies and other large corporations are not fixated on a single sustainability problem such as e-waste. The multidimensional approach is clearly demonstrated by Apple Inc.—the American multinational technology company headquartered in California (Apple Inc. 2017a) that was ranked third on the 2016 Fortune 500 list (D&B Hoovers 2017) and 92nd on the 2017 Best

Corporate Citizens (CR 2017). This electronics giant's global sustainability and CSR activities lead the way on abating environmental conditions that impact public health by helping their partners to minimize carbon emissions, eliminate landfill waste, conserve water, and replace unsafe chemicals throughout their supply chain while switching over to renewable energy resources. Another sustainable strategy the company follows is the creation of a zero-waste manufacturing facility by partnering with local recycling facilities to develop better processes for separating and recycling waste. Apple is also using responsible sourcing by mapping their supply chains in detail to provide the shortest routes to conserve fuel and minimize emissions.

U.S.-based Johnson & Johnson (J&J) is also heavily focusing on the betterment of the environmental conditions by adopting a variety of sustainable strategies. Listed in the 2016 Dow Jones Sustainability North America Index, J&J is increasingly focusing on reducing their greenhouse emissions and controlling supply chains. They joined more than 80 companies nationwide in signing the American Business Act on Climate Pledge (Lane 2015), partnered with the RE100 initiative—which is a global and collaborative initiative of influential businesses that are committed to 100% renewable electricity (RE100 2015), and partnered with World Wildlife Fund (https://www.worldwildlife.org/) to launch the Corporate Renewable Energy Buyers Principles (http://buyersprinciples.org/) (SDG 17). The principles create opportunities to raise awareness of the challenges faced by corporate energy purchasers to improve energy efficiency including the application of cogeneration (on-site generation of electricity and recovery of the wasted heat to increase overall efficiencies); on-site renewable energy that will not produce carbon dioxide (CO_2) emissions; renewable electric purchases; and carbon trading and sequestration. Carbon trading is defined as buying and selling licenses by companies and governments to produce CO_2 (Cambridge 2017) while carbon sequestration is described as processes (natural or deliberate) by which CO_2 is either diverted from the sources of emission or eliminated from the atmosphere and collected in different natural environments, such as ocean, vegetation, sediment, and other geologic formations (USGS 2016) (SDGs 9,12, and14). J&J has also made incremental targets to reduce carbon emissions by 20% by 2020 working toward the objective to supply the power for all their facilities with clean and renewable energy by 2050 reducing emissions by 80% (Richardson 2015, *para* 4) (SDGs 7 and 13).

10.4.2 Corporate Action to Address Employees' Well-being

With the intense growth of globalization, companies function in many different countries employing local citizens in each country they practice. For example, Apple Inc. is responsible for two million jobs only in the United States (Apple Inc. 2017a) and maintains about 500 retail stores in 19 countries (Dunn 2017) with millions of additional workers (SDG 8). Employees' working conditions, their well-being, and continued positive relations with them are important corporate functions that should be paid attention as a part of sustainable roadmap. How they regulate employee working conditions and monitor their progress towards sustainable goals will be in the spotlight here.

10.4.2.1 Employee Working Conditions, Safety, and Health

Multinational corporations operate in many developing nations where the working conditions generally have poor health implications for employees. To fight against this worldwide problem, Apple is committed to a strict internal "Code of Conduct" that requires their suppliers to "adhere to high standards for safe working conditions, fair treatment of workers, and environmentally safe manufacturing" (Apple Inc. 2017b, *para* 2). Consequently, Apple holds a vast and influential role in which rigid adherence to work environment and production standards is a model for the appropriate level of corporate responsibility. Precautions to protect employees in the work environment through the implementation of ethical standards and recognition of child labor restrictions that afford educational opportunities demonstrate the many facets of sustainable business development that promote human health and well-being (SDGs 3, 4, 10, and 16). Similarly, LG Electronics (http://www.lg.com/us) also has internal programs to increase employees' awareness of environmental and social issues demonstrating ethical company communication with their customers, employees, and partners to reach their competitive outcomes.

Like Apple, ensuring employee safety and health is a focal point for Toyota Motor Corporation, one of the largest car companies founded in 1937 with corporate headquarters in Japan employing about 325,000 people worldwide (Toyota 2017a) selling their vehicles in more than 170 countries that are manufactured worldwide in 53 overseas facilities in 28 different countries (Toyota 2017b, *para* 1). This company's focus was reflected in the advice to its employees in 1957 when Eiji Toyoda, Senior Managing Director at the time, advised employees that a "safe work is the gate to all work" (Toyota 2012, *para* 1). The company has a three-pronged approach to safety and health which is the roadmap toward achieving zero accidents. The three prongs are (1) developing people, (2) risk management, and (3) environment and facility preparation (Toyota 2016, p.46). Developing people focuses on ensuring that each person can detect risks. Risk management promotes a safe management system and environment in which preparing the facility and the machinery for workplace comfort and safety has a high priority. Developing strong employee relationships by addressing these conditions can improve employee retention rates, their contentment, and productivity levels—all of which are important management aspects for companies that want to stay competitive in the market.

10.4.2.2 Human Rights

Employee related human rights like initiatives, such as those put in place by Apple and Toyota, have also been successfully adopted by Costco Wholesale Corporation, the second-largest retailer in the U.S. behind Walmart (Bloomberg 2013), ranking number

16 on the Fortune Global 500 list (Fortune 2017). Costco has a global supplier code of conduct which prohibits human rights abuses in the supply chain. They specifically outlaw practices such as human trafficking, physical abuse of workers, confiscation of passports and worker documentation, unsafe work environments, failure to pay adequate wages, excessive and/or forced overtime, illegal child labor, and many other similar practices (Costco 2017a, *para* 1–2). Suppliers are contractually bound to follow the code of conduct, ensure that their sub-suppliers are also in compliance, and are subject to third-party facility audits for product quality and employee safety. This kind of supplier code of conduct has positive implications in other nations establishing that the company does not and will not support suppliers who violate human rights abuses.

10.4.2.3 Keeping Track: Corporate Monitoring and Reporting

Planning and implementing measurement goals are an important aspect of achieving corporate sustainability business objectives. Thus, monitoring and reporting must be embedded into the vision statements, mission statements, and corresponding goals of each company. For example, Apple administers yearly progress reports and assessments on several categories being monitored within the company based on a 100-point scale corresponding to their Code of Conduct. Apple reports indicate compliance rates of 85 or above for these labor and human rights, human health, and environmental indicators (Apple 2017b, *para* 4) while maintaining a profitable business and an ongoing interest to act on community needs by providing employee education, support, and training.

Apple conducted comprehensive site audits of 1.2 million employees at 705 facilities in 2016—the largest in company history, reporting working hours compliance in their manufacturing plants at 98%while reaching a first-time milestone at 100% UL Environment Zero-Waste to Landfill validation for all final assembly sites in China. UL Environment is a business unit of Underwriter's Laboratory (http://industries.ul.com/environment/zero-waste). However, the supplier audit unveiled one instance of underage employment in China and bonded labor at another location in the United Arab Emirates. Apple required the Chinese supplier provide the underage worker safe passage home and to continue paying their wages while the worker participated in an education program. The subcontractor who withheld employee passports, provided lower-then-standard meal allowances, and held the employee accountable to unacceptable rules in the living quarters was removed from the subcontractor supply chain (SDGs 8,10, and 16).

10.4.3 Partnering to Target Specific Public Health Crisis

Some corporations may build partnerships with other organizations to overcome widespread and challenging human health problems, such as pandemics or epidemics, as a part of their CSR and sustainability actions. For example, Apple has partnered with RED group (RED Group n.d.)—a nonprofit organization that is striving to fight HIV/AIDS, tuberculosis, and malaria in Africa (RED Group 2017). The company sells those products under this program named the "RED line" (e.g., Apple Watch Band, iPod Touch, iPod Nano, iPad Air 2 Smart Case, iPhone 6S case, and iPhone 6S Plus) in which a portion of profits gained is donated to the RED group's Global Fund in the fight to cure the HIV epidemic in Africa (SDGs 3 and 17). RED attributed Apple with $100 million in donations from product sales (RED Group n.d.). Through these and other proactive movements, Apple incorporates an element of civic engagement by using their large customer and economic power base to help those who are in need.

10.4.4 Natural Habitat Conservation

Natural habitat conservation is another important activity that many corporations are practicing as one element of their sustainable business strategy demonstrating positive impact on human health, well-being, and suggesting that healthy environments elicit healthy members of society. Toyota is currently using their worldwide brand awareness and strong economic capacity to improve living conditions for people, plants, and wildlife. This well-known giant in car production was ranked number eight on the 2016 Fortune Global 500 list, right before Apple (Fortune 2017) and the number 1 motor vehicle company for the third consecutive year on the Fortune's "World's Most Admired Companies" list (Toyota 2017c).

Toyota utilizes integration with the natural surroundings as a major sustainable objective at production sites that house their global manufacturing facilities. Some of their unique practices are impacting environmental conservation in Belgium and Brazil supporting projects to protect or increase the population of certain endangered or threatened species such as Macaws, preventing desertification and conducting reforestation in China, promoting environmental awareness through farming in Korea, and maintaining the ecological value of self-sustaining principles in the United Kingdom (Toyota 2017d).

10.4.5 Conflict Resources

Toyota expanded the local concept of workplace safety and comfort in 2012 when they invited their suppliers to engage in responsible material procurement. They followed this announcement with a full-scale investigation in 2013 to eliminate suppliers who utilized conflict resources—minerals or other materials mined from a war zone, or one experiencing civil unrest, in which items are sold to support that conflict. Toyota probed more deeply into this problem in 2015 by examining the global supply chain of their tier one suppliers to ensure that they were not unwittingly contributing to social unrest (Toyota 2017f).

Similarly, LG Electronics Inc., South Korean multinational electronics company, designs energy efficient products that limit the use of conflict minerals and hazardous components, and includes more recoverable materials in their products (LG Electronics 2017). Further, Lenovo Group Ltd., the Chinese multinational technology company, continuously works on life cycle management, uses more environmentally sensitive materials in products, puts together programs to promote product and parts recycling, reduces waste to landfills, and uses recycled post-consumer plastic in new designs (Lenova 2017)

10.4.6 Customer Protection and Safety

There are regulations, laws, and standards in place to protect the public against unforeseen risks associated with consumer products. In the U.S., Consumer Product Safety Commission (CPSC) administers and enforces these federal laws (CPSC 2017a). When companies do not comply with these regulations and laws, they may see financial and reputational damages to the company. Children's robes sold on Amazon.com, Inc. in August 2017, for example, were recalled by Belle Investment for failure to meet federal flammability standards posing a risk of children burn injuries (CPSC 2017b).

Some of the corporations who are strongly oriented towards sustainability are aiming to go a step forward in providing customer safety rather than minimally addressing consumer safety standards. An important human health implication of Toyota's business sustainability action is related to their strong customer orientation. Thus, their overarching goal as a prominent manufacturer of vehicles is to achieve zero casualties from traffic accidents in two primary ways: (1) development of safe vehicles, and (2) road safety education for drivers and pedestrians. Therefore, Toyota promotes an integrated three-part system for safety involving people, vehicles, and traffic environments. Consequently, the company has conducted traffic safety education activities continuously since the 1960s (Toyota 2017e). Viewing this activity from the business perspective, this kind of customer-focused business sustainability strategy is important to building a strong corporate image and improving customer value and trust.

10.4.7 Sustainable and Fair Trade

Global value chains of corporations are linking different countries to each other resulting in an increasing emphasis on global international trade. Although growth in trade may offer major opportunities for many countries, a growth-only focus causes some challenges for achieving sustainable development as well as meeting the SDGs (UNEP 2015). Countries that adopt sustainable trade and green global value chains can prosper and grow sustainably with the help of appropriate environmental policy, social policy, and incentives. "Avenues for making trade more sustainable include a focus on enhanced production capacity, use and exchange of environmentally sound technologies, goods and services, increased resource efficiency, and reduced environmental and resource impacts through more sustainable consumption, production and life-cycle approaches" (UNEP 2015, p.2).

Starbucks Company, an American coffee company and coffeehouse chain, has grown to more than 25,000 stores in over 75 countries since 1971 (Starbucks 2017a). Today, the company is listed in the 2016 Dow Jones Sustainability North America Index and is committed to buying coffee beans from 100% ethical sources in partnership with Conservation International (Starbucks 2017b). The company takes a holistic approach to ethically source high-quality coffee using responsible purchasing practices, supporting loans for farmers, and collaborating with forest conservation programs. This kind of ethical sourcing helps foster improvements in sustainable working conditions for farmers and a stable regional natural climate (SDGs 8, 11–13, and 15).

Costco Wholesale Corporation also practices fair trade. This American company is committed to preserving and making a positive impact on the environment with the intention to benefit everyone everywhere. They work towards this by paying attention to how their products are sourced, packaged, and understanding how these products may affect the environment. For instance, they are a member of the Roundtable on Sustainable Palm Oil (RSPO) (http://www.rspo.org/), a product from palm trees used in various products (e.g., soap, cooking oil), promoting the use of suppliers who have been designated RSPO-certified palm oil because they are using responsible agricultural practices. They also are partnered with IDH Sustainable Trade Initiative, Winrock International, and Cargill to support palm oil smallholders where they plan to develop a program to manage peat lands in a sustainable manner, increase market access, and reduce greenhouse gas emissions. Costco also participates in other product certification programs, such as Forest Stewardship Council (FSC) certified teak (Newman 2017) and the Rainforest Alliance (http://www.rainforest-alliance.org/) for rose growers (COSTCO 2017b) signifying their dedication to abate deforestation practices, protect ecosystems and wildlife habitats, conserve water and soil, promote decent and safe working conditions, and ensure that the farms are good neighbors to rural communities and wild lands.

10.5 Management Tools to Assess Sustainable Business Ventures and Corporate Status

Assessing an organization without standard metrics is a task without reward. However, there are numerous nonprofit organizations that examine corporate sustainability activity across the globe. They provide management tools from which to assess progress and performance of corporate social responsibility and to track the perceived character and status of an organization.

10.5.1 Corporate Social Responsibility and Performance Reporting

Global Reporting Initiative (GRI)—a U.S.-based, global nonprofit organization providing guidelines for reporting on corporate social responsibility and performance (e.g., environmental, social, and governance) has a reputation as one of the best guidelines because of the universal application of their metrics to all organizations (O'Rourke 2004). Since the inception of the organization in 1997 in Boston, GRI has refined and improved their guideline through several modifications with contributions from business, civil society, and the labor movement since G1—the first version, debuted as the first global framework for comprehensive sustainability in 2000 (GRI n.d.). In 2011, GRI's Sustainability Disclosure Database was launched to catalog all sustainability reports (GRI and non-GRI based) followed by the release of The Reporting Principles, Standard Disclosures and Implementation Manual with the fourth generation of Guidelines, G4, in 2013. This further supports the preparation of sustainability reports by organizations of any size or sector. Finally, in October 2016, GRI launched the first sustainability reporting global standards. With the help of GRI Standards, organizations can publicly report on their social, environmental and economic impacts, and by so doing, demonstrate their contribution towards sustainable development. (GRI n.d.).

The world's largest database of corporate sustainability reports is provided as a part of the United Nations Global Compact—a voluntary initiative that offers a policy framework for organizing and developing corporate sustainability strategies. Adopted in 2005, the initiative drives business awareness and is a platform to organizations encouraging innovative sustainability actions and partnerships with variety of stakeholders (UN Global Compact 2017a). The UN Global Compact's multi-year strategy needs voluntary commitment by the member corporate Chief Executive Officer to implement universal sustainability principles that contribute to achieving the SDGs by 2030 (UN Global Compact 2017b). These collaborative efforts hold promise as "the GRI, the United Nations Global Compact and the World Business Council for Sustainable Development (WBCSD) have joined forces to mobilize the private sector as a key player in achieving our world's Sustainable Development Goals (SDGs)" (GRI 2014, *para* 1).

10.5.2 Establishing Organizational Status

Assessing the organizational status of companies in terms of their sustainable engagement is made possible by determining their position in the marketplace using a variety of available rankings. One prominent initiative is the RepTrak model for analyzing the reputations of companies and institutions—best known via the Forbes-published Global RepTrak 100, the world's largest study of corporate reputations (Strauss 2017). The Reputation Institute, a reputation management consulting firm founded in Boston in 1997, conducts an annual study and identifies the CSR reputation of the world's 100 most highly regarded and familiar global companies presented annually as the CSR Global RepTrak® 100 list (Reputation Institute 2017). The study covers 15 different countries and produces a list of the best corporate citizens by ranking them based on their weighted averages in relation to their activities on the environment, climate change, human rights, employee relations, corporate governance, philanthropy, and financial scores. Information about the company embedded in the results can become a model for other organizations to emulate.

A similar list comes from Corporate Knights—a Toronto-based magazine and research firm. Since 2005, the firm annually publishes the Global 100 that is a list of the world's most sustainable companies (Corporate Knights 2017). "Using publicly available data, Corporate Knights rates large firms on 14 key measures, evaluating their management of resources, finances and employees" (Kauflin 2017, *para* 1). The Global 100 process includes the conduct of four screening processes beginning each October 1 that establishes a short list followed by analysis of key performance indicators across global industry classification (GICs) standards until top performers emerge as the Global 100. "The Global 100 is calculated by Solactive, the German index provider" (Corporate Knights 2016, *para* 2).

Many corporations cite another important index in their CSR related websites—the Dow Jones Sustainability Indices (DJSI), representing the top ten percent of the world's largest 2500 companies based on their economic, social, and environmental sustainability performance (DJSI World 2017, *para* 1). The methodology encompasses a variety of criteria, such as climate change strategies, energy consumption, corporate governance, human resources, knowledge management, and stakeholder relations. The index was launched as the first global sustainability benchmark for corporations in 1999 (RobecoSAM 2017, *para* 1). The DJSI North America Index, on the other hand, comprises North American sustainability leaders and represents the top twenty percent of the largest 600 North American companies with the same criteria of economic, environmental and social performance (DJSI North America 2017, *para* 1). DJSI North America Index comes from one of the world's largest providers of financial market indices, S&P Dow Jones Indices, and RobecoSAM—a sustainable investment specialist (http://www.robecosam.com/).

10.5.3 The Absence of "Best Companies" Addressing SDG Objectives

Notable is the absence of a single major corporation in the list of a variety of "Best Companies" that is adequately confronting issues identified by the SDGs, such as climate change and resource scarcity. When we examine the lists, we conclude that across multiple areas, such as supply chain management to carbon emissions reductions, a small but growing number of companies rank in the top tiers in terms of their performance. Therefore, identifying those companies that are genuinely working on the sustainability initiatives by establishing best practices as well as ingraining sustainable strategies into their operations is important. However, the key question would be, "Are these best business practices able to capture and work towards resolving the world's prominent SDGs?" Given the nonexclusionary supposition that all companies, regardless of size, can contribute to the SDGs and that the scale and scope of the global goals are unprecedented (UN Global Compact 2017c, *para* 1) thus warranting maximum participation for success, the next key question rests on, "Which companies demonstrate leadership and best practices towards achieving SDGs?" Answering these questions can help us identify the current areas of focus in today's marketplace and will provide governments, organizations, corporations, and policy makers a direction towards a sustainable future. For this purpose, we will look at the best sustainable business ventures that are the leaders of many aspects of sustainable initiatives and have aligned their actions with the SDGs.

10.6 Corporate Business Ventures That Align with SDGs

An appropriate direction for corporate sustainable business initiatives is to link objectives to existing protocols established in the UN SDGs. According to the PwC Global (2015), compared to the general population, SDG awareness amongst the business community is almost three times higher (33% citizens vs. 92% businesses aware of SDGs). Although this is promising, linking and identifying how corporate objectives meet the protocols established in the UN SDGs recommendations with their current sustainability strategies is important to resolving the environmental conditions that impact public health and the ecosystem.

Global sustainability benchmarks and independent third-party sustainability (or CSR) rankings of companies underwent review to identify various corporate sustainability activities and their alignments with relevant SDGs. For this purpose, we used two lists: (1) 100 Best Corporate Citizens compiled annually by Corporate Responsibility Magazine (CR 2017) from metrics in seven data categories with 260 data elements in the CR Magazine Corporate Citizenship database (CR 2016), and (2) Dow Jones Sustainability Indices (DJSI World 2017), representing the top ten percent of the world's largest companies based on their economic, social, and environmental sustainability performance. The following demonstrates how several corporations have successfully embedded the SDGs into their corporate objectives and strategies (Table 10.1).

10.6.1 Campbell Soup Company

The Campbell Soup Company is an American producer of canned soups and related services with manufacturing operations in six countries and products sold in 120 countries. The company employs more than 18,000 people and was ranked tenth in

Table 10.1 Corporate strategies aligning with United Nations Sustainable Development Goals[a]

	Goal brief	Objective	Company
1	No poverty	End poverty in all its forms everywhere	All listed companies provide jobs
2	Zero hunger	End hunger, achieve food security and improved nutrition, and promote sustainable agriculture	Campbell Soup Company: General Mills, Inc.
3	Good health and well-being	Ensure healthy lives and promote well-being for all at all ages	Apple Inc.; Campbell Soup Company; Clorox Company; General Mills, Inc.; Hess Corporation
4	Quality education	Ensure inclusive and equitable quality education and promote life-long learning opportunities for all	Apple Inc.; Clorox Company
5	Gender equality	Achieve gender equality and empower all women and girls	Apple Inc.; General Mills, Inc.
6	Clean water and sanitation	Ensure availability and sustainable management of water and sanitation for all	Apple Inc.; Campbell Soup Company; Clorox Company; General Mills, Inc.; Hess Corporation
7	Affordable and clean energy	Ensure access to affordable, reliable, sustainable, and modern energy for all	Apple Inc.; General Mills, Inc.; Hess Corporation; Johnson & Johnson
8	Decent work and economic growth	Promote sustained, inclusive and sustainable economic growth, full and productive employment and decent work for all	Apple Inc.; Campbell Soup Company; Clorox Company; General Mills, Inc.; Hess Corporation; Nike, Inc.; Starbucks
9	Industry, innovation, and infrastructure	Build resilient infrastructure, promote inclusive and sustainable industrialization, and foster innovation	Apple Inc.; Hess Corporation; Nike, Inc.; Hewlett Packard; Johnson & Johnson
10	Reduced inequalities	Reduce inequality within and among countries	Apple Inc.; General Mills, Inc.
11	Sustainable cities and communities	Make cities and human settlements inclusive, safe, resilient and sustainable	Apple Inc.; Hess Corporation; Starbucks
12	Responsible consumption and production	Ensure sustainable consumption and production patterns	Apple Inc.; Campbell Soup Company, General Mills, Inc.; Hewlett Packard; Johnson & Johnson; Starbucks; Nike, Inc.
13	Climate action	Take urgent action to combat climate change and its impacts	Apple Inc.; General Mills, Inc.; Hess Corporation; Johnson & Johnson; Nike, Inc.; Starbucks
14	Life below water	Conserve and sustainably use the oceans, seas, and marine resources for sustainable development	Johnson & Johnson; Hess Corporation

(continued)

Table 10.1 (continued)

	Goal brief	Objective	Company
15	Life on land	Protect, restore, and promote sustainable use of terrestrial ecosystems, sustainably manage forests, combat desertification, and halt and reverse land degradation and halt biodiversity loss	Apple Inc.; Campbell Soup Company, Hess Corporation; Inc.; Johnson & Johnson; Starbucks
16	Peace, justice, and strong institutions	Promote peaceful and inclusive societies for sustainable development, provide access to justice for all and build effective, accountable, and inclusive institutions at all levels	Apple Inc.; Clorox Company; General Mills, Inc.
17	Partnerships for the goals	Strengthen the means of implementation and revitalize the global partnership for sustainable development	Apple Inc., Clorox Company; General Mills; Johnson & Johnson; Nike, Inc.

Source: [a]United Nations 2017
Notes: This table was created based on the chapter discussion content and company listing on one of the two indices (i.e., CR 2017 or DJSI World 2017). The chart is intended as a representative roadmap of sustainable actions and does not reflect an inclusive assessment of all activity

the annual 100 Best Corporate Citizens List in 2016 and fifth in 2017. Ranking improvements are very important for companies because progress reflects determination, consistency, and advances in CSR activities. Over the past seven years the company was named to the North American index and six times in the World index.

Campbell's sustainability actions focus on reducing energy and water use (SDG 6) and waste generation, increasing recycling and sustainable packaging (SDG 9), practicing sustainable agriculture by addressing the issues of soil health, pesticide use, deforestation, biodiversity, and water use to both improve human health and end hunger (SDGs 2, 3, and 15). They address these goals by optimizing supply chain operations and using their 2008 product portfolio as a baseline to ultimately reduce their environmental footprint by half in relation to food production measured in per tonnes (Campbell 2017). Since 2008, Campbell has reduced their water use by 17.8%, energy consumption by 15.6% and greenhouse gas emissions by 24.3% (Campbell 2017, p.40). The company has targeted the goal of reducing energy use by 35% and sourcing 40% of electricity from renewable or alternative energy sources by 2020. According to Campbell's 2016 CSR report, their global recycling rate is up to 86% and they plan to increase that to 95% within the next three years and have a strategy to derive 100% of their global packaging materials from either renewable, recyclable, or recycled content (Campbell 2017, pp.41–42).

The company also pays great attention to the rise in chronic diseases and takes product related actions in safety, quality and transparency to provide consumers with many healthy product alternatives (e.g., low salt), labeling foodstuffs with genetically modified organisms (GMO), ingredient safety, and extending packaged fresh options. As reported in the 2015–2020 Dietary Guidelines for Americans "rates of chronic diseases related to poor-quality diet and physical inactivity have increased, with half of all US adults having one or more preventable, diet-related chronic diseases, including cardiovascular disease, type 2 diabetes, and overweight and obesity" (Campbell 2017, p.24). Thus, Campbell's goals are to continue to limit negative nutrients and introduce positive nutritional benefits to become more health conscious for their consumers. Their product changes and increasingly transparent farm to table approach aligns with SDG 12 in terms of public information and providing healthy product options that was rewarded by $2.9 billion of total gross sales of healthy foods (i.e., foods with nutritional profiles satisfying the criteria set by the FDA and other global organizations) in 2016 (Campbell 2017, p.26).

SDG 8 is met by Campbell through their inclusive approach to ethical business practices and sustainability activities where employees are actively engaged in the advancement of company Environmental Sustainability Policy. Sustainability Leadership Teams are called upon to observe environmental performance and active participation becomes embedded into the corporate culture resulting in positive employee morale, increased productivity, and improved employee retention. The company also focuses on a variety of human rights activities, diversity, and inclusion to better meet and more accurately reflect the changing demographics in society. Campbell achieves this by building awareness and capability through specific programs and engaging leaders, talents, and creating community. They also encourage the health and safety of not only their employees but each of their stakeholders as well by incorporating global safety standards, technological advances, and communication to increase positive social impacts.

10.6.2 Nike, Inc.

Nike, Inc. is an American multinational corporation engaging in the design, development, manufacturing, and worldwide marketing and sales of footwear, apparel, equipment, accessories, and services. The company is known for its innovative capacities and is now increasing its focus on sustainable initiatives. Mark Parker, President and CEO of Nike, Inc. outlines this effort, "At Nike, we believe it is not enough to adapt to what the future may bring—we're creating the future we want to see through sustainable innovation" (Nike, Inc. 2017). The company ranks number 29 in the Global Best Corporate Citizens list of 2017 with a weighted average score of 88.57 (CR 2017).

Nike reaffirms commitment to environmental and social targets in their new sustainable business report reflecting the company's efforts to create a new business model that enables low-carbon and closed-loop operations (Nike, Inc. 2016). Consequently, reduction of carbon emissions to a level that supports the global carbon budget is their priority and rests on the development and adoption of a business system named "low-carbon growth economy" for product and business model innovations. This company objective aligns with the SDG 13 to combat the impact of climate change. The company sustainable initiatives support the transition from linear to circular business models that move towards closed-loop products by using fewer resources, better materials, and assembly methods allowing ease of reuse in new products. Because Nike considers every stage of the product life cycle including the end of a product's life, they build resilient infrastructures and create sustainable industry practice that foster innovation in line with SDGs 9 and 12, respectively.

The company has identified and focused on two important responsibilities: (1) environmental responsibility that includes chemistry, energy, GHG emissions, water use, nonrenewable resource depletion, and (2) socioeconomic responsibility that includes community impact, employment, excessive overtime, labor compliance, occupational health and safety, total compensation, and workforce development (SDG 8). The company pursues ongoing improvement in these areas and continues to monitor emerging issues. To deliver on their strategy, they also recognize that they must integrate sustainability throughout their business and external partnerships reflecting SDG 17.

10.6.3 Hess Corporation

Founded in 1920, Hess Corporation is an energy company that explores and produces natural gas, oil, and fossil fuel resources. Headquartered in the U.S., Hess was ranked number 26th and 51st in the Global Best Corporate Citizens list in 2016 and 2017, respectively. The company has earned a place on the DJSI North America for seven consecutive years between 2009 and 2015 (Hess 2017a). Hess reports according to the GRI framework and the requirements set forth by several organizations such as the 2010 International Petroleum Industry Environmental Conservation Association, American Petroleum Industry, and the Oil and Gas Industry Guidance on Voluntary Sustainability Reporting. The company focuses on reducing water use, energy consumption, GHG emissions, and the use of pollutants. Activities providing tangential support to these high-level priorities include implementing spill prevention initiatives, conducting biodiversity screenings during site evaluation for operations, and using new drilling techniques to minimize environmental impacts.

The Hess CSR is centered on stakeholder engagement, social risk and impact management, and strategic social investments that facilitate direct and indirect local benefits. Hess demonstrates their global reach in two projects—the agricultural program in Equatorial Guinea and Wau Kite safety in Malaysia. In Equatorial Guinea, Hess provides equipment, financial and technical support, as well as guidance and training tools to locals with the aim of creating two small farming cooperatives for employment, decreasing rural flight and improving the quality of life (SDG 3). With the second project, Hess assists with the annual Kelantan International Kite Festival to increase safety awareness concerning helicopters used in oil and gas operations (SDG 11).

The company has a strong position on climate change resulting from rising greenhouse gas emissions and global temperatures that pose risks to society and ecosystems. Access to affordable energy is an important issue for Hess and for this reason the company is a proponent of cost-effective policy responses that balance mitigation, adaptation and societal priorities (Hess 2017b). The company is eco-sensitive and contributes to the resolution of the world's growing energy needs with variety of projects, such as gas capture and recovery in North Dakota, transparency measures, and Hess greenhouse gas inventory protocol. They continuously monitor, measure, and reduce their carbon footprint (Hess 2017c) addressing SDG 7 for sustainable energy.

10.6.4 General Mills, Inc.

General Mills, Inc. is a U.S.-based company that has been making brand name food products, such as Cheerios, Betty Crocker, Pillsbury, Haagen-Dazs and Cascadian Farm, for customers for over 150 years. The company is located throughout six continents in more than 100 different countries (General Mills 2014) providing over 39,000 jobs and careers to these communities. In 2016, the company's global sales were over 16.6 billion, and in 2017, the company was ranked number 19 in the annual 100 Best Corporate Citizens List with the number one ranking in the human rights category.

General Mills exercises its CSR by focusing on four main categories: health and wellness, sustainability, workplace, and community. Within the health and wellness category General Mills has a commitment to provide convenient, nutritious food (SDG 2) and when combined with diet and exercise this can lead to a healthier life for all (SDG 3). The company promotes environmentally sustainable and socially responsible practices across the entire value chain with the aim of protecting critical resources for the business (SDG 12). There are six main sustainability goals of the company: climate change, sustainable sourcing, water stewardship, human rights, animal welfare, and production operation environmental performance representing key SDGs 6, 7, and 13 to manage resources, sustainable energy, and climate change.

Within the workplace category, General Mills create a safe, ethical, diverse, and inclusive environment laying a foundation for their employees to prosper. For example, General Mills supports all forms and dimensions of diversity, not limited to race, gender, or sexual orientation but also aiming to include other aspects of diversity such as values, preference, beliefs, and communication styles, which is very well aligned with the SDG 8. Lastly, the goals from the community approach are to strengthen communities by increasing food security across the globe by advancing sustainable agriculture to address SDG Goal 2 to end hunger.

The major reason for General Mill's outstanding human rights ranking was because of the Policy on Human Rights launched in 2015. The company believes that societies, economies, and businesses thrive when human rights are protected and respected. Thus, the respect for human rights is a fundamental practice for the company is guided by the principles of human rights, labor, the environment and anti-corruption of United Nations Global Compact (UNGC). General Mills has been a signatory to the UNGC since 2008 aligning with SDG Goals 8 and 16 promoting inclusive employment, accountability, and justice. Finally, the company has also embraced the United Nations Women's Empowerment Principles (General Mills 2015) to address gender equality in SDG Goal 5.

10.6.5 Clorox Company

Founded in 1913, the Clorox Company is a multinational consumer, professional product manufacturer and marketer with approximately 8000 employees worldwide. The company operates in over 25 countries and territories with 2016 reported sales of $5.8 billion. The company is most famously known for their bleach and cleaning products such as Pine-Sol, Fresh Step cat litter, Brita water filtration systems, and Burt's Bees (Clorox Company 2017a). The company was ranked number 12 in the annual 100 Best Corporate Citizens List of 2017 with their best ranking in the climate change category at number 10.

The Clorox Company has a variety of CSR initiatives in place, such as the Safe Water Project, Disaster Relief program, and Public Health education. The Clorox Safe Water Project addresses the issue of unsafe drinking water in Peru (Rosenberg 2017). Through this project, Clorox has donated bleach to 21 different communities in Peru and provided over 100 million liters of safe drinking water annually to more than 25,000 people. The project is a two-step effort with bleach dispensers for water treatment and education sessions to the local communities to teach them the importance of bleach and disinfecting water. Also, in times of disasters, the Clorox company partners with the American Red Cross to provide financial support and product donations (American Red Cross 2017). For example, in recent years, Clorox has donated truckloads of products including Clorox liquid bleach and Glad trash bags to those experiencing flooding (e.g., Texas, Mississippi, South Carolina, Georgia, and Missouri) and the 2016 earthquake in Ecuador. Clorox products reduce virus outbreaks that are common after natural disasters, battle Ebola in West Africa, and Zika outbreaks in the Americas. The company leads education programs establishing methods to use bleach to stay healthy and promote public health. Cumulatively, these efforts by the Clorox Company reflect the SDG Goals 3, 4, and 6 ensuring healthy lives, providing opportunities for life-long learning, and aid in water resource management, respectively.

Clorox demonstrates their strong emphasis on employee relations by matching employee donations and contributing to their volunteer organizations through the employee-led GIFT program. In 2015, Clorox employees donated 123,053 hours of their time to hundreds of nonprofits and raised a little less than 5 million dollars to support more than 3500 nonprofit organizations with the matching contribution from the foundations. Almost half of the of Clorox employees annually (Clorox Company 2017b).

Many companies are "learning that providing employees with opportunities to participate in volunteer projects for the community can build the employees' connection to their organization. Such volunteer projects enhance the employees' pride in improving the community, teamwork in working with their coworkers, and pride in their employer" (Liebowitz 2010, p.54). This is also a good way of improving the awareness and educate the local communities on important sustainability issues. Two of the SDGs align well with these types of initiatives, SDG 8, "Promote sustained, inclusive and sustainable economic growth, full and productive employment and decent work for all" and SDG 17, "Strengthen the means of implementation and revitalize the global partnership for sustainable development."

10.7 Conclusion

"Business should be neither harmful to nor a parasite on society, but purely a positive contributor to the wellbeing of the society" (Garriga and Mele 2004, p.62). Following this insight, sustainable business development has prompted a notable shift in the way emerging and developed nations extend their business goals to include concern for the global ecosystem and human development guided by the UN SDGs. The adoption of business practices that include CSR and TBL to profit objectives are important to building public trust and achieving corporate status. This is especially critical when corporations respond to consumer demand to advance material acquisition and processing methods that improve public health.

Consequently, these activities also position responsible corporations in the marketplace generating a loyal customer base. Thus, the effect of sustainable business practices presents an opportunity to address global environmental conditions, such as carbon emissions, e-waste, and natural habitat conservation while progressing business objectives. Key aspects of incorporating a socially responsible plan include understanding the impact of business environmental sustainability on public health and utilizing management tools to assess sustainable business ventures and corporate status. Another prominent aspect of this chapter is the recommendation to establish business ventures that align with SDGs as demonstrated by several case examples. The "common good" approach founded on the UN SDGs may be the best path to achieve the betterment of society across the globe.

Glossary

Carbon sequestration Processes (natural or deliberate) by which CO_2 is either diverted from the sources of emission or eliminated from the atmosphere and collected in different natural environments, such as ocean, vegetation, sediment, and other geologic formations (USGS 2016).

Carbon trading Buying and selling licenses by companies and governments to produce CO_2.

Circular economy System with the objective of reducing energy and material consumption in which the resource inputs and waste generated by production can be regenerated minimizing resource depletion through a system of multiple strategies for reutilization.

Conflict resources Natural resources mined in a zone experiencing social or civil unrest where profits are used to support continued aggression.

Equity An ethical and balanced attention to a problem, product, plan, or service.

Feasibility Realistic; acceptable viable options.

Financing Providing monetary support for a project, plan or product.

Global Reporting Initiative (GRI) A global independent nonprofit standards organization providing guidelines for reporting on corporate social responsibility aspects and performance (e.g., human rights, climate change, corruption).

Halogenated The appearance of chemicals called halogens (e.g., bromine, chlorine, fluorine) in other substances, such as carbon, that have a long-term environmental impact due to their characteristic stable structure; highly restricted use in production, banned in most countries.

Shareholder An entity (person or company) that owns a company stock share.

Stakeholder All those impacted by an organization's activities including businesses, competitors, government, community members, environment, and others.

References

American Red Cross. The Clorox company. 2017. http://www.redcross.org/disasterresponder/Clorox. Accessed 9 Aug 2017.

Apple, Inc. Two million U.S. jobs. And counting. 2017a. https://www.apple.com/job-creation/. Accessed 11 Jul 2017.

Apple, Inc. Supplier responsibility. 2017b. https://www.apple.com/supplier-responsibility/. Accessed 11 Jul 2017.

Bloomberg. Costco CEO Craig Jelinek leads the cheapest, happiest company in the world. 2013. https://www.bloomberg.com/news/articles/2013-06-06/costco-ceo-craig-jelinek-leads-the-cheapest-happiest-company-in-the-world. Accessed 11 Jul 2017.

Boxer L. Sustainability perspectives. Phil Manag. 2007;6(2):86–98.

Breivik K, et al. Tracking the global generation and exports of e-waste. Do existing estimates add up? Environ Sci Technol. 2014;48:8735–43.

Cambridge. Cambridge dictionary. 2017. http://dictionary.cambridge.org/dictionary/english/carbon-trading. Accessed 6 August 2017.

Campbell. 2017 corporate sustainability report. 2017. http://www.campbellcsr.com/_pdfs/Campbells_2017_CSR_Report.pdf. Accessed 9 Aug 2017.

Cannon T. Corporate responsibility. 1st ed. London: Pitman; 1992.

Carroll AB, Shabana KM. The business case for corporate social responsibility: A review of concepts, research and practice. Int J Manag Rev. 2010;12(1):85–105.

Ceres. The 21st century corporation: a ceres roadmap to sustainability. Boston: Ceres; 2010.

Cernansky R. How HP and Dell are reducing the toxics in their electronics. 2016. https://www.greenbiz.com/article/how-hp-and-dell-are-reducing-toxics-their-electronics. Accessed 30 Jun 2017.

Chen A, et al. Developmental neurotoxicants in e-waste: an emerging health concern. Environ Health Perspect. 2011;119:431–8. https://doi.org/10.1289/ehp.1002452.

Clorox Company. Who we are. 2017a. https://www.thecloroxcompany.com/. Accessed 9 Aug 2017.

Clorox Company. Employee volunteerism. 2017b. https://www.thecloroxcompany.com/corporate-responsibility/social-impact/employee-volunteerism/. Accessed 9 Aug 2017.

Corporate Knights. The results for the 2016 Global 100 most sustainable corporations in the world index. 2016. http://www.corporateknights.com/magazines/2016-global-100-issue/2016-global-100-results-14533333/. Accessed 7 Aug 2017.

Corporate Knights. Corporate knights about us. 2017. http://www.corporateknights.com/us/about-us/ Accessed 7 Aug 2017.

Costco Wholesale Corporation. Costco disclosure regarding human trafficking and anti-slavery. 2017a. https://www.costco.com/disclosure-regarding-human-trafficking-and-anti-slavery.html. Accessed 11 Jul 2017.

Costco Wholesale Corporation. Environmental impacts. https://www.costco.com/sustainability-environment.html. 2017b. Accessed 11 Jul 2017.

Corporate Responsibility (CR) Magazine. 100 best methodology: how we determine the winners. 2016. http://www.thecro.com/100-best/100-best-methodology-how-we-determine-the-winners/. Accessed 7 Aug 2017.

Corporate Responsibility (CR). CR's 100 best corporate citizens. 2017. http://www.thecro.com/wp-content/uploads/2017/05/CR_100Bestpages_digitalR.pdf. Accessed 9 Aug 2017.

D&B Hoovers. Apple Inc. company information. 2017. http://www.hoovers.com/company-information/cs/company-profile.apple_inc.4c9baa063908dbd8.html. Accessed 11 Jul 2017.

Dow Jones Sustainability Indices (DJSI) North America. DJSI North America composite index. 2017. https://us.spindices.com/indices/equity/dow-jones-sustainability-north-america-composite-index. Accessed 7 Aug 2017.

Dow Jones Sustainability Indices (DJSI) World. DJSI world composite index. 2017. http://us.spindices.com/indices/equity/dow-jones-sustainability-world-index. Accessed 13 Aug 2017.

Dunn J. Here's how Apple's retail business spreads across the world. 2017. Business Insider. http://www.businessinsider.com/apple-stores-how-many-around-world-chart-2017-2 Accessed 30 Jun 2017.

Eccles RG, et al. The impact of corporate sustainability on organizational processes and performance. Manag Sci. 2014;60(11):2835–57.

Elkington J. Cannibals with forks. Gabriola Island: New Society; 1998.

Fombrun C, Van Riel CBM. The reputational landscape. Corp Reputation Rev. 1997;1(1–2):5–13.

Fortune (2017) Global 500. http://fortune.com/global500/. Accessed 11 Jul 2017.

Frederick WC. Toward CSR3; why ethical analysis is indispensable and unavoidable in corporate affairs. ? Cal Manag Rev. 1986;28:126–41.

Frederick WC. From CSR1 to CSR2. Bus & Soc. 1994;33:150–66.

Friedman M. The social responsibility of business is to increase its profits. The New York Times Magazine. 1970, September 13;13:32–33, 122, 124, 126.

Garriga E, Mele D. Corporate social responsibility theories: mapping the territory. J Bus Ethics. 2004;53:51–71.

General Mills, Inc. Businesses. 2014. https://www.generalmills.com/en/Company/Businesses. Accessed 9 Aug 2017.

General Mills Inc. Policy on human rights. 2015. https://www.generalmills.com/en/News/Issues/human-rights. Accessed 9 Jun 2017.

Grant K, et al. Health consequences of exposure to e-waste: a systematic review. Lancet Glob Health. 2013;1(6):e350–61. https://doi.org/10.1016/S2214-109X(13)70101-3.

Global Reporting Initiative (GRI). Joining forces for business action on SDGs. 2014. https://www.globalreporting.org/information/news-and-press-center/Pages/Joining-Forces-for-Business-Action-on-Sustainable-Development-Goals.aspx. Accessed 30 Jun 2017.

Global Reporting Initiative (GRI). GRI's history. n.d. https://www.globalreporting.org/information/about-gri/gri-history/Pages/GRI's%20history.aspx. Accessed 11 Jul 2017.

Hess. Hess named to Dow Jones Sustainability Index North America for seventh consecutive year. 2017a. http://www.hess.com/company/news-article/2016/09/09/hess-named-to-dow-jones-sustainability-index-north-america-for-seventh-consecutive-year. Accessed 9 Aug 2017.

Hess. Climate change and energy. 2017b. http://www.hess.com/sustainability/climate-change-energy. Accessed 9 Aug 2017.

Hess. Social responsibility. 2017c. http://www.hess.com/sustainability/-social-responsibility. Accessed 9 Aug 2017.

Hewlett Packard (HP). Global citizenship, employee gallery, Dr. Paul Mazurkiewicz. 2017. http://h41112.www4.hp.com/test-globalcitizenship/global-citizenship/pages/society/employees/paul-mazurkiewicz.html. Accessed 6 Aug 2017.

Kauflin J. The world's most sustainable companies 2017. 2017, January 17. Forbes. https://www.forbes.com/sites/jeffkauflin/2017/01/17/the-worlds-most-sustainable-companies-2017/#33f1c2ca4e9d. Accessed 07 Aug 2017.

Kahn M E. Requiring companies to disclose climate risks helps everyone. 2017. Harvard Bus Rev [online]. https://hbr.org/2017/02/requiring-companies-to-disclose-climate-risks-helps-everyone. Accessed 7 Aug 2017.

Kurdve M, et al. Waste flow mapping to improve sustainability of waste management: a case study approach. J Clean Prod. 2015;98:304–15.
Laff M. Managing organizational knowledge. Triple bottom line: creating corporate social responsibility that makes sense. 2009. https://www.td.org/Publications/Magazines/TD/TD-Archive/2009/02/Triple-Bottom-Line-Creating-Corporate-Social-Responsibility-That-Makes-Sense. Accessed 30 Jun 2017.
Lane J. 81 Companies sign American business act on climate change pledge. 2015 http://www.biofuelsdigest.com/bdigest/2015/10/25/81-companies-sign-american-business-act-on-climate-change-pledge/. Accessed 11 Jul 2017.
Lenova. Think green products: materials. 2017. http://www.lenovo.com/social_responsibility/us/en/materials/. Accessed 11 Jul 2017.
LG Electronics. Hazardous substances management: LG Electronics is researching and developing technology for the management and replacement of hazardous substances. 2017. http://www.lg.com/global/sustainability/environment/management-of-hazardous-substances. Accessed 11 Jul 2017.
Liebowitz J. The role of HR in achieving a sustainability culture. J Sust. Dev. 2010;3(4):50–7.
Lundgren K. The global impact of e-waste: addressing the challenge. International Labour Office, Programme on Safety and Health at Work and the Environment (SafeWork), Sectoral Activities Department (SECTOR). Geneva: International Labour Office. 2012. http://www.ilo.org/wcmsp5/groups/public/---ed_dialogue/---sector/documents/publication/wcms_196105.pdf. Accessed 27 Jun 2017.
Mukherjee A, et al. Business strategies for environmental sustainability. In: Sarkar D, et al., editors. An integrated approach to environmental management. Hoboken: Wiley; 2016. p. 195–229.
Myler L. Acquiring new customers is important, but retaining them accelerates profitable growth. 2016. https://www.forbes.com/sites/larrymyler/2016/06/08/acquiring-new-customers-is-important-but-retaining-them-accelerates-profitable-growth/#7af825766711. Accessed 6 Aug 2017.
Newman S. The great outdoors. Constructing Costco's outdoor furniture program. 2017. https://www.costco.com/patio-connection-outdoor-furniture-march-2017.html. Accessed 11 Jul 2017.
Nidumolu R, et al. Why sustainability is now the key driver of innovation. Harvard Bus Rev. 2009;87(9):56–64.
Nike, Inc. Sustainable innovation. 2017. http://about.nike.com/pages/sustainable-innovation. Accessed 9 Aug 2017.
Nike, Inc. Sustainable business report. 2016. http://www.sustainablebrands.com/digital_learning/csr_report/next_economy/nike_inc_fy1415_sustainable_business_report. Accessed 9 Aug 2017.
Norman RE, et al. Environmental exposures: an underrecognized contribution to noncommunicable diseases. Rev Environ Health. 2013;28:59–65.
Onel N, Mukherjee A. Consumer knowledge in pro-environmental behavior: an exploration of its antecedents and consequences. World J Sci Technol Sustain Dev. 2016;13(4):328–52.
O'Rourke D. Opportunities and obstacles in CSR reporting in developing countries. Berkeley: University of California; 2004.
Osborn D et al Universal sustainable development goals. Understanding the transformational challenge for developed countries. Report of a study by Stakeholder Forum. 2015. https://sustainabledevelopment.un.org/content/documents/1684SF_-_SDG_Universality_Report_-_May_2015.pdf. Accessed 30 Jun 2017.
Pollach I. Strategic corporate social responsibility: The struggle for legitimacy and reputation. Int J Bus Gov Ethics. 2015;10(1):57–75.
Porter ME, Van der Linde C. Toward a new conception of the environment-competitiveness relationship. J Econ Perspect. 1995;9(4):97–118.
PwC Global. Make it your business: engaging with the Sustainable Development Goals. 2015. http://www.PwC.com/gx/en/sustainability/SDG/SDG%20Research_FINAL.pdf. Accessed 30 Jun 2017.
RE100. Interview: Paulette Frank, vice president, environment, health, safety and sustainability. 2015. http://there100.org/johnson-johnson. Accessed 11 Jul 2017.

RED Group. Our proud partners. n.d. https://red.org/our-partners/. Accessed 30 Jun 2017.
RED Group. Working together to end AIDS. 2017. https://red.org/what-is-red/. Accessed 30 Jun 2017.
Reputation Institute. Global REPTRAK 100®. 2017. https://www.reputationinstitute.com/research/Global-RepTrak-100.aspx. Accessed 11 Jul 2017.
Richardson J. Health & wellness: Johnson & Johnson commits to new energy and climate goals. 2015. https://www.jnj.com/health-and-wellness/johnson-johnson-commits-to-new-energy-and-climate-goals. Accessed 11 Jul 2017.
RobecoSAM. DJSI investment objective. 2017. http://www.sustainability-indices.com/index-family-overview/djsi-family-overview/. Accessed 7 Aug 2017.
Rosenberg A. Corporate responsibility. Clorox 360-degree video tells safe water story. 2017. https://www.thecloroxcompany.com/blog/improving-access-to-safe-drinking-water-in-peru/#FksGXUQHB9qt7xLz.99. Accessed 9 Aug 2017.
Samy M, et al. Corporate social responsibility: a strategy for sustainable business success. An analysis of 20 selected British companies. Corp Gov. 2010;10(2):203–17. https://doi.org/10.1108/14720701011035710.
Schaefer BP. Shareholders and social responsibility. J Bus Ethics. 2008;81:297–312.
Starbucks Corporation. What is the role and responsibility of a for-profit, public company? 2017a. https://www.starbucks.com/responsibility. Accessed 11 Jul 2017.
Starbucks Corporation. Ethical sourcing: coffee. 2017b. https://www.starbucks.com/responsibility/sourcing/coffee. Accessed 11 Jul 2017.
Strauss K. The world's most reputable companies in 2017. 2017. https://www.forbes.com/sites/karstenstrauss/2017/02/28/the-worlds-most-reputable-companies-in-2017/#3ecfbd042fe3. Accessed 11 Jul 2017.
Toyota Motor Corporation. Safety and health. 2012. http://www.toyota-global.com/company/history_of_toyota/75years/data/automotive_business/production/safety/index.html. Accessed 11 Jul 2017.
Toyota Motor Corporation. Toyota Sustainability data book, basic philosophy regarding employees. 2016, pp. 46-60. http://www.toyota-global.com/sustainability/society/employees/sdb16_so06_en.pdf. Accessed 11 Jul 2017.
Toyota Motor Corporation. Company profile. 2017a. http://www.toyota-global.com/company/history_of_toyota/75years/data/conditions/company/toyota/index.html. Accessed 30 Jun 2017.
Toyota Motor Corporation. Toyota global newsroom: worldwide operations. 2017b. http://newsroom.toyota.co.jp/en/corporate/companyinformation/worldwide. Accessed 11 Jul 2017.
Toyota Motor Corporation. Toyota again named the 'World's Most Admired' motor vehicle company. 2017c. http://corporatenews.pressroom.toyota.com/releases/toyota+fortune+2017+most+admired.htm. Accessed 11 Jul 2017.
Toyota Motor Corporation. Toyota sustainability. 2017d. http://www.toyota-global.com/sustainability/index.html. Accessed 11 Jul 2017.
Toyota Motor Corporation. Aiming for a society with no traffic accident casualties to promote an integrated three part initiative: "people/vehicles/traffic environment." 2017e. http://www.toyota-global.com/innovation/safety_technology/three_part/. Accessed 30 Jun 2017.
Toyota Motor Corporation. Toyota's approaches to conflict minerals issues. 2017f. http://www.toyota-global.com/sustainability/society/human_rights/conflict-minerals-issues/. Accessed 30 Jun 2017.
United States Consumer Product Safety Commission (CPSC). Regulations, laws & standards. 2017a. https://www.cpsc.gov/Regulations-Laws--Standards. Accessed 12 Aug 2017.
United States Consumer Product Safety Commission (CPSC). Richie House children's robes recalled by Belle Investment due to violation of federal flammability standard; sold exclusively at Amazon.com. https://www.cpsc.gov/Recalls/2017/Richie-House-Childrens-Robes-Recalled-by-Belle-Investment. 2017b. Accessed 12 Aug 2017.
United Nations Environment Programme (UNEP). Sustainable trade and investment: achieving the sustainable development goals. 2015. https://wedocs.unep.org/bit-

stream/handle/20.500.11822/7602/-Sustainable_trade_and_investment_Achieving_the_sustainable_development_goals-2015Sustainable_trade_and_investment_.pdf.pdf?sequence=3&isAllowed=y. Accessed 30 Jun 2017.

United Nations (UN) Global Compact. About the UN global compact. 2017a. https://www.unglobalcompact.org/about. Accessed 7 Aug 2017.

United Nations (UN) Global Compact. The world's largest corporate sustainability initiative. 2017b. https://www.unglobalcompact.org/what-is-gc. Accessed 7 Aug 2017.

United Nations (UN) Global Compact. Global goals for people and planet. All companies can play a role. 2017c. https://www.unglobalcompact.org/sdgs/about. Accessed 7 Aug 2017.

United Nations (UN). Sustainable development knowledge platform. 2017. https://sustainabledevelopment.un.org/sdgs. Accessed 9 Aug 2017.

United States Geological Survey (USGS). Climate and land use change. Carbon sequestration. 2016. https://www2.usgs.gov/climate_landuse/carbon_seq/carbonseq.asp. Accessed 6 Aug 2017.

Werbach A. Strategy for sustainability: a business manifesto. Harvard Bus Press [online]. 2013.

Further Reading

Crane A, Matten D. Business ethics: managing corporate citizenship and sustainability in the age of globalization: Oxford University Press; 2016.

Karabell Z, Cramer A. Sustainable excellence: the future of business in a fast-changing world. New York: Rodale; 2010.

McDonough W, Braungart M. Cradle to cradle: remaking the way we make things. New York: North Point Press; 2010.

Werbach A. Strategy for sustainability: a business manifesto. Boston: Harvard Business Press; 2009.

Willard B. The new sustainability advantage: seven business case benefits of a triple bottom line. Gabrioloa Island: New Society; 2012.

Chapter 11
Upstream Policy Recommendations for Pakistan's Child Mortality Problem

Samina Panwhar and Beth Ann Fiedler

Abstract Policymakers in Pakistan continue to face challenges in reducing mortality in children under the age of five. Leading causes of death in this age category—(1) neonatal tetanus and severe infection, (2) pneumonia, (3) diarrheal disease, (4) measles, (5) injury, and (6) malaria—have been generally attributed to social, economic, and environmental factors. These include poverty, malnutrition/undernutrition, poor hygiene, unsafe water and sanitation. The nation has a legacy of commitments to achieving public health goals and demonstrated their desire to improve conditions by working towards the 2015 Millennium Development Goals (MDG) reducing the child mortality rate by approximately 42% by 2015. However, the dismal progress towards addressing child mortality and morbidity in Pakistan can be attributed to the current downstream approach. Therefore, an upstream preventive approach, considering the root causes of child injuries and death, is recommended. This chapter provides a snapshot of the nation's current health policy, recent history and encounters with natural disasters, current healthcare funding, and health profile with an emphasis on children under the age of five. The chapter puts forth policy recommendations grounded in the concept of upstream approaches in health policy that encompass social, economic, environmental, and structural factors that must be addressed to achieve a sustainable solution to child mortality in the country.

S. Panwhar (✉)
Oregon Health Authority, Salem, OR, USA

B. A. Fiedler
Independent Research Analyst, Jacksonville, FL, USA

B. A. Fiedler (ed.), *Translating National Policy to Improve Environmental Conditions Impacting Public Health Through Community Planning*,
https://doi.org/10.1007/978-3-319-75361-4_11

11.1 Parable of Upstream and Downstream Approach to Public Health

Parables are stories that reflect an analogy of a situation and present an opportunity to increase learning. In public health field, there is a parable that explains the upstream and downstream approach in addressing health problems (Meili 2013):

> Imagine you're standing on the edge of a river. Suddenly a flailing, drowning child comes floating by. Without thinking, you dive in, grab the child, and swim to shore. Before you can recover another child comes floating by. You dive in and rescue her as well.
>
> Then another child drifts into sight… and another… and another. You call for help, and people take turns fishing out child after child. Hopefully before too long some wise person will ask: Who keeps chucking these kids in the river? And they'll head upstream to find out.
>
> Every time we have to clean up an environmental disaster, every time a young person winds up in jail, every time people have to take medicines to make up for the fact that they couldn't afford good food, we're suffering from the results of downstream thinking.

The parable illustrating attempts to save drowning children downstream represents the widely used approach that is apparent in Pakistan's curative approach towards child health policy. The downstream strategy limits Pakistan's ability to address underlying causes of child mortality and recurrence of the childhood health problems that warrants a directional change. The upstream approach signifies the thinking where the focus is to identify the root causes of the problem and address those before they lead to child mortality and morbidity. Saving the children before they are underwater will require a fundamental shift at addressing environmental, economic, and social conditions that elicit positive health outcomes using prevention strategies.

11.2 Introduction

The current health policy in Pakistan, a developing region in southeast Asia, has been characterized as both committed to improving public health and one in which little priority public health funding is evident to address the urgent needs of the sixth most populous country in the world with 190 million residents. The most pressing concern is the child mortality rate that prematurely takes the lives of over half million children under the age of five placing Pakistan as the fourth leading nation in child mortality behind India, Nigeria, and China (WHO 2017a). Geographically, the country is surrounded by the Arabian Sea at the southern border and four countries—Iran, Afghanistan, China, and India—a mix of culturally and religiously divergent nations with their own aspirations to improve upon their national status and quality of life. Even within her own borders, an influx of immigrants from Afghanistan, four regionally defined provinces and a federally administered tribal area compete for limited national funds across diverse and often treacherous terrain.

Before understanding the scope of the problem of child mortality, taking into consideration the nation's geopolitical concerns, recent history and encounters with natural disasters are key to understanding the difficulties in translating a national commitment and expanding capacity to improve public health under these pressing circumstances.

11.2.1 Commitment to Public Health

Pakistan was a signatory to Alma Ata Declaration of 1978 (WHO 1978), based on the principle of the health as a right, promoting financial allocation as the major commitment towards achieving public health goals. During this time, the Pakistani policymakers visited China and other developing countries to seek effective health policies that would lead to achieving the declaration goals.

The treaty did establish some important definitions and human rights considerations beginning with health as a "state of physical, mental, and social well-being, and not merely the absence of disease and infirmity." The idea of the social determinants of health was rooted in this declaration and the People's Health Charter which evolved at the first People's Health Assembly at Gonoshasthaya Kendra (GK)—Savar in Bangladesh on 8th December 2000 (Khan 2006; WHO 2017c). The charter also endorsed the principles and practice of universal, comprehensive primary healthcare as outlined in the Alma Ata Declaration.

Promoting a framework to move commitment to practical application, the World Conference on Social Determinants of Health was held in Switzerland in 2012 where World Health Organization (WHO) member states adopted the Rio Political Declaration focusing on five key areas (WHO 2017c):

- Adopt improved governance for health and development
- Promote participation in policy-making and implementation
- Further reorient the health sector towards promoting health and reducing health inequities
- Strengthen global governance and collaboration
- Monitor progress and increase accountability

Together, these fundamental commitments provide a common platform from which to draw national and international public health policy. Several decades after Pakistan's engagement in these promising global efforts, their health sector remains void of policies that address the root causes of the most prevalent diseases that lead to child morbidity and mortality.

11.2.2 Recent Geopolitical Concerns and Political History

Pakistan's political history has been volatile since their independence in 1947 (Khan 2006). With the majority of its 70-year history under military rule, both the military and democratic governments have been generally focused on either strengthening the military or advancing personal gains and ideologies. As a result, underprivileged segments of society have suffered causing the social indicators to drop much lower than other developing countries of similar economies.

Geographic location and population density are often the impetus for geopolitical tension and activity. Such is the case for Pakistan and two of her neighboring countries—India and Afghanistan. Since the partition in 1947, Pakistan and India have been involved in several major conflicts and wars mainly over the possession of Kashmir. The war of 1971, which originated in East Pakistan, resulted in the formation of Bangladesh rendering economic loss and further weakening of the political system. During the Soviet invasion of Afghanistan and the United States intervention from 1978 to 1980, Pakistan being the border country was used as a buffer state in the fight against Soviet occupation of Afghanistan (Khan 2006). This conflict resulted in thousands of refugees migrating into the country from Afghanistan, which further added complexity to the social fabric of the country (Mohiuddin 2006). More recently, home-grown terrorism and an influx of religious fundamentalists from neighboring Afghanistan have created havoc in many parts of the country jeopardizing security and well-being of the citizens. Frequent bomb attacks in populated areas have rendered scores of people dead including young children.

The country is also a land of contrasts with greatly varying climatic zones and topography: "towering mountain ranges, jagged and snow-capped peaks, vast glaciers, gushing rivers, dry plateaus, fertile plains, lush valleys, arid deserts, and hundreds of miles of almost uninhabited sandy beaches" (Mohiuddin 2006, p.6). This ecological and cultural diversity is reflected in varying levels of social development in the country as well as the urban-rural divide in each province. The overall urban population of the country is about 33%, but there are huge variations between the provinces—merely 17% in NWFP and almost 50% in Sindh, which is mainly attributed to the urban population of Karachi accounting for 30% of the Sindh's population and approximately 7% of the total population of the country (Mohiuddin 2006, p.22).

However, the need to maintain a large military budget should become apparent from these cursory examples. Further, military expenditures are one reason why healthcare expenditures and services to the poor continue to have a low priority (Khan 2006). Another problem that emerges is the dispersal of the population throughout the nation with various topography creating a barrier to services. Accounting for additional costs to transport vaccines and other goods into areas with limited infrastructure adds a significant cost to distribution and is often prohibitive in most circumstances.

Despite these immense challenges throughout the history of the country, Pakistan has managed to maintain a high growth rate—close to 6%, with sustained growth projected in the next 10 years (Zahid 2017, *para* 1). This economic indicator, however, is not reflected in the social indicators of the country.

11.2.3 Encounters with Natural Disasters

Pakistan has suffered from several major natural disasters (e.g., droughts, floods, earthquakes) since the country was established 70 years ago. During the drought of 2000 lasting over 10 months, about 1.2 million people were affected including over 100 lives lost and millions of animals perished because of dehydration in Balochistan

(IRIN 2010). In 2005, a mega earthquake hit the Kashmir region on the border of Pakistan and India and parts of northwestern Pakistan killing 73,000 people and leaving 3.3 million homeless. Most recently in 2010, heavy floods affected over six million people and caused 1600 deaths. Conditions following natural disasters leave scores of people displaced without proper shelter, food, water, and sanitation, worsening an already problematic situation. Further, notable spikes in diseases after these incidents disproportionately impact children.

11.3 Scope of Pakistan's Child Mortality and Their Social Determinants

While the under-five child mortality rate (per 1000 live births) declined from 139 in 1990 to 81 in 2015, the numbers fell short of the MDG target of 46 by 2015 (World Bank 2017). Numerous research studies and data collected on the subject have established that the underlying causes for most childhood illnesses and deaths are factors related to the social conditions of health referring to the conditions in which people are born, live and grow (WHO 2017c). Key aspects of these conditions include poverty, malnutrition/undernutrition, poor hygiene, unsafe water and sanitation, and other social, economic, and environmental factors.

The major cause of child mortality in Pakistan is neonatal tetanus and severe infection followed by preventable diseases such as pneumonia, diarrhea, measles, injury, and malaria (Fig. 11.1) According to WHO estimates, 83% of under-five deaths are caused by infectious, neonatal, and nutritional conditions (WHO 2017a). Neonatal disease classification has several underlying causes of death including severe infection, birth asphyxia, preterm birth, neonatal tetanus, congenital abnormalities, diarrheal diseases, and others.

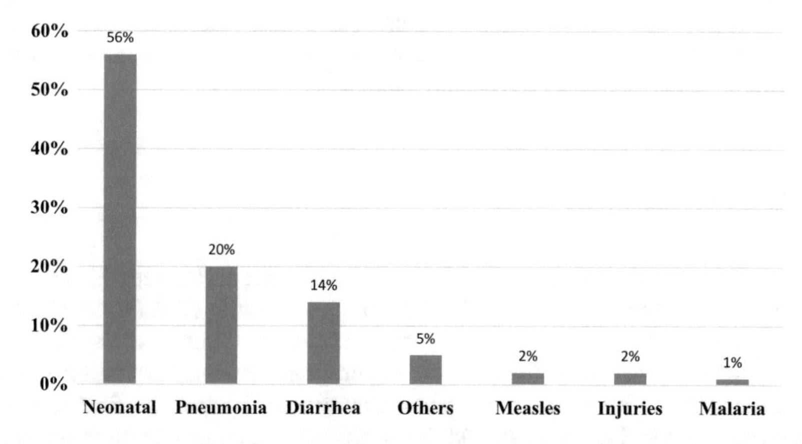

Fig. 11.1 Causes of under age five mortality in Pakistan, 2014. Source: The World Bank Group 2017

11.3.1 Neonatal Causes of Morbidity

Pakistan had the third highest rate of neonatal mortality in the world in 2004 with a rate of 55 deaths per 1000 live births (Nisar and Dibley 2014, p.1) down one notch to fourth with a reported rate of 45.5 deaths per 1000 live births in 2015 (WHO 2017a; WHO 2016). Consequently, Pakistan has incorporated newborn care into national health policy at all hospitals as one measure to address this dismal situation. In the conventional three-tier health system, there are currently 965 tertiary and secondary hospitals and 13,051 primary care facilities in the country. Access to these facilities, however, is very low due to distant/inconvenient locations of the healthcare facilities, restricted hours of operation, poor infrastructure within and outside healthcare facilities, lack of staff, equipment, and drugs, and affordability (Nisar and Dibley 2014). These limitations prevent the households from gaining access to preventive healthcare measures such as immunization against tuberculosis, polio, measles, neonatal tetanus, and smallpox. Availability of healthcare facilities and services, however, is a partial solution to this problem. High rates of neonatal mortality are linked with social determinants which are now well established by several studies on the subject. For instance, the level of education of parents (Nisar and Dibley 2014) plays a major role in dictating the neonatal health and mortality outcomes. In the absence of education and health awareness, parents are unable to make informed decisions about timely immunization and other health and well-being requirements for their children. Furthermore, less educated parents are less likely to communicate to their children simple preventive measures, such as handwashing, that can lead to improved health conditions.

Other factors such as the housing conditions or a lack of housing, access to nutritious food, availability of clean water and adequate sanitation, and access to healthcare are dependent upon the economic status of a household (Mahmood 2002). Maternal factors such as the age of mother and birth order and interval also have a significant impact on the survival of neonates. The significance of breastfeeding is well recognized as the most important factor in neonate health and survival; however, breastfeeding remains underutilized due to factors such as parental education, mother's nutrition, and other household conditions.

11.3.2 Pneumonia

Pakistan is among the top five countries in the world that account for 99% of pneumonia cases leading to more than 92,000 children annually (The Express Tribune 2015). Although Pakistan has the "Extended Program on Immunization" that offers free pneumonia vaccination for children, the program remains underutilized to the extent that about 46% of the child population are not immunized. Prevalence of malnutrition is considered as an additional obstacle when providing treatment to children affected with pneumonia (The Express Tribune 2015).

Many of these deaths occur in underserved parts of the country due to several primary reasons including the lack of parental education, women's dependency on men for taking the children to see the health provider, transportation constraints, and access to quality health services (Hazir 2008). Most households in Pakistan do not own personal vehicles, and instead they rely on public transportation, such as buses, or may own motor bikes presenting an additional risk for children riding without helmets. Cultural restrictions do not generally allow women to access public transportation unescorted and thus rely on male family member to accompany them.

11.3.3 Diarrheal Disease

Diarrhea is one of the leading causes of child mortality globally, accounting for 9% deaths among children under the age of 5 years old or about 526,000 children each year (UNICEF 2017). Deaths resulting from diarrhea in Pakistan, about 125,000 annually, account for nearly one-fourth of the global deaths placing the nation in the top five countries facing the devastation resulting from this problem. Standard diarrhea treatment protocol in Pakistan is managed by providing patients with a combination of zinc and Oral Rehydration Salts (ORS). Research studies have shown that zinc and ORS reduce the severity and duration of diarrhea by more than 40% (Dawn 2013, *para* 7). However, the implementation of these healthcare programs is not widely adopted and is prevalent only in about 5% of the country.

The Integrated Global Action Plan for the Prevention and Control of Pneumonia and Diarrhea (GAPPD) put forth an integrated framework with key evidence based interventions to address these children's health problems (UNICEF and WHO 2013). These interventions include providing breastfeeding in the first 6 months of life, complementary nutritious feeding, vitamin A supplements, immunization against rotavirus, and most importantly safe drinking water, sanitation, and hygiene. Around 60% deaths are attributable to unsafe drinking water, lack of proper sanitation, and hygiene globally. Handwashing alone can reduce the risk of diarrhea by 40%, according to the GAPPD, but access to water in many regions remains problematic (UNICEF and WHO 2013).

11.3.4 Measles

Measles virus is highly contagious virus and spreads through the air through coughing and sneezing. Measles, mumps, and rubella (MMR) vaccine is quite effective in preventing measles. More than 14, 000 reported cases of measles in Pakistan affecting mostly children resulted in 210 deaths in 2012 (Niazi and Sadaf 2014, p.1). Measles vaccination is administrated in two doses in Pakistan, at 9 months and 2 years of age. The coverage for the first dose has improved but the second dose coverage remains very low. The causes of low coverage have been associated with health sector corruption, weak health management, poor health infrastructure, negligence among parents, influx of unvaccinated refugees, and lack of training of health professionals regarding correct vaccine administration according to defined schedule (Niazi and Sadaf 2014). While measles alone is rarely fatal, the disease can lead to serious complications, such as meningitis and pneumonia, especially in children with malnutrition and low immunity (Galpin 2013).

11.3.5 Injuries

Injury is the sixth leading cause of death in Pakistan for children under the age of 5 with 39.5 deaths per 100,000 every year (Razzak et al. 2013, p.1) and the third major cause of mortality for children ages 1–5 years old (Razzak et al. 2013, p.1). The total injury related deaths are around 9800 per year for the under-five population (Razzak et al. 2013, p.3). The most common injuries include drowning, road traffic accidents, burns, and falls.

Injury-related child mortality is significantly higher in rural areas, 32 per 100,000 compared to 15 per 100,000 in urban areas (Razzak et al. 2013, p.1). All these injuries are preventable with intervention strategies that are widely used in other parts of the world. Some of the simple interventions include securing water bodies, creating childproof containers for hazardous household substances/drugs, speed control near schools and other sensitive areas, securing staircases and roofs against falls, securing household cooking stoves to prevent burns, and helmet laws for bicyclists and motorcycles. Educating parents about child safety is another step to decreasing injuries.

11.3.6 Malaria

Pakistan is categorized in Group 3 countries of the WHO Eastern Mediterranean Region with estimated 95% or 1.5 million annual cases of malaria in that sector. Other countries include Afghanistan, Djibouti, Somalia, South Sudan, Sudan, and Yemen. Over 500,000 individuals are infected causing 50,000 deaths each year in the country. Approximately 95 million of the total 160 million Pakistan's 2010 population lived in malaria endemic regions, the prevalence varies by province and between districts within provinces (Khattak et al. 2013, p.1). Of the total, 37% of the disease burden occurs along the international borders with Afghanistan and Iran (Kakar et al. 2010, p.1).

The main causes of the diseases are associated with mass movement of population within the country, mainly from rural to urban areas; low immune status of the population; climate changes; socioeconomic conditions; poor health infrastructure; resource constraints; lack of access to preventive and curative services; and increasing drug and insecticide resistance in parasites and vectors. Monsoon rains and vast irrigation networks also contribute to breeding grounds for disease carrying mosquitos in many regions. Children, especially under the age of five, are prone to malaria with 86% deaths occurring in this age group (Hussain et al. 2013, p.343).

11.4 Low Health Expenditures

Pakistan spends very little, i.e., about 1% of GDP on health despite overwhelming evidence that supports the need for increased funding, recognition of the value of health as a right, and increasing health budgets in the last 2 years (Bilal 2017, *para* 17). While eight of every 100 children die before reaching the age of 5 years, Pakistan continues to spend 18% of its budget on the defense and almost 32% on debt servicing while less than 1% on health (Bilal 2017, *para* 9).

In the 1980s, the WHO made a minimum health spending recommendation of 5% of GDP that represented the highest global percentage spent on health at the time (Savedoff 2007). In the last few decades, however, the health spending in some countries has surpassed that recommendation while Pakistan remains one of the few countries in the world with <3% health expenditure (WHO 2017b) illustrated in Fig. 11.2. These budget priorities reflect a disproportionate appropriation for military defense and debt servicing when compared to the concern for public health and well-being of their vulnerable population.

The problem of the cost of debt servicing is important to the number of debts, amount of debts, and the high interest costs associated with repayment that further

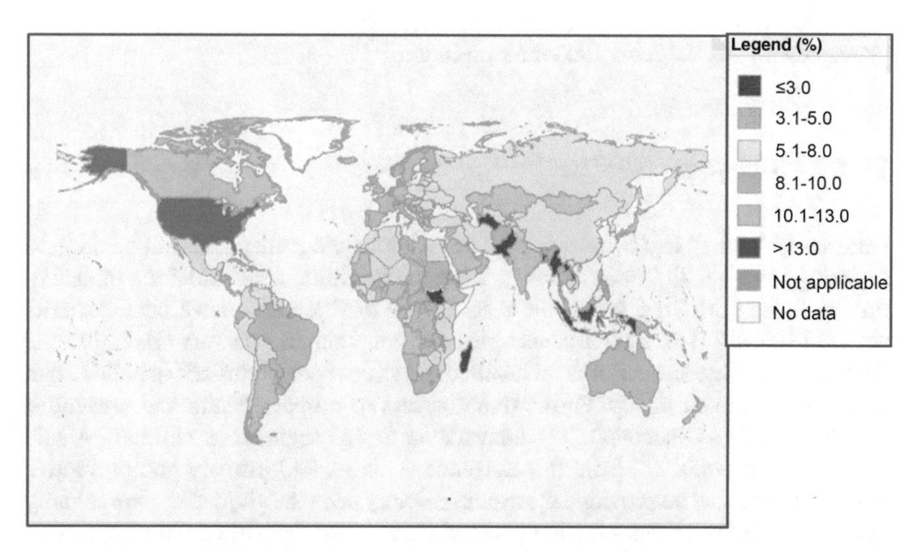

Fig. 11.2 Total expenditure on health as a percentage of the gross domestic product (%), 2014 (WHO 2017b, used by permission)

decrease health funding. Thus, the problem of child mortality in Pakistan is not solely associated with the dearth of resources; it is due to lack of innovation in government resource strategy, broken healthcare systems, and inefficient allocation of health resources.

11.5 Discussion and Upstream Policy Recommendations

Pakistan has taken a "downstream approach" in addressing child mortality and morbidity. The causes of most of the health issues leading to this plight are preventable or can be mitigated to some extent improving the present situation. Educating parents in their communities and incorporating interventions related to antenatal care and training to healthcare providers to manage childbirth-related complications are two essential steps to improving health outcomes.

Numerous regional, national, and international efforts and millions of dollars invested in different programs have not yielded promising results. Most of these efforts are curative (downstream) rather than preventive. Furthermore, most of these programs are incoherent and only function in isolation. Recommendations that utilize an "upstream approach" focusing on the social, economic, environmental, and institutional determinants of the health may provide the foundation for an improved strategy in combating child mortality. Initiating an upstream approach requires that Pakistan invest in the future generation and overall quality of life by allocating more funds towards public health by decreasing spending on defense and other areas that do not benefit the people. The introduction of intersectoral collaboration and cooperation could be at the center of child health policies to meet the immediate population needs through adequate shelter, nutrition, water and sanitation, solid waste management, and reducing indoor air pollution.

11.5.1 Adequate Shelter

Pakistan is "home" to 1.5 million children without adequate shelter. In addition to suffering from health issues resulting from malnutrition, heat/cold, lack of sanitation and clean drinking water, more than 90% of these kids have been sexually abused (Styles 2014). Sexual abuse presents compounding factors leading to the destruction of physical and mental health that has not been addressed in child health or law enforcement policy. Furthermore, access to primary health and preventive measures, such as vaccination, is unavailable to this segment of children. A safe shelter can protect them from this horrendous abuse, and primary and preventive healthcare can also be provided more conveniently once the child is in a community setting. Providing shelters for homeless children must be part of the discourse in devising child health policies in Pakistan and may include the development of a foster care system to more easily transition children to safe havens.

11.5.2 Nutrition

Nutrition is a major factor in defining child health. There are various avenues to ensuring sufficient nutrition for children, especially those that are under the age of five. Most diseases leading to child mortality and morbidity are due to malnutrition and low immunity. For instance, diarrhea in a child concurrently suffering from malnutrition will most likely lead to a more serious health condition or mortality because of lower resistance to disease. Although policies around nutrition can be complex in a resource deficient country like Pakistan, some practical approaches can be implemented. Free lunch programs in schools have shown encouraging results in many countries such as Sri Lanka (Riley 2008). Providing free meals at school not only provides adequate nutrition to children improving their immunity towards disease but also encourages them to stay in school and continue their education producing long-term positive effects.

11.5.3 Water and Sanitation

Access to adequate water is immensely critical and one of the most challenging elements to address. Although the literature shows 97% Pakistan's population as having access to improved water, the data is misleading for several reasons. First, the water supply infrastructure is in disrepair. Second, in those areas where there is an intermittent supply, sporadic water supply pulls contaminants into the line delivering water that is unsuitable for human consumption. Third, while the middle and upper class can purchase bottled water, many must rely on the tap water or wells and lakes in rural areas. Fourth, while home water supplies may undergo some sort of treatment to reduce contaminants, the ad hoc methods may not be sufficient to permit safe consumption contributing to recurring and increasing cases of diarrhea in children.

Numerous local nonprofit and international programs are engaged in addressing the problem of improved water and sanitation; however, they lack a concerted and sustainable effort. Considering the existing resource limitations, repairs of the entire infrastructure may not be a feasible option for Pakistan. Instead, the focus should be to develop community level, small-scale water treatment systems. Several examples of the small-scale water treatment systems have proven to be successful and sustainable.

Poor sanitation including open defecation leads to numerous health problems in children living in those areas. Recurring episodes of diarrhea in children and chronic issues, such as stunting and malnutrition, are associated with poor sanitation and contaminated drinking water. Approximately 41 million in Pakistan do not have access to a household toilet leading to complex health problems including violence against women and girls who may unintentionally expose themselves in public. A concerted effort is needed that focuses on educating the population on the significance of proper sanitation, hazards of open defecation, and health benefits of constructing low-cost toilets in their homes. Additionally, public schools should be equipped with toilets for boys and girls to help improve regular attendance of children in schools.

11.5.4 Solid Waste Management

Pakistan generated more than 20 million tons of solid waste annually and that number is growing exponentially with increasing population and rapid urbanization. Regulation of solid waste management is void despite the existence of an environmental ministry and environmental laws. The problem is reflected in the piles of waste seen on most streets and roadsides. Burning of waste in streets and public areas is very common which leads to the release of toxins into the air. The major victims of this situation are the homeless people including young children who are exposed to fecal matter, improperly disposed medical waste, and other hazardous materials. Most of the street children spend their day scavenging the piles of this waste collecting glass, plastic, copper, aluminum, and other metals to sell for food but the earnings are insufficient for daily nutritional requirements. Consequently, these children suffer from diarrhea, respiratory diseases, infected wounds, and numerous other health problems. About 4 million children die each year from waste-related diseases in Pakistan (Zahidi 2014).

Management of waste is the number one step towards improving public health without which management of complex services (e.g., advanced healthcare, education, transportation) cannot achieve an acceptable level of sustainable effectiveness (World Bank 2012). Local governments, under new federal directives and government support, should consider public awareness and education initiatives that focus on the proper collection and disposal of waste supporting improved population health.

11.5.5 Indoor Air Pollution

Surprisingly, about two-thirds of Pakistan's nearly 200 million people live in rural areas where the average household size is 6.8 persons (Fatmi et al. 2010). Biomass (e.g., wood, charcoal, agricultural residues, dung) is the main source of fuel for cooking and heating in Pakistan. The process of burning biomass, coupled with small house sizes and a lack of ventilation, contributes to indoor air pollution leading to more than 50,000 deaths in under-five children in the country (Fatmi et al. 2010, p.3). The problem is further exasperated in households when natural fuels are unavailable due to the practice of burning plastic bottles and polythene bags resulting in additional hazardous materials in the air.

Several nongovernmental organizations have introduced safer stoves for the rural population that have proven to be smoke free and more efficient (Ebrahim 2010).

Design elements have also been reported to be very simple enabling women to build them using local materials. Scaling up these efforts will require concerted efforts from government and nongovernmental organization (NGO) groups. But something as simple as smoke-free stoves can save lives of thousands of children downstream.

11.6 Conclusion

Reevaluating and revising Pakistan's child health policies to promote improved health outcomes should become a priority in view of the half million annual deaths that occur in the under-five years old age category. Numerous local and international efforts have been underway to address various aspects of child health but all with meager results. The reasons for the lackluster performance include insufficient budget allocation, lack of concerted efforts, and a lack of focus on the social determinants of health which are at the root of morbidity and mortality in children. Instead of the current downstream approach which mainly focuses on the treatment of disease, an upstream approach is needed that considers the root causes of the health issues. Based on the discussion above, three key policy directions are highly recommended:

1. Increase budget allocation to health and social determinants of health. WHO recommends 5% of country's budget towards health; Pakistan currently allocates about 1% of the budget.
2. Intersectoral coordination considering social determinants of health as discussed above. Child health policy goes beyond the realm of the health department. Due to the strong impact of social determinants on health, a broad collaborative approach is critical in addressing the problem.
3. A coordinated effort involving local, national, and international actors must be implemented to realize the optimum benefits. The current ad hoc activities involve numerous local and international NGOs as well as government providing sporadic solutions with disappointing results.

Glossary

Biomass Animal or plant based material such as wood and coal used as fuel

Neonatal The first 4 weeks of life after birth

Social determinants of health Conditions in which people are born, grow, live, and work; examples include economic status, environmental quality, access to healthy food and clean water, and access to green spaces.

Three-tier health system of Pakistan Pakistan's health system is three-tiered with management of responsibilities divided between federal, provincial, and district governments.

References

Bilal Z. Understand the federal budget 2017-18 [Online]. The Daily Times. 2017. http://dailytimes.com.pk/pakistan/07-Jun-17/understand-the-federal-budget-2017-18. Accessed 19 June 2017.

DAWN. 2013. Pakistan among top five diarrhoea death victims [Online]. https://www.dawn.com/news/1077426. Accessed 19 June 2017.

Ebrahim Z. Pakistan: smoke-free stoves a godsend for village women [Online]. Inter Press Service News Agency. 2010. http://www.ipsnews.net/2010/02/pakistan-smoke-free-stoves-a-godsend-for-village-women/. Accessed 18 June 2017.

Fatmi Z, et al. Situational analysis of household energy and biomass use and associated health burden of indoor air pollution and mitigation efforts in Pakistan. Int J Environ Res Public Health. 2010;7:2940–52. https://doi.org/10.3390/ijerph7072.

Galpin R. Fighting Pakistan's measles epidemic [Online]. BBC News. 2013. http://www.bbc.com/news/world-latin-america-22724080. Accessed 18 June 2017.

Hazir T. Pneumonia: no. 1 killer of Pakistan's children. Bull World Health Organ. 2008;86(5):330–1. https://doi.org/10.2471/BLT.08.040508.

Hussain K, et al. Seroprevalence of pediatric malaria in Quetta, Balochistan, Pakistan. Iranian J Parasitol. 2013;8(2):342–7.

IRIN. The top 10 natural disasters since 1935 [Online]. 2010. http://www.irinnews.org/news/2010/08/10. Accessed 18 June 2017.

Kakar Q, et al. Malaria control in Pakistan: new tools at hand but challenging epidemiological realities. East Mediterr Health J. 2010;16:S54–60.

Khan KS. Social determinants of health in Pakistan: the glass is more than half empty. 2006. https://assets.publishing.service.gov.uk/media/57a08c29ed915d622c00117d/Khan_Socialdeterminants.pdf. Accessed 18 June 2017.

Khattak AA, et al. Prevalence and distribution of human *Plasmodium* infection in Pakistan. Malar J. 2013;2:297. https://doi.org/10.1186/1475-2875-12-297.

Mahmood MA. Determinants of neonatal and post-neonatal mortality in Pakistan. Pak Dev Rev. 2002;41(4 Part II):723–44.

Meili R. Upstream: talking differently about health. 2013. http://www.thinkupstream.net/upstream_talking_differently_about_health. Accessed 19 June 2017.

Mohiuddin YN. Pakistan: a global studies handbook. Santa Barbara, CA: ABC CLIO, Inc.; 2006.

Niazi AK, Sadaf R. Measles epidemic in Pakistan: in search of solutions. Ann Med Health Sci Res. 2014;4(1):1–2. https://doi.org/10.4103/2141-9248.126600.

Nisar YB, Dibley MJ. Determinants of neonatal mortality in Pakistan: secondary analysis of Pakistan Demographic and Health Survey 2006–07. BMC Public Health. 2014;14:663. https://doi.org/10.1186/1471-2458-14-663.

Razzak JA, et al. A child an hour: burden of injury deaths among children under 5 in Pakistan. Arch Dis Child. 2013;98(11):867–71. https://doi.org/10.1136/archdischild-2013-303654.

Riley JC. Low income, social growth, and good health: a history of twelve countries. (California/Milbank Books on Health and the Public.). Berkeley/Los Angeles: University of California Press, with Milbank Memorial Fund; 2008.

Savedoff WD. What should a country spend on healthcare? Health Aff. 2007;26(4):962–70. https://doi.org/10.1377/hlthaff.26.4.962.

Styles R. Why thousands of Pakistani children are falling prey to paedophiles [Online]. Daily Mail. 2014. http://www.dailymail.co.uk/femail/article-2739799/Why-millions-Pakistani-children-falling-prey-vicious-paedophiles.html#ixzz4kSol75nL. Accessed 19 June 2017.

The Express Tribune. 92,000 children die of pneumonia in Pakistan every year [Online]. 2015. https://tribune.com.pk/story/988945/92000-children-die-of-pneumonia-in-pakistan-every-year/. Accessed 19 June 2017.

The World Bank. What a waste: a global review of solid waste management. 2012. http://documents.worldbank.org/curated/en/302341468126264791/pdf/68135-REVISED-What-a-Waste-2012-Final-updated.pdf. Accessed 19 June 2017.

The World Bank Group. Mortality rate, under-5 (per 1,000 live births). 2017. http://data.worldbank.org/indicator/SH.DYN.MORT?locations=PK. Accessed 18 June 2017.
United Nations Children's Fund (UNICEF). Diarrhoea remains a leading killer of young children, despite the availability of a simple treatment solution. 2017. https://data.unicef.org/topic/child-health/diarrhoeal-disease. Accessed 19 June 2017.
United Nations Children's Fund (UNICEF) and World Health Organization (WHO). Integrated global action plan for the prevention and control of pneumonia and diarrhoea. 2013. https://www.defeatdd.org/global-action-plan-pneumonia-diarrhea. Accessed 14 Aug 2017.
World Health Organization (WHO). Declaration of Alma-Ata international conference on primary health care, Alma-Ata, USSR, 6–12 September 1978. 1978. http://www.who.int/publications/almaata_declaration_en.pdf. Accessed 18 Jun 2017.
World Health Organization (WHO). Global Health Observatory country views, Pakistan statistics summary (2002 - present). [Last updated 19 Jul 2017]. 2016. http://apps.who.int/gho/data/node.country.country-PAK. Accessed 14 Aug 2017.
World Health Organization (WHO). Global health observatory (GHO) data: child health. 2017a. http://www.who.int/maternal_child_adolescent/epidemiology/child/en/index.html. Accessed 18 June 2017.
World Health Organization (WHO). Total expenditure on health as a percentage of gross domestic product (US$). 2017b. http://www.who.int/gho/health_financing/total_expenditure/en/. Accessed 18 June 2017.
World Health Organization (WHO). What are social determinants of health? 2017c. http://www.who.int/social_determinants/sdh_definition/en/. Accessed 18 June 2017.
Zahid W. Pakistan's GDP growth rate is even higher than that of China: Harvard study [Online]. The Express Tribune. 2017. https://tribune.com.pk/story/1452332/pakistans-gdp-growth-rate-even-higher-china-harvard-study/. Accessed 14 Sept 2017.
Zahidi F. Worries pile up as waste grows in Pakistan [Online]. Alzazerra. 2014. http://www.aljazeera.com/indepth/features/2014/08/solid-waste-pakistan-karachi-2014867512833362.html. Accessed 19 June 2017.

Further Reading

United Nations Children's Fund (UNICEF). Levels and trends in child mortality. Report 2015. Estimates developed by the UN inter-agency group for child mortality estimation, New York. 2014. http://www.childmortality.org/files_v20/download/IGME%20Report%202015_9_3%20LR%20Web.pdf. Accessed 14 Aug 2017.
World Life Expectancy. Health profile: Pakistan. 2017. http://www.worldlifeexpectancy.com/country-health-profile/pakistan. Accessed 14 Aug 2017.
Beyond health care: the role of social determinants in promoting health and health equity. 2015. http://www.kff.org/disparities-policy/issue-brief/beyond-health-care-the-role-of-social-determinants-in-promoting-health-and-health-equity/. Accessed 10 Sept 2017.

Chapter 12
Water Quality: Mindanao Island of the Philippines

Angelo Mark P. Walag, Oliva P. Canencia, and Beth Ann Fiedler

Abstract The Philippines is an archipelagic country dominated by water and inland water sources. Water quality has been the subject of attention for the country and specifically, Mindanao Island, because of the role this natural resource plays in agriculture. Water supply and usage for the island and the nation are identified and discussed in relation to the scarcity of potable water. Potential threats and pollution hotspots bring forth the various health and environmental impact attributed to the water system accessibility, distribution, and quality. Strategies addressing water resources problems are taken into consideration side-by-side the numerous national laws, policies, standards, and guidelines in addressing water quality control and management. Therefore, the legal framework for various agencies to carry out these policies on quality control, usage, and water management are pivotal to recommendations on revision of certain provisions that rely on embedding local community involvement to lessen the environmental impact that is causal to poor population health. The World Bank has been instrumental in prompting local activity with initiatives first established in relation to the United Nations Millennium Development Goals that are being carried forward today in the Sustainable Development Initiatives. This chapter extends the recent UN and World Bank initiatives to demonstrate how further community involvement can continue to improve quality of life for Philippine citizens through education and participation.

A. M. P. Walag (✉)
Department of Science Education, University of Science and Technology of Southern Philippines, College of Science and Technology Education,
Cagayan de Oro, Misamis Oriental, Philippines

O. P. Canencia
Research Division, University of Science and Technology of Southern Philippines, College of Science and Mathematics, Cagayan de Oro, Misamis Oriental, Philippines

B. A. Fiedler
Independent Research Analyst, Jacksonville, FL, USA

B. A. Fiedler (ed.), *Translating National Policy to Improve Environmental Conditions Impacting Public Health Through Community Planning*,
https://doi.org/10.1007/978-3-319-75361-4_12

12.1 Introduction and Background

Living on an island nation with multiple natural water resources did not guarantee access to clean water for the 75% of the Philippine population that has low socio-economic status and live in rural villages called barangays (United Nations 2017, *para* 2). However, global concern generated by the introduction of the United Nations (UN) Millennium Development Goals (MDGs) (United Nations 2015) and a steady flow of financial support from the World Bank at $638.1 million (United Nations 2017, *para* 7; World Bank 2014) provides guidance and funding that led to the development of important national legislation and the enactment of institutions to respond to these and other community needs. Stronger institutions represent greater opportunities for citizen engagement through community-driven development (CDD) initiatives prompted by the UN. CDD is a platform for citizens to "make their own decisions in identifying, developing, implementing, and monitoring development initiatives based on their priorities" (United Nations 2017, *para* 2).

The progression of moving policy decision-making process from global initiatives to national initiatives began first with the UN establishing internal partnerships with existing Philippine government institutions, such as the Department of Social Welfare and Development and the National Statistical Coordination Board, providing community access and local monitoring. The UN also had external development partnerships, such as the Japan Social Development Social Fund and several governments, which were instrumental in developing important internal mechanisms and metrics based on monitoring the MDGS (United Nations 2017). These metrics establish empirical evidence for decision-making with the long-term goals of a healthy environment and population. "The monitoring of the MDGs taught us that data are an indispensable element of the development agenda," and that "what gets measured gets done" (United Nations 2015, p.10).

Monitoring at the turn of the millennium quickly brought forth data indicating the leading water consumers, the problem of scarcity of water resources, and other threats to the availability of potable water that remains problematic in the nation. The baseline established the disproportionate use of agricultural consumption for irrigation and fisheries (Greenpeace 2007) accounting for 85.27% of the total water supply followed by the industrial sector (7.46%) and the remaining 7.27% for domestic consumption (World Bank 2004, p.29). Further, differentiating groundwater and piped-water supply systems sources was instrumental in revealing harmful practices in which groundwater extraction is done without permit. This indiscriminate and unregulated method of withdrawal led to the enactment of Executive Order No. 123 Series of 2012. The order mandates the transfer of National Water Resources Board (NWRB) from the Department of Public Works and Highways (DPWH) to the Office of the President then to the Department of Environment and Natural Resources' (DENR) jurisdiction. Furthermore, the NWRB was tasked to immediately review the implementing rules and regulations of the Water Code of the Philippines (Barba 2004). These modifications to multiple water agencies and the introduction of new legislation were brought into action to regulate, monitor, and redistribute usage of water resources but distribution remains the same

Table 12.1 Total population served by different water service providers by region as of 2007 (Israel 2009)

Region	Water district	LGU[a]	RWSA[b]/BWSA[c]	Cooperatives	Total population served
Region 9[d]	135,000	109,590	7208	510	252,308
Region 10[e]	190,435	159,930	40,146	0	388,511
Region 11[f]	285,596	47,932	28,586	27,151	389,265
Region 12[g]	149,002	4842	0	0	153,844
ARMM[h]	123,455	35,740	0	0	159,195

[a]Local Government Units
[b]Rural Water Supply Associations
[c]Barangay Water Supply Associations
[d]Zamboanga Peninsula
[e]Northern Mindanao
[f]Davao Region
[g]Soccsksargen
[h]Autonomous Region in Muslim Mindanao

today. Further, the water agencies struggle with interagency integration, manpower shortages, and lack of financial resource allocation at the local levels often rendering their mandated efforts ineffective (Rola et al. 2015).

The success of the UN MDG targets in the Philippines were evident meeting goals to improve access to drinking water up from 85% of the population in 1990 to 92% in 2010 (Fehr et al. 2013, p.638) but several challenges remain. Improved water sources (e.g., bottled, regulated water refilling stations) (Israel 2009; Madrazo 2002; Magtibay 2004; UNICEF and WHO 2012), an adequate freshwater supply and high rate of precipitation contributed to improvements (see Table 12.1). However, several factors such as biased geographic distribution, seasonal variations, and water shortages based on population distribution remain problematic (Barba 2004; Dumlao 2016; Ranada 2015). Damage to infrastructure due to civil unrest (Malapit et al. 2003) and the long history of the southern part of the Philippines being disenfranchised and underrepresented in the government is apparent in the lack of infrastructure projects there (Clausen 2010; Silva 2005) providing a historical basis leading to the present conditions. Furthermore, investments and policies crafted to better provide water access have been greatly affected by these conflicts (Clausen 2010). Earlier analysis of these political factors (e.g., institutional deficiencies, weak regulatory policies, lack of government leadership and political will, and lack of an integrated water resources management system) (Madrazo 2002) continue to pose additional barriers to the water crisis. Therefore, the legal framework on water quality, use and management are important factors for any proposed solutions.

The National Water Resources Board (NWRB) and Japan International Cooperation Agency (JICA) identified nine urbanized areas in the country, three of which are in Mindanao Island (Davao, Cagayan de Oro City, and Zamboanga City), facing water demand challenges in the next several years (JICA 1998). Health hazards associated with the shortage include an increasing number of gastrointestinal diseases caused by unpotable water and new housing developments that alter the balance of supply of and demand (Cortes-Maramba et al. 2006; Tacio 2014).

Consequently, these areas establish the basis for a growing concern for a national water crisis by 2025 (JICA 1998). Striking a national balance between the water supply and demand, especially in the areas limited by infrastructures and facilities, is vital to optimizing, producing, and distributing potable water.

This chapter unfolds the problem scope and legal framework for surface and ground water management, the important aspects of assessing water quality, and the health and environmental impact of contaminated water. Then, several water quality initiatives will be discussed followed by a series of recommendations promoting civic engagement to support local community involvement in government organized projects. The chapter concludes with a high-level summary.

12.2 Water Scarcity Problem Scope

The scope of water scarcity in the Philippines still rests on systemic problems brought forth at the onset of baselining the nation's status in relation to UN MDGs by the World Bank in 2003. Several major and tangential issues remain the foremost, of which access to clean water is important to population health. Ranked number 5 in the overall causes of death for the nation in 2010 analysis was preventable diarrhea attributed to unsanitary water at a rate of 354.5 per 100,000 population (DOH 2012, p.14). Therefore, the location of natural resources in the form of surface and groundwater provide geographic references demonstrating regional water availability and the problem location poses to access in areas of need.

Major issues concerning the use and scarcity of water include: (1) inconsistency of water supply and demand (Barba 2004; Madrazo 2002), (2) lack of water allocation system and distribution formula (Barba 2004), (3) NWRB weak regulation, permit monitoring, and enforcement of water use due to insufficient manpower and low operating budget (Barba 2004), (4) outdated principles mandated in the Water Code of the Philippines "first in time priority in right" and discretion is vaguely granted to a deputized government agency to investigate violations (Barba 2004, p.2), and (5) unsustainable water pricing that does not properly reward efficient water users with economic incentives (Barba 2004). Other threats to water availability are linked to (1) outdated research and framework plans, and (2) hampered policy decision-making due to insufficient data collection in certain areas, lack of data sharing protocols governing inter-agency access, and lack of a common integrated knowledge management database (Barba 2004).

Natural water-related disasters and environmental degradation are persistent threats to most of the watersheds in Mindanao impacting water access and quality. A super typhoon Bopha (Pablo) struck significant part of Mindanao in 2012 and super typhoon Sendong (Washi) in Cagayan de Oro caused watershed damage leading to high rates of erosion (Franta et al. 2016; Rodolfo et al. 2016). In 2015, the Butuan City Council approved the Resolution declaring a city-wide water crisis due to low water supply to 200,000 residents attributed to the damaged facilities and infrastructures of Butuan City Water District after onslaught of tropical storm Seniang.

Table 12.2 Water resource potential by region in Mindanao Island in million cubic meters (MCM) (World Bank 2003)

Region	Surface water	Groundwater	Total
Southwestern Mindanao	12,100	1082	13,182
Northern Mindanao	29,000	2116	31,116
Southeastern Mindanao	11,300	2375	13,675
Southern Mindanao	18,700	1758	20,458

However, investigation later revealed that the water crisis was a result of the neglect, callousness, and inefficiency of the officials of the local water district (Serrano 2015).

Man-made activities, such as deforestation or denudification, also spur on water-related disasters that degrade watersheds. DENR representatives cited three such watersheds due to the urgent need for rehabilitation from excessive deforestation (BusinessWorld 2011). Reducing nonrevenue water, the water that is lost from leaks, pilferage through illegal connections, and wastage, is another aspect in the problem scope of water scarcity.

While the problem of water scarcity spans several areas (e.g., policy, poor oversight, natural disasters, environmental degradation), there some are cases of emerging solutions. For example, Cagayan de Oro City and USAID partner to implement water-saving measures by reducing the percentage of nonrevenue water. The local water district of Cagayan de Oro estimates that they lose 53% (80,000 m^3) of their water supply as nonrevenue water and aim to reduce to acceptable levels ranging from 20 to 30% (Jerusalem 2016). Upon completion of the project, water recovered in the process was slated to serve areas still lacking a water service connection.

12.2.1 *Mindanao Water Source Potential*

The water resources of the Philippines are composed of inland freshwater, coastal, bay, and oceanic water (Raymundo 2015). The portion of potential supply of water both surface and groundwater of Mindanao Island per region is shown in Table 12.2 demonstrating the uneven distribution of these resources that favor the Northern and Southern regions. Water resources differ also from province to province based on several factors like population density, rainfall patterns, watershed quality, and the rate of groundwater recharge (Senate Economic Planning Office 2011).

12.2.2 *Mindanao Surface Water Resources*

The Philippines have five principal river basins and two are found in Mindanao—the Agusan and Pulangi River Basins (Tan et al. 2012). The surface water resource of the nation is primarily the inland freshwater resources occupying 1830 km^2 of the

Philippine area (World Bank 2003) with an estimated 262 watersheds (Tan et al. 2012). Eight of the 18 significant rivers covering an area greater than 1000 km^2 are in Mindanao (World Bank 2003) which makes up watersheds or river basins that further drains into the bays in the north, east, and south.

12.2.3 Groundwater Resources

Mindanao houses two of the four major groundwater reservoirs in the Philippines, the Agusan Groundwater Reservoir (8500 ha) and Pulangi Groundwater Reservoir (estimated at 6000 ha). These groundwater resources lie beneath Mindanao's vast watersheds or recharging zones—the Agusan and Ligawasan Marshes (Tan et al. 2012) establishing Southeastern and Northern Mindanao as the highest potential groundwater resources (World Bank 2003).

A 5.3% annual increase in total demand for groundwater resources (e.g., domestic, industrial, and commercial) throughout the Philippines also saw a decline in precipitation reducing recharge by an average 3.7% annually and a steady decline in the volume of groundwater at an average annual rate of 1.4% from 1988 to 1994 (Philippine Statistics Authority 2016, *para* 4). This reveals that there is a continuing trend towards depletion of the country's groundwater resource stock making Mindanao Island, heavily reliant on the agricultural and industrial sectors for economic development, highly susceptible.

12.3 Legal Framework and Policies on Quality Control, Regulation on Water Usage, and Water Management

Understanding the existing national legal policy and framework on water use establishes important systemic factors in the existing protocols and presents an opportunity to apply analysis techniques to generate novel responses to the water scarcity problem. This section introduces government agencies, national laws, quality and emission standards, and presents problems associated with enforcement of existing guidelines.

12.3.1 Government Agencies

The water resources management of the Philippines is divided into several components performed by multiple government agencies and offices (Table 12.3) mandated by law and their charter, to perform roles in water supply, hydropower, irrigation, pollution, flood control, and watershed management (Dayrit 2001). The foremost agency in water management is the National Water Resources Board

Table 12.3 Philippine regulatory agencies and their primary enacted water resource function[a] (Madrazo 2002; Dayrit 2001)

Agency	Function	URL
Supply and water distribution		
Department of Interior and Local Government (DILG)	Local government unit-run water supply, sewerage, and sanitation systems	http://dilg.gov.ph/
Department of Public Works and Highways (DPWH)	Flood control and drainage regulation	http://www.dpwh.gov.ph/dpwh/
Local Water Utilities Administration (LWUA)[b]	Local water districts managing water supply and sewerage systems	http://www.lwua.gov.ph/
Policy formulation and planning		
National Economic Development Authority (NEDA)	Highest socioeconomic planning agency and policy advisor to Congress and the Executive Branch	http://www.neda.gov.ph/
National Water Resources Board (NWRB)	Policy formulation, administration (water permits), and enforcement of the Water Code of the Philippines	http://nwrb.gov.ph/
Water resource regulation		
Department of Environment and Natural Resources (DENR)	Watershed regulation and quality; mandated to enforce environmental protection and pollution control regulations	http://www.denr.gov.ph/laws-and-policies.html
Department of Health (DOH)	Water sanitation, potability, and safety	http://www.doh.gov.ph/
Other relevant regulatory agencies		
Bureau of Soils and Water Management (BSWM)	Irrigation regulation	http://www.bswm.da.gov.ph/
National Power Corporation (NPC)	Hydropower regulation	http://www.napocor.gov.ph/
National Irrigation Administration (NIA)	Irrigation regulation	http://www.nia.gov.ph/

[a]Various local government units (LGUs) participate in each of the designated categories and are mandated to perform regulatory functions as stipulated in the Local Government Code of 1991 (Republic Act No. 7160)
[b]Also participates in Policy Formulation and Planning

(NWRB), responsible for policy formulation, administration, and enforcement of the Water Code of the Philippines (Madrazo 2002). The overlapping duties of the agencies and their regulatory framework can create a complex and competitive environment hindering effective water resource management.

12.3.2 National Water Use, Management Laws and Policies

The adoption of National Water Code of 1976 (Presidential Decree of 1067) is the first attempt by the national government to systematically manage the water resources of the Philippines. The main purposes of this policy are to (1) provide basic principles and structural framework for the appropriation, control, conservation, and protection of water resources to achieve optimum development and efficient use to meet present and future needs; (2) determine the scope of the rights and obligations of water users and provide for the protection and regulation of such rights; and (3) the necessary and essential administrative machinery and systems. Several related laws and policies are enumerated below.

- *Republic Act No. 8041 or National Water Crisis Act of 1995*. Water supply, distribution, finance, privatization of state-run water facilities, conservation and protection of watersheds, and wastage and pilferage of water including the matters of graft and corruption in all water agencies.
- *Presidential Decree No. 198 or Provincial Water Utilities Act of 1973*. Mandates to create, operate, maintain, and expand local water districts (LWDs); direct and administer economically viable and sound provincial water supply and wastewater disposal systems.
- *Presidential Decree No. 1586 or Environmental Impact Statement System of 1978*. Mandates the administration of environmental impact assessment for all investments undertaken by the government of private sectors.
- *Presidential Decree No. 424 or Creation of National Water Resources Council*. Mandates the creation of a National Water Resources Council; primary duty of coordinating and regulating national water resource development; planning and policy for social and economic development.
- *Republic Act No. 7160 or Local Government Code of 1991*. Mandates the LGUs to enforce water-related laws and policies for sanitation, water supply, and flood control (Chan Robles Virtual Law Library 2015).

12.3.3 Water Quality Control Laws, Classification, and Assessment

The main document establishing and defining the basic regulatory programs (e.g., discharge standards, issuance of permits, monitoring of compliance) is the Philippine Environment Code (Presidential Decree No. 1151). Several national laws have also been passed and established defining policy on abatement, control, and water quality management. These laws are summarized below.

- *Republic Act No. 9275 or Clean Water Act of 2004*. Mandates the protection, preservation, and revival of the quality of the country's freshwater, brackish, and marine waters; pollution abatement; market-based instruments that charges fees based on effluent discharge volume impacting applications for permitting; and strengthens enforcement by imposing stiffer penalties for violations of standards.

- *Commonwealth Act 383 or Anti-Dumping Law of 1934*. Early legislation addressing environmental pollution (e.g., solid waste dumping) in rivers causing water levels to rise and/or streamflow blockage.
- *Presidential Decree No. 984 or Pollution Control Law of 1976*. Guideline for water pollution control water from industrial sources; establishes penalties for noncompliance and violation; requires industries to acquire necessary permits before operation.
- *Presidential Decree No. 856 or Sanitation Code of the Philippines*. Establishes the standards for collection and disposal of sewage, refuse, excreta covering both solid and liquid wastes; mandates cities and municipalities the responsibility to furnish efficient and proper waste disposal systems and to manage nuisance and offensive trades and occupations.
- *Republic Act No. 9003 or Ecological Solid Waste Management of 2000*. Mandates the systematic implementation of a national program that will govern the transfer, transport, processing, sorting, and disposal of the country's solid waste; establishes the criteria and standard for identifying landfill sites ensuring that their operation does not affect the groundwater sources in nearby aquifers.
- *Republic Act No. 6969 or Toxic Substances and Hazardous and Nuclear Wastes Control Act*. Establishes the standards in the control and management of the importation, manufacturing, processing, distribution, utilization, treatment, transportation, storage, and disposal of toxic, hazardous, and nuclear wastes and substances (Chan Robles Virtual Law Library 2015).
- *DENR Administrative Order No. 34 Series of 1990 or Revised Water Usage and Classification*. Establishes the categories and classification of water bodies in terms of their best usage; defines the minimum required for different water quality parameters per type of water classification.
- *DENR Administrative Order No. 35 Series of 1990 or Revised Effluent Regulations*. Stipulates the national standards for the discharge of effluents for the different classifications of water bodies.
- *DENR Administrative Order No. 26A Series of 1994 or Philippine National Standards for Drinking Water*. Establishes the national standard values for the different water quality parameters; guidelines and methodologies accepted for assessing the drinking water quality.
- *DENR Administrative Order No. 38 Series of 1997 or Chemical Control Order for Mercury and Mercury Compounds*. Establishes the policies on regulation and control of the importation, manufacturing, distribution, and use of mercury and mercury compounds; defines the accepted procedures on storage, transportation, and disposal of mercury and mercury compound wastes.
- *DENR Administrative Order No. 39 Series of 1997 or Chemical Control Order for Cyanide and Cyanide Compounds*. Establishes the requirements and procedures for importing, manufacturing, distributing, and using cyanide

Table 12.4 Number of classified inland surface waters and the classification criteria (Environment Management Bureau 2014)

Class	Beneficial use	Number in Class
AA	Public water supply class I. Intended primarily for waters having watersheds which are uninhabited and otherwise protected; require approved disinfection to meet the Philippine National Standards for Drinking Water (PNSDW)	5
A	Public water supply class II. For sources of water supply that will require complete treatment (e.g., coagulation, sedimentation, filtration, and disinfection) to meet the PNSDW	234
B	Recreational water class I. For primary contact recreation such as bathing, swimming, and skin diving. (particularly those designated for tourism purposes)	197
C	1. Fishery water for the propagation and growth of fish and other aquatic resources 2. Recreational water class II (e.g., boating) 3. Industrial water supply class I (for manufacturing processes after treatment)	333
D	1. For agriculture, irrigation, livestock watering. 2. Industrial water supply class II (e.g., cooling) 3. Other inland waters as determined by their quality belong to this classification	27

and cyanide compounds; determines protocol for the storage, transport, and waste disposal for these compounds.

- *DENR Administrative Order No. 58 Series of 1998 or Priority Chemical List/ DENR Administrative Order No. 27 Series of 2005 or Revised Priority Chemical List.* Determines the potentially harmful substances which pose unreasonable health risks to the public and even to the environment. The order requires companies, industries, distributors, importers, and manufacturers of chemicals listed to submit reports twice a year (DENR 2017; Chan Robles Virtual Law Library 2015).

Many of the water resource problems relate to quality rather than the quantity (Senate Economic Planning Office 2011) as water pollution affects island marine waters, fresh and groundwater sources. Surface water quality in the Philippines is classified in terms of its beneficial use (Table 12.4) and different portions of a water body can have several uses with multiple classifications. One example is the Lipadas River in Region 11 which has four classifications; Class AA upstream, Classes A and B midstream, and Class C downstream (EMB 2014). Notable is that two of the five Class AA inland waters can be found in Mindanao Region 11—the Lipadas River (upstream) and Baganga-Mahan-Ub (upstream).

Mindanao has 236 classified inland waters as of 2013 which were based on data monitored and collected by the EMB from 2006 to 2013 as shown in Table 12.5 (EMB 2013). Based on the data available, further efforts must be employed to

Table 12.5 Number of classified inland water of Mindanao per region (EMB 2013)

Region	Class AA	Class A	Class B	Class C	Class D
Region 9[a]	0	32	33	6	0
Region 10[b]	0	40	1	11	0
Region 11[c]	2	9	12	10	3
Region 12[d]	0	9	13	15	5
Caraga[e]	0	11	1	12	9
ARMM[f]	0	0	0	2	0
TOTAL	2	101	60	56	17

[a]Zamboanga Peninsula
[b]Northern Mindanao
[c]Davao Region
[d]Soccsksargen
[e]Caraga Administrative Region
[f]Autonomous Region in Muslim Mindanao

classify the remaining inland waters to provide additional information and for further management and rehabilitation if needed, especially in the case of Autonomous Region in Muslim Mindanao (ARMM).

The assessment of water quality is based on the number of samples taken from the body of water meeting the DAO 1990–34 water quality criteria per parameter (EMB 2014, p.9). Only bodies of water with at least four sampling events, representing both the dry and wet seasons, were included (EMB 2014). Please refer to the EMB (2014) for details on assessment methodologies used to rate water bodies for optimum levels of various particulate matter based on DENR formulations of ambient standards. DENR standards emphasize parameters such as dissolved oxygen (DO), biological oxygen demand (BOD), total suspended solids (TSS), total dissolved solids (TDS), and heavy metals to assess inland water quality. The standard value in each parameter serves as the benchmark data for monitoring and assessing water quality in their respective classification.

12.3.3.1 Dissolved Oxygen

Dissolved oxygen (DO) is a parameter used to indicate level of water pollution and the capacity to support aquatic plants and animal life (Greenpeace 2007). Water movement, temperature, and pollution can also affect the concentration of DO in a body of water. High levels of DO are observed in water bodies with these activities.

Only 138/164 (84%) of the inland waters monitored by the EMB met the required sampling events from 2006 to 2013 while 81/138 (59%) were deemed to have "good" water quality (EMB 2014, p.9). Most of these are Class A or C designated bodies of water located in Regions 10, 12, and 13 of Mindanao (EMB 2014).

12.3.3.2 Biological Oxygen Demand

Biological oxygen demand (BOD) is a measure of the amount of oxygen consumed by microorganisms in decomposing organic matter from a pollution source (EMB 2014). Higher levels of BOD manifest downstream where decomposition occurs and not where the effluent is directly discharged (EMB 2014).

Only 75/131 (57%) if the inland waters that met the sampling requirements are considered "good" (EMB 2014, p.11). They were from Class A or Class C water bodies in Cordillera Administrative Region (CAR) and in Regions 10, 12, and 13 of Mindanao.

12.3.3.3 Total Suspended Solids

Total suspended solid (TSS) is a measure of undissolved solid in water (e.g., silt, decaying plant and animal matter, domestic and industrial wastes) (EMB 2014). A body of water with high TSS value has lower capability of supporting aquatic life due to reduction of the light penetrating the body of water.

Only 40/138 (29%) Class AA and Class A water bodies met the sampling requirements while only 13/40 (33%) bodies of water manifested "good" quality (EMB 2014, p.12). Two out these water bodies were just shy of reaching 100% compliance rating—(1) Mindanao, upper portion of Taguibo River (99%), and (2) Lake Mainit (98%) (EMB 2014, p.12). Several water bodies from Mindanao received a "poor" rating including the Davao River (upper reach) in Region 11, Lun Masla River in Region 12, and Iponan River in Region 10.

12.3.3.4 Total Dissolved Solids

Total dissolved solids (TDS) refers to a broad array of chemical contaminants coming from agricultural runoff, leaching soil contamination, and point source pollution from industrial or domestic sewage (EMB 2014).

Only 17 (55%) bodies of water manifested "good" quality out of 30 Class AA/A bodies of water monitored which are mostly concentrated in Region 3 and only Marilao River in Bulacan had a "poor" quality level (Greenpeace 2007, p.16).

12.3.3.5 Heavy Metals

Heavy metal ions are soluble in water that forms toxic sediments at the bottom of bodies of water. These are considered harmful to aquatic life and to humans who consume seafood contaminated with high concentrations of heavy metals. Monitoring heavy metals is important to maintaining healthy waterways especially in water bodies that are near mining industries, electroplating, tanning, and other similar activities (Appleton et al. 1999; Baharom and Ishak 2015; Canencia et al. 2016).

Additional findings in the EMB report include results from 63 inland surface water bodies that were monitored in terms of total mercury, cadmium, and lead from

2006 to 2013. These monitored rivers exhibited 100% total mercury compliance except for Agno, Malaguit, Panique, and Tubay Rivers (Mindanao) (EMB 2014, p.16). Tubay River (Class A) did not meet the criterion in two sampling events out of 56 conducted. However, the presence of mercury there could remove the Tubay River as potential source of potable water.

Similarly, the maximum limit of cadmium was present in 10/18 bodies of monitored waters from 2006 to 2013. Of these ten, the lower part of the Davao River (Class B) is found in Mindanao. Although this river did not completely meet the compliance standard, notable is that of the ten rivers, the Davao River exhibited the highest compliance rating with 93% (EMB 2014, p.17).

Lead monitoring indicates that only 7/18 bodies of water monitored met the maximum limit demonstrating a 100% compliance rating. The Davao River in Mindanao, both upper and lower sections did not meet the maximum limit and both sections failed some aspect of sampling collection event (EMB 2014, p.18). These findings are particularly alarming for the upper section of Davao River, because of the Class A designation as a source of potable water.

12.3.4 Standards Overview: Ambient Water Quality, Wastewater Emission, and Enforcement

Various Philippine legislations cover different water quality parameters. This section provides an overview of major evaluation protocol for surface water, groundwater used to produce drinking water, bottled water, and wastewater. Then we present some high-level issues of enforcement relating to these standards.

12.3.4.1 Ambient Water Quality

Ambient water (e.g., lakes, rivers, oceans) quality is defined as the average water purity distinguished from discharge measurements taken at the source of the pollution as defined by the Clean Water Act of the Philippines (Greenpeace 2007). DENR Administrative Order No. 34 Series of 1990 sets forth 33 water quality assessment for minimum and desired levels for drinking water, water purification, polyvinyl chloride, and bacteria. Five key parameters determine classification and reclassification of surface water bodies: (1) pH, dissolved oxygen (DO), biological oxygen demand (BOD), and total coliforms.

12.3.4.2 Drinking Water

For drinking water, the Philippine National Standards for Drinking Water (DOH 2007) holds criteria for bacteriological, physical, chemical, radiological, and biological qualities across 56 parameters used to assess groundwater source quality.

Only three measures—fecal coliform, salinity or chloride content, and nitrates (EMB 2014) are highly relevant. Chloride and nitrates constitutes the total dissolved solids (TDS) with a maximum limit of 500 mg/L while no total coliform must be detectable in 100 mL sample for the fecal coliform parameter (World Bank 2003).

12.3.4.3 Bottled Water

Standards for bottled water are stipulated in Bureau of Food and Drugs (BFAD) Administrative Order No. 18-A Series of 1996. The BFAD stipulates assessment of several parameters including the levels of bacteria, viruses, parasites, fertilizers, pesticides, hydrocarbons, detergents, phenolic compounds, heavy metals, radioactive substances, and other soluble organic and inorganic substances. Source quality, production processes and facilities, and handling and proper labeling are also part of the BFAD order.

12.3.4.4 Wastewater

The protocol for wastewater effluent emission standards are gathered in DENR Administrative Order No. 34 and 35 Series of 1990 as they apply to the different classifications of water bodies. Several standards dictate maximum corresponding numerical values coming from any point source for any effluent discharge but target toxic and deleterious substances which can affect the quality of the receiving body of water. Discharge of effluents in bodies of water categorized as Class AA is strongly prohibited to ensure protection of public health while for other categories, industrial discharges and effluents should not contain toxic substances greater than the indicated value in the said order (Greenpeace 2007). Standard values on conventional and other pollutants which affect the aesthetic and oxygen demand are also established in these administrative orders. Some researchers have suggested that despite the number of governing policies, standards, and guidance, these assessment parameters appear to be relatively insensitive to the actual ambient standards due the utilization of concentration-based standards (Luken 1999).

Current wastewater standards do not reflect the proliferation of toxic chemicals used for and as a byproduct of modern industrial and commercial processes especially in electronics and semiconductor industry, such as beryllium, nickel, copper, tin, zinc, vanadium, and many other volatile organic compounds (VOCs).

12.3.4.5 Enforcement

Enforcement of existing laws and regulations are another prominent issue. Several researchers have identified the problematic nature of government institutions due to inefficient and/or ineffective activities. For example, overlapping, or in some cases competing, water resource management function and enacted responsibilities across various levels of government challenging leaders to agency realignment (Rola et al. 2015). Because of this problem of variance in policy and implementation mechanisms, consistent enforcement remains a challenge for the national and local governments (USAID and AECEN 2004). The problem becomes transparent when a new law is enacted but then adopts a new or different strategy, giving varied powers and responsibilities to existing government agencies like the EMB, LGUs, and other especially constituted multisectoral management and regulatory bodies.

Several challenges in the enforcement of existing regulations, such as an unclear reporting structure, accountability, enforcement responsibilities, and nonstandardized inspection procedures, have been identified by the EMB (2014). The EMB faces their own challenges in reporting structure as staff in the provincial and community offices are categorized as reassigned personnel reporting to the DENR regional offices and not directly to the EMB hierarchy as prescribed by the EMB mandate. Additionally, these EMB personnel are in the DENR Regional offices and depend on their resources. This crease results in the delay of submissions of reports, determination of accountable personnel, and mandate enforcement.

Another prevailing enforcement issue is that most local government officials are unaware of their responsibilities with regards to the enforcement of the Ecological Solid Waste Management Act and other pertinent policies. Most of the responsibilities and obligations LGU require significant technical capability aside from financial investments. However, training conducted by the DENR and internal training conducted by the LGU do not reflect this. While a good strategy to address this challenge is for the DENR to facilitate compliance of LGUs through capacity building activities, workshops, and penalties exacted on LGU officials that violate or fail to meet their mandated responsibilities, DENR budgets do not currently allocate for training or monitoring of LGUs. EMB annual budgets for training, monitoring and inspection are annually exceeded and do not receive a steady revenue source. This creates a challenge of allocating enough budget for the DENR to be able to provide a comprehensive program for capacity building to prepare LGUs for the enforcement of certain provisions of the law.

Another enforcement problem is the lack of cohesive, standardized procedures in various EMB field offices. Instead, field agents often establish and practice their own procedural strategy when conducting inspection and monitoring tasks. Although several attempts have been made to produce unofficial field guides, manuals, and checklists for the standard conduct of inspection, these items were unsuccessful. First, they were considered impractical to actual field situations, and second, they failed to garner support because they were not backed by official administrative orders reinforcing their implementation.

Demand to address certain limitations of current and existing laws, standards for water quality and effluents, and enforcement is apparent. While policies are presumably adequate, agencies face limitations on enforcement that may only be ameliorated by institutional influence.

12.3.5 Groundwater Quality Assessment

The country's groundwater resources provide most of the water needs for households, agricultural activities, commercial, industrial processes, and others. Therefore, preventing groundwater contamination and remediating contaminated groundwater are important considerations that warrant testing and other associated expenses.

In assessing the country's groundwater quality, the Philippine National Standard for Drinking Water (PNSDW) is referenced. This standard includes relevant parameters indicating the level and degree of pollutants such as fecal coliform and nitrates. Other common parameters (e.g., salinity, chloride content) are used to indicate the level of seawater intrusion.

12.3.5.1 Fecal Coliform

The PNSWD prescribes that drinking water should contain less than 1.1 Most Probable Number per 100 mL (MPN/100 mL) using the method of Multiple Tube Fermentation Technique (EMB 2014). The EMB conducted a program in 2008 to consolidate the results of analyses on tap water samples for Total and Fecal Coliforms submitted by different regional laboratories across the country. Under this program, 59 shallow wells were monitored in selected areas of the country and 6 were found to be potable, 23 failed to meet the fecal coliform standard, and the remaining 30 sites require further testing (EMB 2014). Sites found not potable in Mindanao are in Zamboanga City and Davao City (Greenpeace 2007).

12.3.5.2 Nitrates

Environmental nitrates are found in the salts of ammonium, sodium, potassium, and calcium from soil fertilizers during agricultural runoff, wastewater treatment, confined animal facilities, and from sewage discharge of septic systems (EMB 2014). No major study has been conducted to determine the nitrate levels of various groundwater sources in Mindanao except in the agricultural regions of Northern and Central Luzon (Tirado 2007).

12.3.5.3 Salinity or Chloride Content

Excessive withdrawal of groundwater causes the natural groundwater gradient to reverse and allow seawater to contaminate and intrude the aquifers in coastal areas (Pinder 1981). Seawater intrusion can affect the potability of drinking water and the quality of water in irrigation wells leaving some areas unfit for continued agricultural activities (EMB 2014).

Table 12.6 Standard rates for evaluation of groundwater and surface water quality (World Bank 2003)

Parameter	Satisfactory	Marginal	Unsatisfactory
DO (mg/L)[a]	>5	5	<5
BOD (mg/L)[b]	<5	5	>5
TDS[c]	Less than 10% of wells tested did not meet standard	N/A	10% or more of wells tested did not meet standard
Coliform	No wells found positive for coliform (0%)	N/A	Wells found positive for coliform (>0%)

[a]Dissolved oxygen
[b]Biological oxygen demand
[c]Total dissolved solids

No current study assessing the degree of seawater intrusion in the groundwater resources of Mindanao Island to date. However, some studies were conducted in the areas of Luzon (Insigne and Kim 2010) and Visayas (Scholze et al. 2002).

12.3.5.4 Pollution Hotspots

The Philippine Government maintains the quality of water bodies according to intended and beneficial use (DENR 1990). In 2003, pollution hotspots of surface water were assessed by the World Bank and evaluated by province using DO and BOD criteria while groundwater sources tested TDS and coliform. Water quality status of surface waters was categorized and rated as Satisfactory (S), Marginal (M), and Unsatisfactory (U) while groundwater quality status was rated either Satisfactory (S) or Unsatisfactory (U) (Table 12.6).

Results of the 3-year monitoring project conducted by the World Bank reported on the Water Quality Scorecard for Surface Waters from Regions 9–11 and 13 are satisfactory with marginal ratings for the Mercedes River (Region 9), Manicahan River (Region 9) and Agusan River (Region 13) (World Bank 2003, p.36). Several surface water bodies on the island were rated as unsatisfactory including the Saaz River (Region 9) and the Padada, Tuganay, and Agusan Rivers in Region 11 (World Bank 2003, p.36). There were no available data for Region 12 and ARMM.

There were further gaps in analysis. No groundwater data were available for Regions 12, 13, and ARMM for both TDS and coliform while for Region 9 and 11, no coliform data were available (World Bank 2003). Zamboanga del Sur (Region 9) and Misamis Oriental (Region 10) groundwater sources were rated unsatisfactory for TDS while Misamis Oriental (Region 10) was rated unsatisfactory for coliform (World Bank 2003, p.37).

12.3.5.5 Point and Nonpoint Sources

Water pollution can be classified in terms of its source—(1) point source pollution, and (2) nonpoint source pollution. Point source pollution refers to any pollution with an identifiable pollution source with a specific and known discharge point. On the other hand, nonpoint source pollution refers to pollution with no known or identifiable source (World Bank 2003).

Point source pollution can be categorized into three main sources—domestic wastewater discharges, agricultural wastewater discharges, and industrial wastewater discharges. Pollution load is calculated using BOD as the measuring parameter indicating pollution contribution from point sources is 24% from Industrial discharges, 31% from Domestic or Municipal discharges, and 45% from Agricultural discharges (EMB 2014, p.24) The calculations for domestic, agricultural, and industrial BOD can be seen in the documents published by World Bank (2003), EMB (2014), Economopoulos (1993).

Domestic discharges contain the most organic waste with suspended solids and coliforms from common household and kitchen activities (World Bank 2003). The problem is attributed to the lack of appropriate domestic sewage treatment system allowing allows 90% of inadequately treated domestic sewage discharged into surface waters (Greenpeace 2007, p.19). Major areas that generate BOD are Metro Manila and Region 4A (18% and 15%, respectively) while only small levels of BOD are generated in Mindanao regions (World Bank 2003, p.7). In Mindanao, regions 10, 11, and 12 went above the 50 thousand megaton mark for BOD load while areas within regions of 9, 13 and ARMM were below 50 thousand megaton marks (World Bank 2003).

In terms of agricultural BOD, Regions 4 and 1 contributed the most BOD in the country (13% and 12%, respectively). In Mindanao, region 10 is ranked fourth in BOD attributed to active animal and vegetable farming in this region, while Region 13 and ARMM (1.2% and 3.0%, respectively) had the least agricultural BOD contribution (World Bank 2003, p.21). Notable is that Region 13 also has the least agricultural BOD contribution for the whole country.

Industrial BOD contribution depends on the volume and characteristics of industrial effluents which vary by industry type. Water-intensive industries discharge huge amounts of waste water (Canencia and Walag 2016; World Bank 2003). Most of the water-intensive industries are in Luzon in the National Capital Region, Regions 3 and 4, thus having the most BOD contribution (42.5%, 9.0%, and 14.1%, respectively) while other regions, such as 11 (6.6%), 9 (3.3%), 10 (2.2%), and 8 (1.1%), have relatively smaller contributions. Finally, ARMM reports 0% BOD contribution due the absence of or an insignificant number of large industries (World Bank 2003, p.21).

Nonpoint source pollution depends generally on the land use thus it is calculated and estimated based on the different land uses. Several technologies are now available to help monitor, control, and mitigate the effects of point source pollutions but there remains difficulty in these activities for nonpoint sources (Greenpeace 2007). The difficulty in monitoring is evident in the lack of information and scarcity of monitoring on the contribution of solid waste, a major source of nonpoint pollutants (World Bank 2003).

12.4 Health and Environmental Impact

Human population and the surrounding environment are at risk when bodies of water like rivers, streams, and lakes are polluted with wastewater or spillage. These source bodies of water, in turn, contaminate nearby groundwater making humans susceptible to environmentally-related illness and disease resulting in mortality and morbidity (Cabral 2010; Grimes et al. 2015). Specifically, inadequate sanitation and hygiene brought about by lack of clean, safe, and comfortable facilities could promote the risk of acquiring diarrhea (Pfadenhauer and Rehfuess 2015) "which is second to pneumonia as the leading cause of morbidity in the Philippines" (DOH 2012, p.63) in diseases related to the environment. Several studies discussed in this section have firmly established the relationship between polluted water supply and disease in the Philippines (WEPA n.d., *para* 7):

> Untreated wastewater... makes water unfit for drinking and recreational use, threatens biodiversity, and deteriorates overall quality of life. Known diseases caused by poor water include gastro-enteritis, diarrhea, typhoid, cholera, dysentery, hepatitis, and more recently, severe acute respiratory syndrome (SARS).

Water bodies in urban areas are the most susceptible to contamination due to the direct and indirect pollution caused by unprecedented development. However, rural surface waters are endangered due to farming, animal production, and other food sector industries that release organic pollutants into the water system. Consequently, the environmental impact of improper sewerage leading to unsanitary water causes a variety of debilitating health effects on living creatures—land-dwelling animals, aquatic life and humans.

12.4.1 Water Supply Contamination and Diseases in Humans

Excessive levels of fecal coliform organism and *E. coli* indicative of surface water contamination was detected in a recent study of Cagayan de Oro River upstream. The contamination was attributed to improper disposal of animal wastes, human wastes which are discarded directly to the river, and poor sewerage in nearby communities (Lubos et al. 2013; Lubos and Japos 2010).

Several studies confirm the need for increasing attention to watershed management and sanitation. The Labo and Clarin Rivers are considered important to the different communities in Misamis Occidental, where both tested positive for coliforms; the site along the agroforest and agricultural areas had the highest total coliform (Labajo-Villantes and Nuneza 2014) confirming the need for increasing attention to watershed management. Several problematic physicochemical and bacteriological qualities were also reported in several rivers—the Aligodon, Misamis Oriental, Daveo River, and Talomo (Ido 2016; Laud et al. 2016).

Morbidity from outbreaks of diarrhea continue to be a major health problem stemming from groundwater contamination of wells on farmland in villages in

North Cotabato (Pelone 2014a) and the application of herbicides on cornfields that are washed down to river systems (Bacongco 2014). One death and 32 instances of mortality was consequent to contamination through leakage of distribution pipes in Zamboanga City (Pelone 2014b) where 14/19 residents there later tested positive for norovirus (Radyo Natin 2016).

12.4.2 Fish Kills and Red Tide Occurrences

Low DO levels in water, abrupt and abnormal shifting water temperature, and deteriorating water quality are common environmental conditions that kill aquatic life (EMB 2014). Several fish kills were documented and recorded throughout the island including the 1 km long algal bloom of *Cochlodinium* sp. in the coastal area Jasaan, Misamis Oriental in 2003 (Jabatan 2004). The bloom occurs because of high surface temperature, favorable transport, radiation available for photosynthesis, and enrichment for organic nutrients (Kim et al. 2016; Lee and Choi 2009; Tomas and Smaydab 2008).

Several fish kills were reported in the island to have been caused by oxygen depletion due to overcrowding and harmful algal blooms Lake Sebu and Lake Seloton in South Cotabato and Iligan bay (Fernandez 2017; Vicente et al. 2002). Consequently, government representatives of Maguindanao took precautionary measures to ensure the balance of environment and marine life in the Lake Buluan by regulating the number of fish pens (Sarmiento 2017).

The health of humans and marine species are both continuously threatened by occurrences of Red Tide. Mindanao's affinity for red tides, shown on the data from the Incidences of Red Tide in Coastal Areas in 2016, has been credited to northeast monsoon-driven upwellings (EMB 2014). Balite Bay in Mati, Davao Oriental was exposed to red tide from January to March 2016, posing significant threats to aquatic life until finally deemed toxin free in early March (Bureau of Fish and Aquatic Resources 2016).

12.4.3 Improper Sewerage and Sanitation

In the Philippines, 76.8% of families have sanitary toilet facilities but only less than 10% are connected to piped sewerage system while the rest rely on septic tanks, pit latrines, or open defecation (EMB 2014, p.28). Both the existence of unsuitable sewerage systems or absence thereof greatly impacts the quality of different bodies of water because this type of contamination may give rise to various water-borne diseases caused by various microorganisms (EMB 2014).

While incidents of diarrhea have been deadly several other viral infections can result from unsanitary water. Instances of hepatitis in Surigao del Sur (Crisostomo and Serrano 2006) and leptospirosis in Davao City (Zapanta et al. 2014) were all attributed to poor sanitation and improperly maintained sewage system. Rural areas are typically affected where water systems, such as traditional wells and rivers, contain fecal matter that contaminates the source (Bain et al. 2014).

12.4.4 Mine Tailing Spillages and Siltation

Several activities and sources of mercury and heavy metals that pollute water bodies can be attributed to mercury mining, gold mining, chemical industry, metal smelting, coal combustion, and metropolitan and agricultural runoffs (Li et al. 2009). Several mining industries are in the eastern and western sections of Mindanao where reports of spillages, heavy metal pollution, and siltation of nearby bodies of water have taken place (Appleton et al. 1999; Cortes-Maramba et al. 2006).

The gold mining industry has a strong presence in Eastern Mindanao near the Agusan River where the gold-rush town of Diwalwal has a foothold. Initial analysis revealed that the Diwalwal drainage, evident downstream of the river system, was characterized by extremely high levels of mercury in solution and sediments downstream (Appleton et al. 1999) exceeding multiple international guidelines.

Different kinds of organisms were also recorded as having been contaminated with mercury from different main tailings. Contaminations were also found in rice, fish and mussels from Naboc River (Appleton et al. 2006; Drasch et al. 2001) and in three species of fish in Davao del Norte (Akagi et al. 2000). Population and biodiversity of damselflies and dragonflies in Surigao del Sur (Quisil et al. 2014) and oyster production in Zamboanga Sibugay Province (Lim and Flores 2017) have also been drastically affected by mine tailing ponds.

12.5 Efforts to Address Water Quality

Water quality is a physical and chemical problem. Several projects have been conducted both by the government and nongovernment agencies to address recurring and perennial challenges regarding the protection and conservation of water resources. Programs on the enhancement of water quality in the Philippines are spearheaded by the DENR with the support of various nongovernment organizations, financing institutions, and development partners (EMB 2014).

12.5.1 Environmental Management Bureau Projects and Programs

The DENR is mandated, through the EMB, to be the national authority responsible for the prevention and control of pollution and assessment of environmental impact. Aside from the enforcement and compliance activities of EMB in 12.3, the EMB also take part in projects and activities to enhance and rehabilitate water quality throughout the country.

12.5.1.1 Designation of Water Quality Management Area

The Water Quality Management Area (WQMA) is established by the NWRB together with DENR to assign water quality management areas using appropriate physiographic units to protect water bodies and its tributaries (EMB n.d.b). The WQMA follows a two-step process by first initiating an assessment followed by the development of an agency Action Plan crafted to improve the quality of a certain body of water. Mindanao has ten bodies of water were designated as WQMAs in 2016.

12.5.1.2 Philippine Environment Partnership Program

The Philippine Environment Partnership Program (PEPP) was created to support self-regulation among industries towards improved environmental performance. The voluntary industry partnerships with DENR promote mandatory self-monitoring and compliance with environmental standards (DENR 2003). Under this program, PEPP evaluates and classifies establishments according to tracks. Industries classified as Track 1 are companies driven by competitiveness that go beyond compliance while Track 2 classified industries are companies that are currently unable to comply with regulations. Several companies have been awarded the Seal of Approval from Mindanao, but the first honor went to the San Miguel Brewery, Inc. in Darong, Davao Del Sur, Region 11. Other companies who received this recognition include many food, materials, and energy suppliers from Regions 10, 11, and 12 (DENR n.d.).

12.5.2 Financing Institutions and Development Partners

Financing institutions and development partners aid various projects aiming to promote, conserve, rehabilitate, and manage water quality. While the World Bank, Development Bank of the Philippines, JICA, and USAID all contributed to various national projects to protect, conserve, manage and rehabilitate the water bodies in the Philippines, we emphasize support for projects on Mindanao Island.

12.5.2.1 Land Bank of the Philippines

The Land Bank of the Philippines, together with the DENR, implemented the "Adopt-a-Watershed Project" restoring 14 hectare (ha) total area of denuded forestlands in six pilot areas nationwide (EMB 2014). (1 ha is equal to 10,000 m^2.)

Two major watersheds in Mindanao were covered in Phase 1(2006–2011) of this project, Lasang River in Davao Del Norte and Silway River in South Cotabato. In Phase 2 (2012–2015) of this project, 10 ha total watershed was covered in Mindanao, these are Paquibato, Davao City and Olympog in General Santos City. In the last Phase (2015–2018), and additional 14 ha of Mindanao watersheds found in Zamboanga Sibugay, Lanao del Sur, Davao del Norte, and South Cotabato will undergo restoration (Land Bank of the Philippines 2014).

12.5.2.2 Asian Development Bank

The Asian Development Bank (ADB) provided technical assistance to Cebu and Davao cities to improve access to water supply and sanitation services. The Urban Water Supply and Sanitation Project (2011–2014) aimed to increase continuous water supply in Cebu and Davao City by 2022 from 50 to 80% of the population while the coverage for clean and hygienic sanitation was targeted to improve from 10 to 50%. Furthermore, marine biodiversity ecosystems in the provinces of Cagayan de Oro and Davao Oriental were also allocated funds by ADB to enhance coastal services and reduce poverty among fisher folks (EMB 2014).

12.5.3 Research and Development Initiatives

Various research and development initiatives and programs conducted by DENR and Department of Science and Technology (DOST) have been reported to address water quality problems nationwide. DENR conducted leachate characterization study from various solid waste disposal facilities from 2005 to 2007 assessing the impacts of leachate on groundwater and studies on toxicity testing to assess the harmful effects of substances like cyanide, cadmium, mercury, arsenic, and nitrates with fish and invertebrate test organisms. The collected data from the tests were used in the formulation of parameters for environmental quality assessment and monitoring (EMB 2014).

The DOST also conducted various research and development initiatives geared towards prevention and control of water pollution under a five-year plan from 2011 to 2016 entitled, "Science & Technology Water Environment Roadmap." Various programs and projects are investigating and implementing water technologies. They include water treatment technological improvement and innovation, wastewater treatment and remediation technologies, and space technology applications on water resources such as Light Detection and Ranging (LiDAR) technology and photonics for aquatic resource assessment (EMB 2014).

12.6 Recommendations to Improve Quality, Control, and Management

The environmental impact and negative health consequences elicited from water scarcity and pollution aid in refining the existing legal framework and policies on quality control, regulation on water usage, and water management. Major recommendations include policy amendments to the Philippine Water Code and Clean Air Act and various methods to further enhance local community involvement in government organized activities.

12.6.1 Policy Amendments

Major policy recommendations include the development of an institutional framework under the purview of the Philippine Water Code and amending the Clean Air Act to eliminate the use of concentration-based standards through the introduction of a two-tiered permit system. Suggestions include providing clarification of the roles and responsibilities of the various enacted national and local government units.

12.6.1.1 Centralized Regulation

A central regulatory body mandated within the main Philippine Water Code would provide an essential reporting structure that legally defines the framework for extraction, allocation, and management of the country's water resources. The transition to central control recognizes the presumably adequate existing law but may afford the necessary opportunity to successfully address the constant challenge of policy enforcement resulting from government institutions having overlapping functions and responsibilities (Rola et al. 2015). Thus, an institutional framework where all water users understand their roles and responsibilities should be enacted under the Philippine Water Code. The NWRB, currently enforcing the Water Code of the Philippines, is a prime candidate for transition. The existing organizational chart of NWRB allows conferring of water right but much of the proportion of water right is freely held by other public institutions like DENR (watershed management), LWUA (domestic water supply), and National Irrigation Administration (NIA) (irrigation water supply) as shown in Fig. 12.1.

This proposal reinforces the technical capacity and administrative function of NWRB by restructuring agency responsibilities to become the country's water resources management authority. Hence, a single, independent, and autonomous regulatory board will ensure the protection of water consumers, enshrine accountability and transparency throughout the water resource management of the coun-

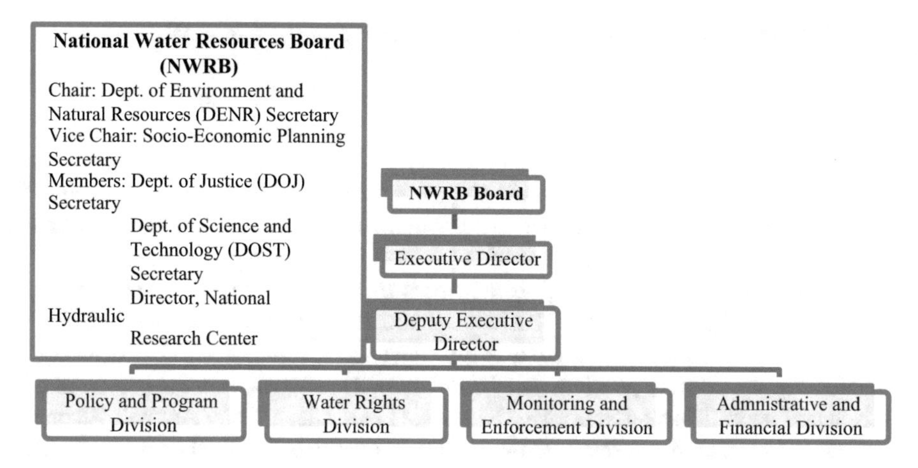

Fig. 12.1 Current organizational chart of National Water Resources Board (National Water Resources Board n.d., Used by Permission of Public Domain)

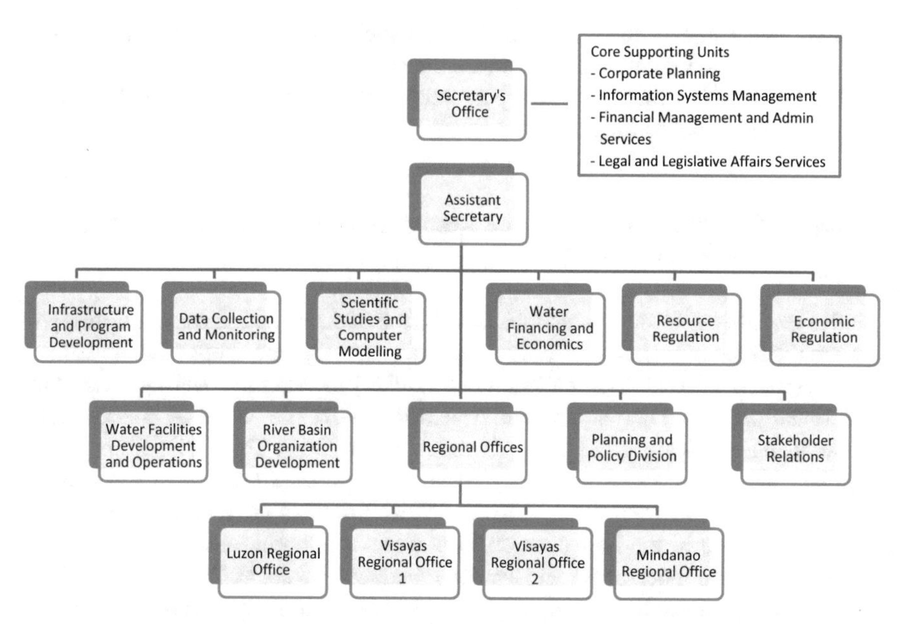

Fig. 12.2 Organizational chart of proposed National Water Resources Management Office (Tabios III 2014; Rola et al. 2015, Used by Permission)

try, and implement an honest and dynamic tariff policy. Further, these steps would streamline all projects and activities geared towards water quality improvement, sustainable allocation, and distribution among all users. The proposed central agency would carry the name National Water Resources Management Office (Fig. 12.2) having the mandate to manage and protect the country's water resources.

12.6.1.2 A Two-Tiered Discharge Permit System in the Clean Water Act

The current policy on effluent standards, as mandated by Republic Act 9275, appears to be relatively insensitive to the real ambient conditions due to the use of concentration-based standards unconsciously allowing industries to dilute their effluent by over extraction of groundwater (Madrazo 2002). A two-tiered system for discharge permits mandated in the Clean Water Act should alleviate this problem. The proposed system charges industries for both the volume and concentration of water discharged thus encouraging industries to meet water quality standards to avoid paying higher environmental fees. Although many industries meet the standards set by law, the fees they pay will reflect the volume of effluent discharge addressing the dilution problem (Madrazo 2002). This revision on the provision of discharge permits has three primary benefits: (1) the Clean Water Act will become stringent in terms of reinforcing ambient water quality and effluent standards, (2) better water quality in receiving bodies of water, and (3) water quality improvements to communities' dependent on receiving bodies for livelihood and domestic purposes. Additionally, the environmental user's fee would produce additional benefits when disbursed to support data enhancing local water quality research, production of modern water treatment technology, implementation and enforcement of local ordinances through added personnel and equipment, and special training monitoring and inspection personnel.

12.6.1.3 Clarification of Roles and Responsibilities of National and Local Government Units

Under the current Clean Water Act, DENR is mandated with the responsibility to enforce various provisions under the said law. Although the agency is capable and competent, the current budget allocation is unlikely to increase covering the cost for additional personnel and equipment even when duties are added as prescribed by existing and new legislations (USAID and AECEN 2004). Thus, DENR operations will be hampered. To address this issue, a revision of the Clean Water Act must be made to devolve some of the functions of DENR to local government units. Local governments are in the best position to perform monitoring and inspection tasks because of existing personnel and available budget (Rola et al. 2015). Further, they can also more easily link monitoring to enforcement in their own new permitting system. Nevertheless, the LGUs require technical training which the DENR can provide. The revision for the Clean Water Act shall be based upon the reorientation of the task of DENR from reinforcement and implementation of the act to provision of standards, training, and oversight over LGUs. In this setup, LGUs will be empowered to effectively manage their own water resources, efficiently resolve local issues and concerns cutting the long delay of bureaucracy, and sustainably provide support and monitoring services for industries to forward local development. Furthermore, since LGUs are empowered they can easily identify issues and challenges and implement programs for the improvement of water quality involving local communities and barangays.

12.6.2 Local Community Involvement in Government Organized Activities

The civil society in the Philippines is very strong and vocal particularly in respect to the environment. National and local nongovernment organizations (NGOs) are very keen in monitoring proposed projects or activities that may pose serious deleterious effects to the environment. For this reason, tapping local community involvement and public participation in various government projects and activities is beneficial to the government, environment, and population. Recommendations encompass a series of local community involvement in government organized activities spanning the important aspect of citizen engagement in environmental impact assessments prior to development and community-managed services, among others.

Public participation in environmental impact assessment (EIA) activities is very significant not only in the process of consultations but also in the process of issuance and renewal of Environmental Compliance Certificates (ECC) (EMB 2007). Certain provision in the EIA requires the creation of a multisectoral monitoring team especially for major development projects. This provision allows public participations to ensure compliance with environmental standards by companies and industries as stipulated in the ECC.

EcoWatch Program is a private sector initiative listing and publicizing major polluters. DENR has adopted this initiative and encourages public participation in monitoring major polluters (EMB n.d.c). This system creates negative publicity for the involved firms since they are "color-coded" according to their compliance with environmental regulations. EcoWarch also allows public recognition and praise to firms and companies categorized as green, silver, and gold.

The Kapitbisig Laban sa Kahirapan-Comprehensive and Integrated Delivery of Social Project (KALAHI-CIDSS) is a World Bank project working with different impoverished communities in the Philippines. The project utilizes a community-driven development approach by enabling villagers to make their own decisions in identifying, developing, implementing, and monitoring development initiatives based on their current need (World Bank 2014). Public participation was very significant due to clearly established guidelines on participation, accountability, and transparency. Furthermore, an impact study revealed that the income of the household beneficiaries who participated in the project rose significantly by 12% as measured in terms of consumption (World Bank 2014, *para* 4).

There are numerous waterless municipalities around the country and about 213 are found in Mindanao (Llanto 2013). SALINTUBIG Project was conceived in 2011 by the DILG, DOH, and National Anti-Poverty Commission (NAPC). Their common objective is to provide water supply systems to the 455 waterless municipalities, barangays, health centers, and resettlement sites in the Philippines. To reach their goals community members and LGU personnel were given technical training in terms of planning, implementation, and operation of water supply facilities. This program emphasizes the capacity building mechanisms and the provision of technical assistance to LGUs in the pursuit of sustainable and efficient water supply services in the country (National Anti-Poverty Commission n.d.).

Cagayan de Oro City through the Cagayan de Oro Water District (COWD) sought the private sector to implement a design-build-operate contract for their septic facility. Through this setup, the private proponent will design and construct the treatment facility, purchase and operate desludging trucks, and implement a program for desludging septic tanks around the city. The local government on the other hand will approve a comprehensive citywide septic management ordinance, develop and targeted promotional campaign (USAID 2010).

The Philippine Center for Water and Sanitation (PCWS) assists in the creation of institutions providing technical assistance for the effective community management of water supply and sanitation systems. The formation of the Provincial Water and Sanitation Center in Agusan del Sur facilitated the capacity building of the municipal-level project implementers, providing sustainable support to community water and sanitation associations (Asian Development Bank 2006).

Lack of access to clean, potable water and improved sanitation is still a longstanding issue in most rural areas in the Philippines. Climate Resilience in Water Stressed Communities (CREST) is a project funded by USAID, local governments and communities in the Philippines to bring potable water to these areas and conflict-affected regions of Mindanao (USAID 2016). This project utilized a community-based, participatory approach to bring safe and potable drinking water through innovative water and water sanitation technologies resilient in the face of climate change.

Finally, the Estero Program is a collaborative effort among estero community members, local government units, private company donors, and DENR through EMB, to clean up waterways that empty into rivers and other bodies of water (EMB n.d.a). This is an effort to mobilize members of the community to actively engage in clean up, planning and implementation of continued plans to keep the estero clean in continuous projects. Immediate of their initial efforts that were observed by residents and other locals include less flooding due to unimpeded water flow and reduction of water-borne diseases.

12.7 Summary

Clean water is essential to improving the quality of public health. Therefore, maintenance and improvement of the quality of water is important to achieving this objective. In the Philippines, several legal frameworks and policies have been established with the mandate of quality control, regulation of water use, and water supply management. National government agencies, taskforces, and committees have been established in response to the implementation of laws and departmental administrative orders. These government agencies through various consultative meetings and research developed ambient water and wastewater emission standards for the protection of water bodies in the country. Although these legal framework and policies are in place, several obstacles are still presently challenging the realization of providing clean and potable water for all Filipinos. These challenges are apparent in the fragmented establishment of legal policies cascading into weak reinforcement that, in turn, is ineffective in preventing pollutants from contaminating fresh and groundwater sources that impacts public health. Efforts must be made to address problems on water quality and pollution, shortage and scarcity of water, and the health and environmental impacts. This could begin in the development of a unified inter-agency and multisectoral taskforce on the management of water bodies. The system of rewards and incentives to improve environmental compliance of firms and industries must be further strengthened. Although several government agencies are mandated with the task of improving the water quality, this requires a multisectoral approach which necessitates the involvement of local government units and communities.

Initiatives by different civic societies and community associations are crucial in the improvement of the water quality throughout the island. Attention should also be given in the capacity building of local communities especially in their involvement on monitoring the compliance of different firms and industries. A good amount of investment must also be made in locally developed and produced sanitation and sewerage systems to introduce public accountability among every citizen. A community association must also be encouraged to manage water distribution and management of wastewater treatment facilities. These efforts to involve and engage local communities would address the challenge on the financial and personnel constraint of both the EMB and DENR. Together with the National Government, the rights and powers stipulated by legislative policies, support from various international and local Nongovernment Organizations, and active and responsible participation from local community members, the dream of providing clean, safe, and accessible water resources is possible. The rich resources of the Philippines must not be taken for granted and action must be taken before it's too late. The community, an untapped resource, must be involved in the various efforts to conserve and preserve the very foundation of life—water. Therefore, now is the time to revise and translate national laws and policies through the involvement of community to better the environmental condition of the Philippines.

Acknowledgment The authors would like to acknowledge the United Nations, World Health Organization, and the World Bank for access to their outstanding resources. The authors accept responsibility for all analysis and interpretation.

Glossary

Biological oxygen demand (BOD) Amount of oxygen dissolved in water required for the survival of microorganisms.

Coliforms Bacteria commonly found in soil, water, and in the guts of animals, which indicate that the water supply may be vulnerable to contamination.

Dissolved oxygen (DO) Amount of diatomic oxygen dissolved in water.

Domestic Refers to the utilization of water for drinking, washing, cooking, bathing, and other household chores and needs.

Effluent Wastewater discharged from a sewage treatment facility or an industrial plant.

Industrial Utilization of water for the needs of factories, industrial plants, and mines.

Irrigation Controlled application of water for agricultural uses through man-made systems to supply water requirements not satisfied by precipitation.

Municipal Utilization of water for supplying the water needs of the community.

Potable water Water that is safe for consumption or food preparation with no risk to health.

Seawater Intrusion The natural phenomenon where freshwater is contaminated with seawater because of overdraft—extracting too much water that leads to an unsafe imbalance in water quality.

Sewerage Collective term used for drains, canals, manholes, pumping stations, and screening chambers for disposal of sewage and surface water.

Volatile Organic Compounds (VOCs) Synthetic chemical compounds dissolved in water which can be vaporized at low temperatures.

Wastewater Water that has been used for various purposes in homes, industries, businesses that is not meant for reuse unless it is treated for contaminants.

Water Quality Management Area Certain water bodies and its tributaries identified by the Department of Environment and Natural Resources (DENR) to be prioritized for protection and conservation.

Water Right The right granted by the government to appropriate and use water.

References

Akagi H, et al. Health assessment for mercury exposure among schoolchildren residing near a gold processing and refining plant in Apokon, Tagum, Davao del Norte, Philippines. Sci Total Environ. 2000;259(1–3):31–43. https://doi.org/10.1016/S0048-9697(00)00547-7.

Appleton JD, et al. Mercury contamination associated with artisanal gold mining on the island of Mindanao, the Philippines. Sci Total Environ. 1999;228(2–3):95–109. https://doi.org/10.1016/S0048-9697(99)00016-9.

Appleton JD, et al. Impacts of mercury contaminated mining waste on soil quality, crops, bivalves, and fish in the Naboc River area, Mindanao, Philippines. Sci Total Environ. 2006;354(2–3):198–211. https://doi.org/10.1016/j.scitotenv.2005.01.042.

Asian Development Bank. 2006. Country water action: Philippines institutional community-management approach for water supply and sanitation in Agusan del Sur, Quezon City. http://www.itnphil.org.ph/docs/Country%20Water%20Action%20Philippines.pdf. Accessed 10 Aug 2017.

Bacongco K. 2014. Diarrhea outbreak kills 7 in Alamada, MINDANEWS. http://www.mindanews.com/top-stories/2014/05/diarrhea-outbreak-kills-7-in-alamada/. Accessed 13 Aug 2017.

Baharom ZS, Ishak MY. Determination of heavy metal accumulation in fish species in Gales River, Kelantan and Beranang mining pool, Selangor. Procedia Environ Sci. 2015;30:302–25. https://doi.org/10.1016/j.proenv.2015.10.057.

Bain R, et al. Fecal contamination of drinking-water in low- and middle-income countries: a systematic review and meta-analysis. PLoS Med. 2014;11(5):e1001644. https://doi.org/10.1371/journal.pmed.1001644.

Barba PF. 2004. The challenges in water resources management in the Philippines. http://rwes.dpri.kyoto-u.ac.jp/~tanaka/APHW/APHW2004/proceedings/JSE/56-JSE-A519/56-JSE-A519.pdf. Accessed 10 Aug 2017.

Bureau of Fish and Aquatic Resources. 2016. Shellfish Bulletin from January 2016 to December 2016. http://www.bfar.da.gov.ph/bfar/download/redtide2016.pdf. Accessed 15 Aug 2017.

BusinessWorld Manila. 2011. Deforestation in Mindanao deemed an "emergency" case. http://www.bworldonline.com/content.php?section=Economy&title=deforestation-in-mindanao-deemed-an-&145emergency&8217-case&id=35554. Accessed 13 Aug 2017.

Cabral JPS. Water microbiology, bacterial pathogens and water. Int J Environ Res Public Health. 2010;7(10):3657–703. https://doi.org/10.3390/ijerph7103657.

Canencia OP, Walag AMP. Coal combustion from power plant industry in Misamis Oriental, Philippines: a potential groundwater contamination and heavy metal detection. Asian J Microbiol Biotechnol Environ Sci. 2016;18(1):55–9.

Canencia OP, et al. Slaughter waste effluents and river catchment watershed contamination in Cagayan de Oro City, Philippines. J Biodivers Conserv Environ Sci. 2016;9(2):142–8.

Chan Robles Virtual Law Library. 2015. Philippines laws, statutes & codes. http://lawlibrary.chanrobles.com/. Accessed 11 Aug 2017.

Clausen A. Economic globalization and regional disparities in the Philippines. Singap J Trop Geogr. 2010;31(3):299–316.

Cortes-Maramba N, et al. Health and environmental assessment of mercury exposure in a gold mining community in Western Mindanao, Philippines. J Environ Manag. 2006;81(2):126–34. https://doi.org/10.1016/j.jenvman.2006.01.019.

Crisostomo S, Serrano B. 2006. Hepa A outbreak eyed in Surigao town. PhilStar Global. http://www.philstar.com/nation/326292/hepa-outbreak-eyed-surigao-town. Accessed 21 Aug 2017.

Dayrit H. 2001. The Philippines: formulation of a national water vision. http://www.fao.org/3/a-ab776e/ab776e03.htm. Accessed 13 Aug 2017.

Department of Environment and Natural Resources (DENR). 1990. Revised water usage and classification/water quality criteria amending section nos. 68 and 69, Chapter III of the 1978 NPCC rules and regulations, Pub. L. No. Administrative Order 34.

Department of Environment and Natural Resources. 2003. DENR Administrative Order No. 2003-14 creating the Philippine environment partnership program to support industry self-regulation towards improved environmental performance. http://pepp.emb.gov.ph/wp-content/uploads/2016/06/PEPP-DAO-2003-14.pdf. Accessed 28 Aug 2017.

Department of Environment and Natural Resources. 2017. Laws & policies. http://www.denr.gov.ph/laws-and-policies.html. Accessed 11 Aug 2017.

Department of Environment and Natural Resources. n.d. The Philippine environment partnership program: recognizing industries with superior environmental performance 2010–2014. http://pepp.emb.gov.ph. Accessed 28 Aug 2017.

Department of Health. 2007. Philippine national standards for drinking water. http://www.lwua.gov.ph/downloads_14/Philippine%20National%20Standards%20for%20Drinking%20Water%202007.pdf. Accessed 12 Aug 2017.

Department of Health, Republic of Philippines. 2012. National objectives for health 2011-2016. http://www.doh.gov.ph/sites/default/files/publications/noh2016.pdf. Accessed 12 Aug 2017.

Drasch G, et al. The Mt. Diwata study on the Philippines 1999—assessing mercury intoxication of the population by small scale gold mining. Sci Total Environ. 2001;267(1–3):151–68. https://doi.org/10.1016/S0048-9697(00)00806-8.

Dumlao SFJ. 2016. Water supply: a priority concern. Business Mirror. http://www.businessmirror.com.ph/water-supply-a-priority-concern/. Accessed 13 Aug 2017.

Economopoulos AP. 1993. Assessment of sources of air, water, and land pollution. World Health Organization, Geneva. http://apps.who.int/iris/bitstream/10665/58750/1/WHO_PEP_GETNET_93.1-A.pdf. Accessed 21 Aug 2017.

Environmental Management Bureau (EMB). 2007. Environmental impact assessment review manual. http://emb.gov.ph/wp-content/uploads/2016/06/EMB-MC-2007-001.pdf. Accessed 8 Aug 2017.
Environmental Management Bureau (EMB). 2013. Additional list of classified water bodies. http://server2.denr.gov.ph/uploads/rmdd/dmc-2013-03.pdf. Accessed 21 Aug 2017.
Environmental Management Bureau (EMB). 2014. National water quality status report 2006-2013. Quezon City. http://water.emb.gov.ph/wp-content/uploads/2016/06/NWQSR2006-2013.pdf. Accessed 21 Aug 2017.
Environmental Management Bureau (EMB). n.d.-a. Adopt-an-estero/waterbody program. http://water.emb.gov.ph/?page_id=45. Accessed 13 Aug 2017.
Environmental Management Bureau (EMB). n.d.-b. Water quality management area. http://water.emb.gov.ph/?page_id=12. Accessed 13 Aug 2017.
Environmental Management Bureau (EMB). n.d.-c. The industrial ecowatch program fact sheet. http://119.92.161.2/embgovph/eeid/Resources/FactSheets/tabid/1397/aid/183/Default.aspx. Accessed 28 Aug 2017.
Fehr A, et al. Sub-national inequities in Philippine water access associated with poverty and water potential. J Water Sanit Hyg Dev. 2013;3(4):638–45. https://doi.org/10.2166/washdev.2013.115.
Fernandez EO. 2017. Massive fish kill wipes out Lake Sebu's tilapia stock Philippine Daily Inquirer. http://newsinfo.inquirer.net/867809/massive-fish-kill-wipes-out-lake-sebus-tilapia-stock. Accessed 21 Aug 2017.
Franta B et al. 2016. Climate disasters in the Philippines: a case study of immediate causes and root drivers from Cagayan de Oro, Mindanao and Tropical Storm Sendong/Washi. Belfer Center for Science and International Affairs, Cambridge, MA: Harvard University.
Greenpeace. The state of water resources in the Philippines. Quezon City: Greenpeace Southeast Asia; 2007.
Grimes JET, et al. The roles of water, sanitation and hygiene in reducing schistosomiasis: a review. Parasit Vectors. 2015;8:156.
Ido AL. Evaluating the physicochemical and bacteriological characteristics of Aligodon River as source of potable water for new Claveria Water System. Int J Res Eng Technol. 2016;5(5):51–8.
Insigne MSL, Kim GS. Saltwater intrusion modeling in the aquifer bounded by Manila Bay and Parañaque River, Philippines. Environ Eng Res. 2010;5(2):117–21. https://doi.org/10.4491/eer.2010.15.2.117.
Israel DC. 2009. Local service delivery of potable water in the Philippines: national review and case analysis (PIDS discussion paper no. 2009–38). Philippine Institute for Development Studies.
Jabatan LA. 2004. Weekender: environment. BusinessWorld. Manila. Financial Times Information, Global News Wire—Asia Africa Intelligence Wire.
Japan International Cooperation Agency. 1998. Master plan study on water resources management in the Republic of the Philippines final report. Tokyo, Japan. http://open_jicareport.jica.go.jp/pdf/11462777_01.pdf. Accessed 21 Aug 2017.
Jerusalem J. 2016. PH won't escape water crisis, USAID exec warns. Inquirer Mindanao. Cagayan de Oro City. http://newsinfo.inquirer.net/756220/ph-wont-escape-water-crisis-usaid-exec-warns. Accessed 13 Aug 2017.
Kim DW, et al. Physical processes leading to the development of an anomalously large cochlodinium polykrikoides bloom in the East sea/Japan sea. Harmful Algae. 2016;55:250–8. https://doi.org/10.1016/j.hal.2016.03.019.
Labajo-Villantes Y, Nuneza OM. Water quality assessment of Labo and Clarin rivers in Misamis Occidental, Philippines. Int J Biodivers Conserv. 2014;6(10):735–42.
Land Bank of the Philippines. 2014. Gawad Sibol Program. https://www.landbank.com/adopt-a-watershed-program-2. Accessed 13 Aug 2017.
Laud NV, et al. Physical and chemical parameters of selected river waters in Davao City. UIC Res J. 2016;19(2):147–63.

Lee MO, Choi JH. Distributions of water temperature and salinity in the Korea southern coastal water during cochlodinium polykrikoides blooms. J Korean Soc Mar Environ Energy. 2009;12(4):235–47.

Li P, et al. Mercury pollution in Asia: a review of the contaminated sites. J Hazard Mater. 2009;168:591. https://doi.org/10.1016/j.jhazmat.2009.03.031.

Lim VL, Flores VB. Water and soil analyses of Balongis fish cage and Oster (Talaba) farms in Concepcion River, Kabasalan, Zamboanga. Asia Pac J Multidiscip Res. 2017;5(1):139–46.

Llanto GM. 2013. Water financing programs in the Philippines: are we making progress? https://dirp4.pids.gov.ph/ris/dps/pidsdps1334.pdf. Accessed 13 Aug 2017.

Lubos L, Japos GV. Extent of Escherichia coli contamination of Cagayan de Oro river and factors causing contamination: a translational research in Southern Philippines. Liceo J High Educ Res Sci Technol Sect. 2010;6(2):44–59.

Lubos L, et al. A study on the fecal contamination of Cagayan de Oro River along the upstream (Barangay Bayanga) and the factors affecting contamination, August 2008–March 2009. Adv Nurs Res. 2013;5(January):1–22.

Luken RA. 1999. Industrial policy and the environment in the Philippines. United Nations Industrial Development Organization. United Nations Industrial Development Organization, Prepared for the Government of the Philippines under UNDP-financed TSS-1 facility, NC/PHI/97/020.

Madrazo AB. Water issues in the context of sustainable development. Paper presented at the 2nd World Conference on Green Productivity, EDSA Shangri-La, Mandaluyong City, Philippines, 9–11 December; 2002.

Magtibay BB. Water refilling station: an alternative source of drinking water supply in the Philippines. Paper presented at the 30th WEDC International Conference, Vientiane, Lao PDR; 2004.

Malapit HJL, et al. Does violent conflict make chronic poverty more likely? The Mindanao experience. Philipp Rev Econ. 2003;40(2):31–58.

National Anti-Poverty Commission. n.d. Sagana at ligtas na tubig para sa lahat. http://www.napc.gov.ph/projects/sagana-ligtas-na-tubig-para-sa-lahat-salintubig. Accessed 28 Aug 2017.

National Water Resources Board. n.d. Organizational structure. http://www.nwrb.gov.ph/index.php/about/organizational-structure. Accessed 28 Aug 2017.

Pelone R. 2014a. NortCot diarrhea outbreak contained, more doctors coming to town. Businessweek Mindanao. http://www.businessweekmindanao.com/2014/05/14/nortcot-diarrhea-outbreak-contained-more-doctors-coming-to-town. Accessed 13 Aug 2017.

Pelone R. 2014b. Child dies, 32 others hospitalized for waterborne disease in Zambo City's west coast barangay. Businessweek Mindanao. http://www.businessweekmindanao.com/2014/09/09/child-dies-32-others-hospitalized-for-waterborne-disease-in-zambo-citys-west-coast-barangay/#more-6900. Accessed 10 Aug 2017.

Pfadenhauer LM, Rehfuess E. Towards effective and socio-culturally appropriate sanitation and hygiene interventions in the Philippines: a mixed method approach. Int J Environ Res Public Health. 2015;12(2):1902–27. https://doi.org/10.3390/ijerph120201902.

Philippine Statistics Authority. 2016. Water Resources. https://psa.gov.ph/content/water-resources. Accessed 13 Aug 2017.

Pinder GF. Groundwater hydrology. Adv Water Resour. 1981;4(20):96. https://doi.org/10.1016/0309-1708(81)90029-4.

Quisil JC, et al. Impact of mine tailings on the species diversity of Odonata fauna in Surigao Del Sur, Philippines. J Biodivers Environ Sci. 2014;5(1):465–76.

Radyo Natin. 2016. DOH urges public to beef up cleanliness to curb diarrhea, norovirus spread. https://www.radyonatin.com/story.php?storyid=10690 [updated 1 Mar 2017]. Accessed 13 Aug 2017.

Ranada P. 2015. Philippines faces "high" level of water shortage in 2040 – study. Rappler. Manila. http://www.rappler.com/science-nature/environment/104039-philippines-water-stress-2040. Accessed 13 Aug 2017.

Raymundo RB. Challenges to water resource management: ensuring adequate supply and better water quality for the present and future generations. Presented at the DLSU Research Congress 2015, De La Salle, Manila, Philippines; 2015.

Rodolfo KS, et al. The December 2012 Mayo River debris flow triggered by Super Typhoon Bopha in Mindanao, Philippines: lessons learned and questions raised. Nat Hazards Earth Syst Sci. 2016;16(12):2683–95.

Rola AC, et al. Challenges of water governance in the Philippines. Philipp J Sci. 2015;144(2): 197–298.

Sarmiento BS. 2017. 30 hectares of illegal tilapia fish pens dismantled in Lake Sebu. MindaNews. Davao City. http://www.mindanews.com/top-stories/2017/06/30-hectares-of-illegal-tilapia-fish-pens-dismantled-in-lake-sebu/. Accessed 21 Aug 2017.

Scholze O, et al. Protection of the groundwater resources of Metropolis Cebu (Philippines) in consideration of saltwater intrusion into the coastal aquifer. Presented at the 17th Salt Water Intrusion Meeting. Delft, The Netherlands; 2002.

Senate Economic Planning Office. 2011. Turning the tide: improving water resource management in the Philippines (PB-11-03). http://www.senate.gov.ph/publications/PB%202011-08%20-%20Turning%20the%20Tide.pdf. Accessed 13 Aug 2017.

Serrano B. 2015. Butuan under state of water crisis. Philippine Star Global. Butuan City. http://www.philstar.com/nation/2015/01/29/1417754/butuan-under-state-water-crisis. Accessed 13 Aug 2017.

Silva JA. Devolution and regional disparities in the Philippines: is there a connection? Environ Plan C. 2005;23(3):399–417. https://doi.org/10.1068/c051.

Tabios III GQ. 2014. Update on proposed national water resources management office (NWRMO). http://www.nast.ph/index.php/downloads/category/40-water-governance?download=151:update-on-proposed-national-water-resources-management-office. Accessed 28 Aug 2017.

Tacio H. 2014. Water crisis looms in Davao. Philippine EnviroNews. http://environews.ph/ecocities/water-crisis-looms-in-davao/. Accessed 13 Aug 2017.

Tan JML, et al. Managing Mindanao's natural capital: the environment in Mindanao's past, present and future. In: Duplito MS, editor. Pasig City: Brain Trust; 2012.

Tirado R. 2007. Nitrates in drinking water in the Philippines and Thailand. http://www.greenpeace.to/publications/Nitrates_Philippines_Thailand.pdf. Accessed 13 Aug 2017.

Tomas CR, Smaydab TJ. Red tide blooms of cochlodinium polykrikoides in a coastal cove. Harmful Algae. 2008;7(3):308–17. https://doi.org/10.1016/j.hal.2007.12.005.

United Nations. 2015. The Millennium development goals report 2015.TakePart http://www.un.org/millenniumgoals/2015_MDG_Report/pdf/MDG%202015%20rev%20(July%201).pdf. Accessed 11 Aug 2017.

United Nations. 2017. Millennium development goals and beyond 2015. http://www.un.org/millenniumgoals/. Accessed 11 Aug 2017.

United Nations Children's Fund (UNICEF) and World Health Organization (WHO). 2012. Progress on drinking water and sanitation. Joint Monitoring Programme for Water Supply and Sanitation, Philippines. https://www.unicef.org/media/files/JMPreport2012.pdf. Accessed 21 Aug 2017.

United States Agency for International Development (USAID). 2010. Philippine sanitation alliance: 10th quarterly report results. Makati City. http://pdf.usaid.gov/pdf_docs/PA00HWJ4.pdf. Accessed 13 Aug 2017.

United States Agency for International Development (USAID). 2016. Building climate resilience in water stressed communities (CREST). https://www.usaid.gov/philippines/energy-and-environment/crest. Accessed 3 Sept 2017.

United States Agency for International Development (USAID) and Asian Environmental Compliance and Enforcement Network (AECEN). 2004. Environmental compliance and enforcement in the Philippines: rapid assessment. http://www.aecen.org/sites/default/files/PH_Assessment.pdf. Accessed 13 Aug 2017.

Vicente H, et al. Harmful algal bloom in Iligan Bay, Southern Philippines. Sci Diliman. 2002;14(2):59–65.

Water Environment Partnership in Asia (WEPA). n.d. State of water environmental issues: Philippines. http://www.wepa-db.net/policies/state/philippines/overview.htm. Accessed 12 Aug 2017.

World Bank. 2003. Philippine environment monitor 2003. Washington, DC: World Bank. http://documents.worldbank.org/curated/en/144581468776089600/Philippines-Environment-monitor-2003. Accessed 21 Aug 2017.

World Bank. 2004. Philippine environment monitor 2004. Washington, DC: World Bank. http://documents.worldbank.org/curated/en/829241468333075012/Philippines-environment-monitor-2004-assessing-progress. Accessed 21 Aug 2017.

World Bank. 2014. Community-driven development project in the Philippines. http://www.worldbank.org/en/results/2014/04/10/community-driven-development-project-in-the-philippines. Accessed 13 Aug 2017.

Zapanta MJ, et al. An outbreak of leptospirosis in Davao City Philippines, 2013: an investigation of the risky behaviors that led to the resurgence. Outbreak Surveill Investig Rep. 2014;7(4):1–5.

Further Reading

Dwyer L. 2014. This floating grass billboard can suck pollution out of filthy rivers. TakePart. http://www.takepart.com/article/2014/06/03/floating-grass-billboard-can-suck-pollution-out-filthy-rivers. Accessed 28 Aug 2017.

Marks SJ, et al. Community participation and water supply sustainability: evidence from hand-pump projects in rural Ghana. J Plan Educ Res. 2014;34:1–11. https://doi.org/10.1177/0739456X14527620.

Morrison K. Stakeholder involvement in water management: necessity or luxury? Water Sci Technol. 2003;47:43–51.

Osumanu IK. Community involvement in urban water and sanitation provision: the missing link in partnerships for improved service delivery in Ghana. J Afr Stud Dev. 2010;2(8):208–15.

Chapter 13
International Changes in Environmental Conditions and Their Personal Health Consequences

Beth Ann Fiedler

Abstract Earth in the balance must consider the international changes in the physical and social environmental conditions resulting from global climate change, economic development, conflict, and other factors. Regardless of what side of the political fence individuals may land relating to climate change, the mounting evidence of air pollution, hazardous chemicals, water scarcity, land conversion, and biodiversity loss are evident. So too is their link to increased metabolic risk factors that damage human organ systems eliciting negative health outcomes (e.g., asthma, neurobehavioral disorders, and zoonotic infectious diseases) leading to morbidity and mortality. Together, these environmental and consequent health conditions should prompt civic engagement to reduce shared risks and consequences. This chapter reports a broad scope of the health disorders from the leading global environmental causes of death, such as pollution, land degradation and land use, providing an overview of key environmental and social problems and social responsibilities facing less-developed, emerging, and industrialized nations. Then moves on to discuss social considerations in two areas: (1) public participation found in environmental impact assessments, and (2) how income inequality in the social environment and social foundation may impact government structure and capitalism. Finally, the chapter brings forth multi-government levels of environmental and public health resources in the United States to prompt civic engagement, address personal behavior patterns and environmental risks. The chapter concludes with a discussion on the role of individual participation towards resolving environmental conditions and their health consequences.

B. A. Fiedler (✉)
Independent Research Analyst, Jacksonville, FL, USA

B. A. Fiedler (ed.), *Translating National Policy to Improve Environmental Conditions Impacting Public Health Through Community Planning*,
https://doi.org/10.1007/978-3-319-75361-4_13

13.1 Introduction

Two important factors that help to determine the risk of susceptibility to environmental conditions that impact health mortality and morbidity are age and the predominant national economic development status of the country in which you are born and develop. Birth location may have the greatest potential impact on the capacity to obtain basic needs, to improve circumstances through opportunity, and the ability to live in a healthy environment as a predictive measure of quality of life. While environmental impact on health can be felt by all age groups, the World Health Organization (WHO) directs attention to the wide array of environmental risks that disproportionately affect the most vulnerable people in the global population in these primary categories—(1) age (e.g., children aged 5 years or less, adults between the ages of 50 and 75), and (2) economic status (e.g., country populations characterized by low and middle class socioeconomic status prevalent in regions such as Southeast Asia, Africa and the Western Pacific) (WHO 2017a).

The term vulnerable population was introduced at the turn of the millennium to differentiate the global population who were "at risk of poor physical, psychological, or social health" (Aday 2001, p.10). However, the U.S. Global Change Research Program has further described vulnerability in terms that directly relate to climate change for individuals, communities and the institutions that guide them. They are (1) exposure representing contact opportunities in which climate stressors can elicit biological, psychosocial or other responses, (2) sensitivity which is the degree a community may be impacted by environmental stressors, and (3) adaptive capacity of the community and existing institutions to respond to known or emerging predictors (USGCRP 2016). Their key findings indicate with high confidence that, "Social determinants of health, such as those related to socioeconomic factors and health disparities, may amplify, moderate, or otherwise influence climate-related health effects, particularly when these factors occur simultaneously or close in time or space" (USGCRP 2016, p.248).

WHO reports that 12.6 million people die annually from environmental conditions representing "23% of all global deaths" (WHO 2017a, p.1). These population segments represent the growing number of people in the global population who are highly susceptible to the increasing number and variety of environmental contaminants (e.g., air pollution, the built environment, deficient sanitary water supply, and hazardous chemicals and waste) contributing to annual morbidity and mortality. The public health impact of environmental conditions, while prominent in less-developed/emerging nations, is getting personal to a greater span of the global population. Further, developed nations are not immune to the personal impact of environmental conditions. Empirical evidence from studies in the US and the European Union (EU) find that environmental hazards, such as air pollution, are associated with toxic and debilitating effects to the human body organ systems (e.g., endocrine, respiratory, cardiovascular, and reproductive) (Colao et al. 2016). While country of origin may foster a better start, the reality is that the long-term effects of environmental conditions can impede global quality of life.

Table 13.1 The World Bank Group world development indicators: global morbidity vulnerability for under age 5 years and noncommunicable and communicable diseases for all ages

Socioeconomic status[†a]	Under age 5 years Death[a]		Deaths Noncommunicable diseases % of total[††b]		Deaths Communicable diseases % of total[†††c]	
	2000	2015	2000	2015	2000	2015
High income	96,333	67,940	87.19	87.81	6.63	6.59
Upper middle income	1,405,443	714,548	77.62	83.44	12.18	8.14
Lower middle income	5,715,967	3,478,060	46.13	59.02	44.91	31.10
Low income	2,565,058	1,683,991	23.00	36.89	68.49	51.95

Source: [a]The World Bank 2017a; [b]The World Bank 2017b; [c]The World Bank 2017c
Notes: [†]Socioeconomic status is based on the 2015 Gross National Income (GNI) per capita defined as the average income per citizen. Low-income economies was $1,025 or less such as Afghanistan, Uganda, and Liberia; Lower-middle income between $1,026 and $4,035 such as Angola, India, and Micronesia; Upper Middle income between $4,036 and $12,475 such as Brazil, Bosnia and Herzegovina, Russian Federation, and Panama; and High-income was $12,476 or more such as France, Greenland, Ireland, Latvia and New Zealand
[††]Cause of death refers to all ages attributed to chronic conditions such as cancer, diabetes mellitus, hereditary irregularities, and diseases of the skin, cardiovascular system, digestive system, and musculoskeletal system
[†††]Cause of death refers to all ages attributed to communicable (infectious) diseases and maternal, prenatal and nutrition conditions (e.g., infectious and parasitic diseases), respiratory infections, and nutritional deficiencies

Consequently, a prominent United Nations Sustainable Development "Goal 3: ensure healthy lives and promote well-being for all at all ages" (United Nations 2017, *para* 1) is a primary focus. Even though health goals are intended to apply to all age, Table 13.1 demonstrates that there are age and national socioeconomic factors that require more attention. For example, more than 5 million deaths in children 5 years and under occurred in low- and lower middle-income nations in 2015 (World Bank 2017a). "In 2015, the global neonatal mortality rate was 19 per 1000 live births and the under-five mortality rate in 2015 was 43 per 1000 live births, representing declines of 37% and 44% respectively from 2000" (WHO 2017b, *para* 14). Hoping to gain momentum on the downward trend, the WHO has challenged the globe to "reduce neonatal mortality to at least as low as 12 per 1000 live births and under-5 mortality to at least as low as 25 per live births" (2017b, *para* 13).

A simultaneously aging and growing population contributes to the rising percent of the total population struggling with one or more forms of noncommunicable disease (NCD) evident across all national socioeconomic status categories from 2000 to 2015 (World Bank 2017a, b; WHO 2017b). NCDs, historically considered diseases of the elderly, have a growing impact on adults starting at age 30. While "the probability of dying from chronic disease, such as diabetes, cancer, cardiovascular disease and chronic lung disease between ages 30 and 70 is 19%, a 17% decline from 2000" (WHO 2017b, *para* 19), there remains an upward momentum (Table 13.1). WHO targets a one-third global reduction in premature noncommunicable disease mortality through a preventive medicine and holistic approach to physical and mental health (WHO 2017b) to reduce the "15 million people [who] die from a NCD between the ages of 30 and 69 years; over 80% of these 'premature' deaths [about 31 million] occur in low- and middle-income countries" (WHO 2017c *para* 2, 9).

The availability of vaccines and distribution channels contribute to the decreasing percent of total deaths from communicable diseases from 2000 to 2015 (Table 13.1) (World Bank 2017c). However, there remains a need to address continuously emerging strains of infectious diseases often brought forth from ecosystem encroachment that dislodges animal, insect, and plant life habitats with unforeseen impact on the human population (WHO 2017d).

Minimizing these risks and others are key to "protecting children and achieving the Sustainable Development Goals" (WHO 2017a) that includes targeting poverty and preventing associated health risks, such as NCDs. Stroke, ischemic heart disease, unintentional injuries, and cancer are the top four leading NCD causes of adult deaths accounting for nearly two-thirds of deaths attributed to existing environmental risks (WHO 2017a, p.2). The fifth largest global cause of death is chronic respiratory diseases (WHO 2017a, p.2) while respiratory infections are the leading cause of death in children under the age of 5 (WHO 2017e, p.1). Economic inequality is often problematic for pulmonary conditions concurrent with health inequality. Implications for poor respiratory and long-term health problems are also high for impoverished children as well as adults who are exposed to occupational health hazards (The Lancet Respiratory Health 2017). Outdoor air pollution, a composition of harmful airborne particles containing particulate matter such as lead and aerosols, is a contributing factor to these metabolic risk factors (Colao et al. 2016; Solomon 2011). "Exposure to ambient air pollution increases morbidity and mortality, and is a leading contributor to global disease burden" (Cohen et al. 2017, p.1907). Indoor air pollution, a result of hazardous chemicals and building materials, and outdoor pollution in 2012 caused "an estimated 6.5 million deaths globally, or 11.6% of all deaths" (WHO 2017b, *para* 32).

The Global Burden of Disease (GBD) risk factor study reports some improvements in risk factors such as the risk of child undernutrition dropping from rank 3 in 1990 to 18 in 2015 (Cohen et al. 2017, p.1911; Global Burden of Disease Study (GBD) 2016). However, high systolic blood pressure remains the highest risk overall and the leading metabolic risk while smoking remained second overall and the leading behavioral risk. Ambient particulate matter pollution dropped one notch from rank 4 overall in 1990 to 5 in 2015 but remains the highest environmental or occupational risk (Cohen et al. 2017, p.1911; Global Burden of Disease Study (GBD) 2016).

Unavoidably, the existing environmental and social conditions leading to negative health outcomes are linked to where we live, work, and play. Is the cost of economic development a disproportionately high price to pay for an elevation in social status that may increase access to some higher quality products while simultaneously exposing the population to new risks? This chapter provides an overview of the key environmental problems plaguing the globe from the perspective of less-developed/emerging nations and industrialized nations, define key social considerations from various perspectives, and supply public resources promoting informed, civic engagement.

13.2 Key Environmental Problems

The public health ramifications of environmental problems are global. Among the many credible lists of environmental indicators, such as the list generated by the Organization for Economic Development and Cooperation (OECD 2008a, b), there is an overarching short list—pollution, land degradation, and land use from which many other environmental hazards are derived. For example, pollution can describe poor air quality, contaminated freshwater supply, or ocean acidification, and thus endangered fisheries, due to airborne contaminants (EPA 2017a; Solomon 2011). In the same way, land degradation speaks to soil erosion and chemical contamination while land-use decisions continue to destroy rural areas in favor of urban development leading to biodiversity loss and land conversion (OECD 2001, 2017a, b). However, there are distinctions between countries that are less-developed and emerging and those who have already achieved industrialization. Nonetheless, the short-list of three environmental indicators can account for numerous environmental risks, indicate national human and economic development status, and contribute to the primary causes of poor public health.

13.2.1 Environmental Problems in Less-Developed and Emerging Countries

Environmental conditions in lesser developed and emerging countries (e.g., Brazil, India, and Mexico) are exacerbated by poverty where overpopulation destructively taps into increasingly limited natural resources (Anand 2013; Cassar 2005). Another prevailing problem faced by these countries is the lack of infrastructure prohibiting access to clean water and sanitation (Anand 2013). The National Council for Science and the Environment (NCSE 2017, *para* 1) defines sustainable infrastructure:

> Broadly defined, infrastructure is the interconnected system of the physical, natural and social components that societies need to survive and function. To make infrastructure truly sustainable, it must not only provide these services, but also take into account the risks and opportunities it generates arising from the bricks, mortar, and financing required to build and sustain the system as well as the environmental and human impacts of the system itself.

Sustainable infrastructure represents the process of improving existing built systems (e.g., buildings, bridges, waste management, and transportation) and natural systems (e.g., waterways). The process also incorporates new structures to facilitate the needs of a given community.

Lack of national funds and a limited number of trustworthy institutions, if any, to distribute medical, food, and water supplies or to otherwise support social services adds another dimension to the problem. Fundamental logistics, even when funds are available and there are trusted institutions, become problematic because of the difficulties in reaching people due to poor infrastructure and the remote nature of some populations. Thus, the cascading impact of poverty permeates throughout the environment and is evident in multiple and inter-related conditions that cumulatively contribute to poor public health.

Urban population growth and low socioeconomic status often combine to form the "synergistic problems of urban poverty, traffic fatalities and air pollution" (WHO 2017f, *para* 2). Reduced access to open spaces and/or the presence of various pollutions deters urban dwellers from physical activity. In turn, lack of physical activity then contributes to the leading causes of death from NCDs. Further, if you combine the effects of these environmental conditions with the consequences of personal habits of irresponsible alcohol consumption, smoking, and poor eating habits, such as a diet high in sodium or low in whole grains and fruits, risk of early onset of various diseases can rapidly increase the likelihood of the impact on systemic organ systems leading to a decline in function. Granted, some dietary and other choices can be a product of the environment—lack of access to fresh food due to lack of transportation or low income. Nonetheless, the consequences of the human body expending energy to repair the damages from these behaviors weaken the capacity to remove toxins because of these behaviors and environmental conditions.

The burden on natural resources (e.g., forests, minerals, fisheries, wildlife) is evident in developing nations where they are the only source of raw materials, such as wood, that are accessible to the population. Often, these nations do not have any policy in place to limit the level of destruction. Finally, the desire to emerge from poverty places further stress on resources and puts the globe at risk through the introduction of new chemicals and materials, as well as those banned in other countries such as asbestos (Al-Delaimy 2013), as poorer countries reintroduce less expensive but often more dangerous materials and processing methods (WHO 2017c) to keep pace with industrialized production.

13.2.2 Environmental Problems in Developed Countries

One word,overconsumption, characterizes the waste demonstrated in developed nations such as the US and EU member states that have prospered from twentieth-century industrialization. A quick view of the national ecological footprint, the difference between the biocapacity of a nation and what they utilize, demonstrates the global imbalance (Global Footprint Network 2017a). "Overall, the developed world has 23% of Earth's population but consumes two-thirds of the resources" (Anand 2013, p.1). The fundamental problem is clear—an overabundance of goods produced at the expense of natural resources. Industrial consumption—the consequence of production and the multiplicity of products, also "affect the environment through the emission of greenhouse gases and other wastes" (Anand 2013, p.2).

Table 13.2 demonstrates the large per capita carbon dioxide (CO_2) emissions from the countries in North America—Bermuda, Canada, and the United States—at 16.11 metric tons per capita in 2013 (World Bank 2017d). However, there is also a decline of nearly 4 metric tons per capita from 2000 to 2013 while other regions are increasing emissions. Relevant to note is that per capita reporting of statistics

Table 13.2 The World Bank world development indicators for carbon dioxide (CO_2) emissions from burning fossil fuels, cement manufacturing processes, and gas-flaring

Socioeconomic status[a]	Regional associations[b]	Carbon dioxide emission (metric tons/capita)	
		2000	2013
High income		12.27	11.04
Upper middle income		3.56	6.62
Lower middle income		1.07	1.43
Low income		0.03[c]	0.28[c]
	Arab World[1]	3.68	4.64
	Central Europe & Baltics[2]	6.61	6.35
	East Asia & Pacific[3]	3.20	6.34
	European Union[4]	8.00	6.73
	Latin America & Caribbean[5]	2.55	3.05
	Middle East & North Africa[6]	4.65	5.91
	North America[7]	19.93	16.11
	Organization for Economic Cooperation and Development[8]	11.06	9.68
	Sub-Saharan Africa[9]	0.846	0.82[c]

Source: The World Bank 2017d

[a]Socioeconomic status is based on the 2015 Gross National Income (GNI) per capita defined as the average income per citizen. Low-income economies were $1025 or less such as Yemen, Mali, Nepal, and Chad; Lower-middle income between $1026 and $4035 such as Georgia, Armenia, Paraguay, Indonesia, and Sudan; Upper-middle income between $4036 and $12,475 such as Turkey, Costa Rica, Romania, and Peru; and High-income was $12,476 or more such as Austria, Sweden, Canada, Saudi Arabia, and Israel

[b1]Algeria, Bahrain, Comoros, Djibouti, Egypt, Iraq, Jordan, Kuwait, Lebanon, Libya, Mauritania, Morocco, Oman, Qatar, Saudi Arabia, Somalia, Sudan, Syrian Arab Republic, Tunisia, United Arab Emirates, West Bank and Gaza, and Yemen; [2]Bulgaria, Croatia, Czech Republic, Estonia, Hungary, Latvia, Lithuania, Poland, Romania, Slovak Republic, and Slovenia; [3]American Samoa, Australia, Brunei, Darussalam, Cambodia, China, Fiji, French Polynesia, Guam, Hong Kong, Indonesia, Japan, Kiribati, Korea, Lao, Macao, Malaysia, Marshall Islands, Micronesia, Mongolia, Myanmar, Nauru, New Caledonia, New Zealand, Northern Mariana Islands, Palau, Papua New Guinea, Philippines, Samoa, Singapore, Solomon Islands, Thailand, Timor-Leste, Tonga, Tuvalu, Vanuatu, and Vietnam. [4]28 members of EU in 2013: Austria, Belgium, Bulgaria, Croatia, Cyprus, Czech Republic, Denmark, Estonia, Finland, France, Germany, Greece, Hungary, Ireland, Italy, Latvia, Lithuania, Luxembourg, Malta, Netherlands, Poland, Portugal, Romania, Slovakia, Spain, Sweden, and United Kingdom; [5]Antigua and Barbuda, Argentina, Aruba, Bahamas, Barbados, Belize, Bolivia, Brazil, British Virgin Islands, Cayman Islands, Chile, Colombia, Costa Rica Cuba, Curacao, Dominica, Dominican Republic, Ecuador, El Salvador Grenada, Guatemala, Guyana, Haiti, Honduras, Jamaica. Mexico, Nicaragua, Panama, Paraguay, Peru, Puerto Rico, Sin Maarten (Dutch), St. Kitts and Nevis, St. Lucia, St. Martin (French), St. Vincent and the Grenadines, Suriname, Trinidad and Tobago, Turks and Caicos Islands, Uruguay, Venezuela, and Virgin Islands; [6] Algeria, Bahrain, Djibouti, Egypt, Iran, Israel, Iraq, Jordan, Kuwait, Lebanon, Libya, Morocco, Oman, Qatar, Saudi Arabia, Syria, Tunisia, United Arab Emirates, West Bank and Gaza, and Yemen; [7]Bermuda, Canada and the United States; [8] United States, United Kingdom, Turkey, Switzerland, Sweden, Spain, Slovenia, Slovak Republic, Portugal, Poland, Norway, New Zealand,

(continued)

Table 13.2 (continued)

Netherlands, Mexico, Luxembourg Latvia, Korea, Japan, Italy, Israel, Ireland Iceland, Hungary, Greece, Germany, France, Finland, Estonia, Denmark, Czech Republic, Chile, Canada, Belgium, Austria, Australia; [9]Angola, Benin, Botswana, Burkina Faso, Burundi, Cabo Verde, Cameroon, Central African Republic, Chad, Comoros, Congo, Cote d'Ivoire, Equatorial Guinea, Eritrea, Ethiopia, Gabon, Gambia, Ghana, Guinea-Bissau, Kenya, Lesotho, Liberia, Madagascar, Malawi, Mali, Mauritania, Mauritius, Mozambique, Namibia, Niger, Nigeria, Rwanda, Sao Tome and Principe, Senegal, Seychelles, Sierra Leone, Somalia, South Africa, South Sudan, Sudan, Swaziland, Tanzania, Togo, Uganda, Zambia, Zimbabwe

[c]Rounded to two decimal places except for numbers <1 that are listed at three or more decimal places

may require further interpretation beyond face value. For example, the population of China, one of 37 nations in the East Asia & Pacific region, was 1.354 billion in 2013 while Bermuda (65,091), Canada (34,881,000) and the United States (316,103,330) combined for 351, 049, 021 or about 25% of the population of China alone. According to 2014 estimates from research conducted with the Carbon Dioxide Information Analysis Center (CDIAC), a subgroup of the United States Department of Energy, mainland China tops the list of fossil-fuel burning, cement production, and gas flaring emission with 2,806,634 thousand tons of carbon, almost twice the emissions of the US at 1432855 thousand tons of carbon (Boden et al. 2014, 2017) who has been steadily decreasing emissions. Individual consumption in North America is larger per capita but the actual amount of CO_2 emissions emanating from the East Asia & Pacific region is greater. Thus, reporting national emissions per capita when population size is a factor can be misleading. Finally, national governments take the hit for overconsumption and growing consumption that impacts the globe, but the accumulation of individual consumption is critical to the consumption direction of each national population. This brings forth the important element of the individual contribution to international changes in environmental conditions and their personal health consequences.

Nothing brings the problem of overconsumption in developed nations to the fore like the global problem of e-waste. "E-waste refers to all types of electrical or electronic equipment (EEE) and its parts that have been discarded without intention for reuse by the owner" (Heacock et al. 2016, p.550). The largest public health factor in the persistent practice of e-waste recycling is the "elevated concentrations of various industrial-use Persistent Organic Pollutants (POPs), such as polychlorinated biphenyls (PCBs)" (Breivik et al. 2016, p.798). PCBs and other POPs are expected to continue to escalate the problem of global emissions.

Approximately 80% of the 2014 estimated global e-waste of 41.8 million tons (Breivik et al. 2014; Heacock et al. 2016, p.550) was redistributed to less-developed/emerging nations in Africa and China (Heacock et al. 2016, p.551; Lundgren 2012). Developed and some emerging nations illegally send e-waste to less-developed/emerging nations who illegally receive these items under the guise of resale. International shipping guidelines, such as the Basel Convention of the United Nations Environment Program, ban this process of disposal (Heacock et al. 2016). Nevertheless, these nations use these discarded items as a waste recycling resource to recover valuable commodities such as iron, copper, and gold. However, e-waste sites are not regulated and do not offer a safe extraction method or protection against hazardous elements contained in these products, such as mercury and lead, when ad hoc dumping sites draw unprotected workers to disassemble these products. Toxic poisoning resulting from handling materials directly or water consumption drawn from streams where heavy metals (e.g., mercury, lead) have accumulated results in damage to the brain and nervous system. Developing systems are highly susceptible as common routes of lead exposure to youth occur during the first few years of development while pregnant women exposed to mercury can seriously harm the fetus.

China, a consumer and recipient of e-waste, is one of several Asian nations who are remedying the problem with an increase in environmental legislation and in the establishment of institutions that are responsible for monitoring and oversight (Honda et al. 2016). “As a continent, Asia generates the highest volume of e-waste, estimated at 16 million tonnes in 2014. However, on a per capita basis, this amounts to only to 3.7 kgs per inhabitant, as compared to Europe and the Americas, which generate nearly four times as much per capita” (Honda et al. 2016, p.26). (Noteworthy to recognize the impact of population size on reported measures.) While incorporating greater controls is an utmost priority, communicating the health problems associated with this practice to unknowing participants, such as women and children, has brought forth the opportunity to innovate to make less harmful component parts in products, provide protective clothing for workers, and introduce safer processing methods that reduce contact with harmful components.

13.2.3 *Can What Is Good for the Emerging Goose Also Be Good for the Industrial Gander?*

The establishment of the 1997 Kyoto Protocol to the United Nations Framework Convention on Climate Change (UNFCCC 2014), now signed by just over 190 countries minus the US, deemphasizes emissions regulation from newly industrializing nations such as China, India, and Brazil. “Reflecting their circumstances, the focus of low-income countries is on climate resilience rather than emissions” (Nachmany et al. 2017, p.5).

Climate resilience is the process of developing sustainable options in response to environmental stressors intensified by climate change (e.g., limited freshwater supply coupled with drought) while emissions regulation seeks to reduce the number of hazardous contaminants into the environment. But development that contributes to the growing burden of environmental and public health decay appears in stark contrast to the true objective of climate resilience. Today, Chinese citizens in Beijing wear masks to protect their lungs against particulate matter found in smog that is known to impact cardiac health (Guan et al. 2017). The emphasis on climate resilience versus emissions also represents a significant difference in the development of regulation, implementation and adherence upon considering the toxic contribution of greenhouse gas emissions from these emerging nations.

There is a small voice battling the emissions exemption to emerging nations established in the Kyoto agreement in contrast to the cry for global solutions rectifying international environmental conditions. A global solution does not appear possible in the face of clear distinctions between monitoring and accountability in industrialized nations compared to emerging nations. The exemption also represents a nearly unrestricted opportunity to build in nations where there is a lack of regulation. The less-developed/emerging nations may be doomed to repeat history and bring the rest of the world with them unless there is an influx of regulatory constraint and a standard of ethical business practice. Further, the implementation of ethical business standards also applies to corporations who have transferred operations from developed nations to emerging and less-developed countries.

However, there is hope for a less dismal future. The OECD foresees linked interdependencies forming mutually beneficial collaborations between developed and emerging nations (OECD 2008b). The basis of which can address resource management, such as projected increases in fossil fuel consumption by emerging nations as they expand their industrial base, social stability, and strategies to halt pandemics and new methods to transfer technology (OECD 2001, 2017b). Nevertheless, merely transferring the point of origin of pollution does not resolve the mounting global impact on the environment and public health. Thus, the social element is important to addressing global environmental problems.

13.3 Key Social Considerations

Various interpretations of the use of the word "social" are expressed in business, economics, life science and psychology. They include extended terminology such as social issues, social environment, and social foundation. Physical and biological environmental assessments, generally headed under social issues, can be found in any example of an environmental impact assessment for proposed development. They can also appear in a critical assessment of income inequality, one element of the social environment, that could have long-term consequences in the structure of representative government—also known as a social foundation. All three "social" perspectives aid in unravelling the complex nature of business development, environmental conditions and their health consequences, income equality and any other shortcomings in the quality of life that limit progression of those with lower socioeconomic status. Thus, this section reviews some of the social issues targeted in environmental impact assessments and the inclusive element of open forums for public review. Then, we view the topic of income inequality in the social environment and the proposition of exclusionary representation in the social foundation of government with competing literature.

13.3.1 Environmental Impact Assessments: Social Issues

Businesses generate new product ideas all the time by perceiving an unmet customer product or service in an existing market or by innovating new product sectors. Product development often requires new manufacturing space that requires land development. When a business or developer requires land, one of the necessary precautions that businesses must undertake in determining if new development is realistic starts with a perceived unmet customer product or service. The term "customer" may change in other arenas but the premise is fundamentally the same. For example, employment growth is linked to regional economic strength and the customers are the constituents of that region. The perceived customer base translates into viable business or policy objectives that often, in turn, require the addition of facilities. The addition of facilities begins with a process of site review and public forums that engage the community. These activities play a significant role in the economic and political feasibility of any new development, program, project, or plan.

A primary tool in this process is the conduct of an environmental impact assessment (EIA). EIA is "the process of identifying, predicting, evaluating and mitigating the biophysical, social, and other relevant effects of development proposals prior to major decisions being taken and commitments made" (IAIA 1999). While national strategies can differ slightly in process and agency reporting structure within nations—demonstrated by a cursory comparison of the United Kingdom (UK) Department for Communities and Local Government (2014) (WHO Europe 2013) and between nations, such as the United States and Central American and Dominican Republic Free Trade Agreement (CAFTA-DR) (EPA 2017b), they share fundamental objectives to minimize environmental damage.

Multilevel government monitoring and reporting also play a key role in regional, national, and international objectives. For example, Ireland often derives national legislation from shared European Union Member State policy, such as Directive 2014/52/EU implemented in 2017 (EU 2014), to guide development of national objectives with local planning authorities—the Department of Housing, Planning, Community and Local Government, and community members impacted by new development (IEPA 2017).

In another example, the US EPA provides an Environmental Impact Statement (EIS) database portal that is open for public access (EPA 2017c). Further, the United Nations Environmental Programme (UNEP) offers status briefs and tools relating to sustainability including detailed training information on EIA and global monitoring (UNEP-WCMC 2015; UNEP 2002).

These selected EIA tools and resources provide a framework for capacity building in conjunction with concern for the environment. Together they envelop social issues expressed in EIA facets of collaboration between and among institutions and the public, understanding the dynamic and multitiered legal foundation of sustainability, and reporting elements that aid in decision-making embracing the perspective of various stakeholders.

The social, environmental and potential health hazards for various stakeholders become transparent in the required content of EIA reports. The EIA reporting elements consist of public involvement, screening (a preliminary assessment), and scoping (CEIL 2015). Scoping is a public process that has two primary elements—(1) the systematic identification of major obstacles, potential solutions, and impact of each; and (2) the capacity to categorize important problems that require further resource allocation, staging, and planning (CEIL 2015).

Elements of environmental and public safety, spanning beach erosion to waste management, often dominate an EIA report. Some of the many concerns in new development include local, national and international topics. Some local aspects include the visual and actual impact of the development on the natural landscape/seascape including fauna and flora, the ability to maintain cultural heritage for the indigenous population, and the short-term impact of accommodating construction workers. National concerns may entail the long-term impact of tourism including national security relating to international visitors and the contribution of job growth to economic stability. Of course, any one of these items may crossover into other levels of concern including concern for government stability, leading us to the next section.

13.3.2 Income Inequality in the Social Environment and Social Foundation of Government

Income inequality, defined as the unequal measure of national wealth distributed across existing socioeconomic classes (e.g., rich, middle-class, poor), is a common problem in less-developed, emerging, and industrialized nations. Academia is overflowing with decades of literature informing that the answer to income inequality is sustainable capitalism (Barton 2011; Schweickart 2010), could be sustainable capitalism (Bradford 2000; Lambin 2009; Liodokis 2010), or can't possibly be sustainable capitalism (Cervantes 2013; Leech 2015; Rull 2011). "Sustainable Capitalism is a framework that seeks to maximise long-term economic value creation by reforming markets to address real needs while considering all costs and integrating ESG [environmental, social, and governance] metrics into the decision-making process" (Generation Investment Management LLP 2012, p.4). Sustainable capitalism—logical in theory, but perhaps slow to transition to application in the business world where short-term gain is the normative objective.

Meanwhile, the debate continues through these and many other examples, bringing forth both the benefits of development and the disdain for accompanying problems. At this junction, there emerges a link between income inequality in the social environment and social foundation of government. Two opposing didactic extend the problem of income inequality to unequal government representation. The first entails the prediction of the fall of a democratic society while the opposing view underscores some important information relating to the hotly debated problem.

Sitaraman (2017) describes the intent of balanced representation in the US Constitutional policy as teetering towards the wealthy as income inequality has marginalized the lower socioeconomic class in American society due to lack of representation. He suggests that the decay of the foundations of democracy might be averted if adjustments to class representative government were incorporated into the Constitution now that he surmises the US Constitutional premise of equality is waning. Thus, he points to long-standing government structures, such as the United Kingdom's House of Lords/House of Commons, that continue to balance power between the wealthy and less affluent (Sitaraman 2017). The election of billionaire real estate mogul Donald J. Trump to the White House as the 45th President of the US certainly supports the proposition as plausible to some.

On the other hand, those who do not believe there is a threat to the foundation of democratic society based on the growing gap of income equality are quick to respond. They cite two main opposing arguments: (1) the less than dismal circumstances of America's lower socioeconomic class operating within a capitalistic market and (2) lack of evidence to support skewed representation in favor of the wealthy. Few, however, would refute the value of Sitaraman's (2017) historical review on the evolution of the US political structure or his position that the restoration of a middle class will promote greater social stability. Yet, the opposing perspective brings forth some important information to pause some fear generated by the proposition that income inequality and thus, declining political representation of lower socioeconomic class citizens, is a prelude to government failure.

First, the plight of an impoverished American compared to those with lower socioeconomic status in other countries is decidedly different. This standing may attest to the sustainability of existing democratic representation and capitalistic principles that apply to the entire population. On the other hand, poverty is poverty. The author notes the importance of the personal nature of the problem and recognizes indications that the population concentration of those experiencing poverty may be moving out of urban America and into rural/suburban strongholds (Allard 2017; Mirsa 2017) after years of policy targeting urban poverty.

Nevertheless, analysis of the last US Census in 2010 indicates that while the number of poor are increasing in the US, their capacity to obtain basic needs (e.g., food, housing, and medical care) have not been entirely thwarted. Only a small percentage (4%) experience homelessness for a period while about 6% may have to live in overcrowded housing (Rector and Sheffield 2011, p.2). Home ownership, in some cases due to government incentives, is not out of reach for many American's with low socioeconomic status. Neither are amenities such as vehicles, television sets with access to cable, personal computers with access to the internet, and microwaves. The buying power of Americans with low socioeconomic status does not appear to be as greatly subverted but this does not necessarily indicate that their political influence has not been suppressed.

However, other scholars concur that while income inequality exists, the notion that the problem threatens democracy is unfounded. Recent analysis suggests that the relationship between growing gaps in income inequality do not favor the political influence of the wealthy for at least three prominent reasons. First, no statistical evidence supports the notion that income inequality threatens democracy; second, evidence does suggest that, in contrast to popular belief, there is a strong correlation of political perspectives across socioeconomic designations; and third, the number of policies that were enacted into law were divided equally even when that policy had opposing positions expressed by constituents in the upper and middle class (York 2017). Even so, "While income alone is not a good predictor of political influence, it is undeniably true that some have greater access to power" proposing that "reformers should address the undue influence of political insiders and root out cronyism instead of focusing on an unrelated phenomenon of income inequality" (York 2017, p.1).

Nonetheless, while the US may not be suffering to the extent of global citizens experiencing low socioeconomic status, there is a worldwide shortfall of components that represent the individual and community needs that act as a social foundation. The social foundation here consists of equitable access to daily needs, political representation, and social equity represented by the availability of healthcare, education, and employment without undue harm to the natural environment (Raworth 2017a). The natural environment, or ecological ceiling, represents various environmental conditions that complicate success at the social foundation. They include contaminants that provoke climate change, ozone layer depletion, and chemical waste destroying water supplies, animal life, and land used to support the food supply (Raworth 2017a, b). Together, this perspective depicts the shortfall in the capacity to achieve the elements of the social foundation as the empty space in the center of a donut. Thus, the phrase "donut economics" (Raworth 2017b) represents the inner radius of the donut with elements of the social foundation that surround the hole while the outer radius of the donut encompasses the ecological ceiling; the space between the inner and outer radius is designated as the safe objective (balancing resource needs and ecological limits). The author argues that this demonstrates a need to generate new economic alternatives proposing a paradigm shift to humanitarian enterprise versus financial incentives, the reallocation of wealth, and incorporating ecosystem sustainability as a key element in economic development (Raworth 2017a).

But is this what the people want? Consider that there is a nation that has a high-rating in several sustainability categories such as government, agriculture, and the environment (Lewis 2015). Access to elements that comprise the social foundation are clear in provisions for healthcare, food, clothing, housing, and equitable government. The country? Cuba! When the notion of a sustainable nation comes to mind, the small island nation south of the Bahamas and the State of Florida on the east coast of the US is hardly the first nation that comes to mind. However, the nation experienced a cultural revolution in 1991 when their primary importer of oil and other goods, the Soviet Union, fell under the weight of Communism. Cubans faced the immediate need to adjust from mechanized farm and other equipment to an agricultural economy due to the shortfalls of fuel, spare parts, and other goods. The transition was supported by the introduction of oxen to work the fields and permaculture (e.g., urban gardens, raised beds, and soil-enriching composting) but took several years before soil composition could produce sufficient quantities of crops (Alvarez 2012; Quinn 2006) evident in reported weight loss of most Cubans during this time. Fifteen years had passed from the onset of their transition and recognition by the World Wildlife Federation across several as the most sustainable nation in 2006.

Today, Cuba receives slightly more than half of their primary imports of petroleum, food, machinery, and chemical supplies from three nations—China (21.3%), Venezuela (17.7%), and Spain (12.1%) (CIA 2016). But the important takeaway from their sudden supply chain loss was the development of cooperative farming that has now spread to other industries (Alvarez 2012). From their perspective, the cooperative approach may be the continued path to economic stability and sustainability; perhaps the answer to sustainable capitalism in the fight against income inequality. What is clear is that the nation represents an example of what to expect when natural and external resources dry up due to failing political alignments, war, and the natural limit imposed on production due to diminishing supply of raw materials.

13.3.3 Still Havana a Good Time: The Cuban Experience

The Obama Administration in 2016 eased conditions on travel and trade on the more than half-century old US trade embargo to Cuba. The action opened the country to travel bringing insights from American tourists who relay direct observations of the people and the nation. A common theme is the historical charm of vintage automobiles, the prominent sense of equality among the people, and that the basic needs of the people are being equally met by the government. Still, travelers relay how Cubans are fascinated with foreigners and are eager to engage in conversation. Topics vary but some will say that almost all Cubans want to leave but will not discuss specific politics with an outsider. But, there is also a reported sense of "something missing" because of the government role in providing population needs.

> I liken the current Cuban system to placing a tiger and a sloth in separate cages. While the sloth can be comfortable in the confinement of the cage, being well-fed and protected, a tiger requires an outlet for activity. Like the tiger, many Cubans are active, alive with curiosity, ambitious, and seeking an outlet to express their unique gifts," says Brian Gerrits, a Florida small-business owner and inspiring inventor exploring innovation in Cuba in 2016. "My general impression of the people is that there is no incentive to work smarter or otherwise excel because the system offers little to no personal reward as everyone receives the same benefits from the government.

In Cuba, even many skilled craftsmen perform their duties using a limited number of tools and time-consuming manual labor. For instance, an American tourist observed that a construction worker spent 5 days chipping away a layer of material from a cement ceiling. Access to simple tools would have reduced the job time to half a day. When the tourist showed the worker pictures of trade tools, they were unable to recognize some common items (e.g., router, electric plane) because they simply did not have access to them.

Ironically, the lack of modern tools and spare parts is one way for the Cuban people to express some individual creativity. Cubans exhibited their innovation by utilizing parts from abandoned vehicles, such as old car axles and tires, to make horse-drawn carts. Even common objects, such as a 2-liter Cola bottle and pulleys from old appliances, would be transformed into a makeshift gas tank and drive belt for a small motorcycle. While this type of local innovation provides some creative outlet, a recent tourist explains that most Cuban people would like to be in a system where they are unfettered so that they would have the opportunity to shine.

These observations may demonstrate that while basic needs are being met in the highly touted Cuban sustainable economy, there may be a lack of individual incentive that may be difficult to embrace in nations filled with entrepreneurs and inventors. Thus, any transition to business development modeled on the ecosystem approach, or similar, must incorporate methods for tigers to embrace meaningful activity.

13.4 Moving the Public Towards Civic Engagement

The long-standing and growing number of research touched upon in this section confirms the relationship between air quality and heart disease (Brook et al. 2010; CDC 2016a; Solomon 2011), the built environment and mental health (Srinivasan et al. 2003), the impact of birth outcomes and inflammation (Brook et al. 2010; Solomon 2011) and a wide variety of health problems associated with the environment. The ability to access resources to understand the foundation of policy is important at all levels of government. Thus, this section introduces a variety of references at the national, state, and local level to promote civic engagement.

Multiple federal (https://www.usa.gov/federal-agencies/a) and state agencies in the US were enacted to address a variety of environmental conditions (e.g., behavioral risk factors such as smoking or alcohol abuse, manufacturing emissions and waste, air and water quality, national security, traffic safety) that cumulatively impacts public health. (Table 13.3). These agencies have a common objective to provide a wide variety of services that improve quality of life including (1) identification and monitoring the source of pollutants, (2) promoting safe environments, (3) providing affordable housing, and (4) opportunities for employment. These and other social services can incrementally improve public health outcomes.

Federal and state agencies target specific areas of public administration such as public health, transportation, and others. These agencies and institutions represent an opportunity to voice opinions, gather information, and recognize how environmental conditions are personal to your health and quality of life. For example, databases generated from EPA monitoring, such as the SPECIATE (EPA 2017d), serve as a "repository of volatile organic compounds (VOCs) and particulate matter (PM) specification profiles of air pollution sources (Simon et al. 2010, p.196). Regional and local analysis of the SPECIATE database information can present a specific opportunity to address immediate public health hazards and reduce the long-term implications of mortality and morbidity.

Table 13.3 Sample resource list of multilevel US government agencies

Agency	Mission	URL
Agency for Healthcare Administration (AHCA)	Specialized Florida State Agency created in response to need for oversite on health funding, such as Medicaid, clinical licensing, and others	http://ahca.myflorida.com/Inside_AHCA/index.shtml
Centers for Disease Control and Prevention	National Public Health policy, monitor and address hazards such as diseases, air pollution, local preparedness, national health	www.cdc.gov
Department of the Interior	National Land use; Bureau of Land Management	https://www.blm.gov/
Environmental Protection Agency (EPA)	National Environmental and Public Health policy including National Ambient Air Quality Standards (NAAQS)[a]	www.epa.gov/
State Department of Health	State Health Agencies	https://www.ehdp.com/links/us-shas.htm
State Department of Transportation	State Transportation Agencies; Infrastructure	https://www.fhwa.dot.gov/about/webstate.cfm
Office of Disease Prevention and Health Promotion (ODPHP)	National Public Health; noncommunicable diseases such as HealthyPeople2020 initiatives[b]	https://health.gov/; www.healthpeople.gov

[a]EPA (2012)
[b]ODPHP (2017)

The US Centers for Disease Control and Prevention (CDC) considers the span of hazards, such as the detailed health effects of multiple air pollutants (CDC 2017a), as well as the relevance of local public health preparedness. Their national approach to public health recognizes that “Every response is local” (CDC 2017b, p.12). The CDC’s annual report demonstrates how they react to local community problems, such as the ZIKA virus in Florida and water contamination in Flint, Michigan, to halt the spread of disease and to assess/address the damage to public health. Access to interim resources through the CDC’s Strategic National Stockpile also acts as a central distribution warehouse to accommodate local populations with medical and physical needs (e.g., food, beds, temporary shelters) during emergency situations (CDC 2017b). The CDC National Center for Environmental Health (CDC 2017c) targets prevention for preventable noninfectious and nonoccupational diseases, engages in laboratory sciences such as biomonitoring and research, and provides environmental toolkits promoting public education on various topics (CDC 2016b).

An agency familiar to most US citizens is the State Department of Health (DOH). The Florida DOH, for example, “works to protect, promote & improve the health of all people in Florida through integrated state, county, & community efforts” (Florida DOH n.d.). In addition to monitoring clinical and other healthcare professional licenses (e.g., audiologist, registered nurse, optician), the agency regulates health-care facilities (e.g., emergency medical service systems, dental laboratories, and pharmacies). One agency that is less familiar to the general population is the Agency for Healthcare Administration (AHCA), enacted by Florida Statute, Chapter 20, to monitor state Medicaid funding, generate state health policy, and work with the Florida Center for Health Information and Policy Analysis to secure and share health care data (AHCA 2017).

The impact of the Florida Department of Transportation (FDOT 2017) is prominent in the development of an interconnected and safe transportation system for citizens and tourists in the state. FDOT addresses various problems by meeting the needs of a variety of modes of transportation including people who drive automobiles on interstate highways, depart on cruise ships from various ports, bicycle along park or roadway paths, walk across bridges, or arrive by rail or air.

Of course, Florida and other states have many agencies with a variety of enacted duties that describe their area of responsibility through state legislation. The Official Portal of the State of Florida demonstrates the wide span of agencies including education, juvenile justice, fish and wildlife conservation (State of Florida 2017). Additionally, this list provides multilevel state information (e.g., county, region) about specialized committees, water management districts, and regional planning councils to allow each citizen to increase their awareness of local problems and engage in decision-making.

The element that all agencies share is a public notification system to invite stakeholders to participate in the decision-making process before new development is approved. While some provide posted agendas and a board meeting calendar, others offer the opportunity to receive announcements, newsletters and to sign up to receive digital news feeds directly to email or through text messaging via cell phone. Often the topics involve results from various reports, such as environmental impact assessments (EIA), and proposed plans that require the attention of those in the community who may be affected by changes.

There are also many national, nonprofit organizations that offer a repository of environmental knowledge. For example, National Council for Science and the Environment (NCSE) (https://www.ncseglobal.org/) advocates scientifically-based empirical research to inform environmental decision-making for the public, educators and international policymakers. Others, such as the Association of State and Territorial Health Officials (ASTHO 2017), provide leaders of public health agencies (e.g., state, territorial) with legal interpretation of multilevel government compliance legislation that impact their decisions for developers, planners, and other regulators.

Together, this small sampling of multilevel government agencies and nonprofits represents multiple institutions and public policies whose mission is to positively impact environmental and public health. They provide an opportunity for each citizen to engage in public discourse, generate awareness through education, provide tools and resources to address a variety of concerns and emergency situations, and establish data and other information to assist in the policy decision-making process.

13.5 Discussion

Literature is streaming with multiple suggestions for national governments and now large businesses to act in the fight against hunger, environmental destruction, and other worthy causes. But the average citizen may seem out of touch from this directive, or worse, feel unaffected because they are not aware of the impact of their own personal consumption choices and lack of civic engagement contributing to legacy decisions and policy leading to climate change and poor public health.

The impact of international changes in environmental conditions and their personal health consequences are a major incentive to engage in opportunities for public discourse on development and other problems, such as unemployment or healthcare, that impact the quality of life. Citizens have a place at the table to participate in EIA through publicly held meetings. But they must take the first step by being willing to reach out to obtain informative resources, increase community awareness, and make a personal commitment to engage in the decision-making process. Through nonhostile active engagement, informed citizens may begin to find the chasm between attaining income equality and protecting natural resources narrowing as stakeholders take the opportunity to introduce safer alternatives with new innovations. This inclusive process will also strengthen governance as input is obtained from a larger representation of the citizen demographic securing public health and representative government.

Remember that each of us are part of a business, nation, and ultimately a global representative, who are being called to action. The international changes in environmental conditions and the decisions that permitted them are also personal because they are affecting your health. It is not someone else's problem, it is everyone's problem to solve. Take a moment to ask the questions, "How much do I contribute to environmental decay," and "What can I do to make this world a better place?" The first step is to conduct a personal account of your individual ecological footprint (Global Footprint Network 2017b).

Contributing to a public meeting may be a scary place to start. If the thought of public speaking is too much for your personality, then start out small. Use internet search engines to find ways you can easily save the planet through tips designed to help the environment. Leave small sections of your landscape natural to attract bees and other insects that are valuable to the ecosystem (Fig. 13.1). Or you can bring the outdoors inside and improve your indoor air quality with several plants that improve respiratory health (Clean Air Gardening 2017) by filtering contaminants such as benzene, trichloroethylene, and formaldehyde.

The legacy of e-waste is one area in which individuals can become more cognizant of their habits in consumer spending, recycling, and charitable donations. But improving recycling should not stop with electronics. Many other items, such as construction material and landscaping waste, often end up in the local landfill. Instead, get creative. Broken sidewalk pavers can become a new rock garden to stabilize soil and permit healthy saturation (Fig. 13.2). Composting yard waste can restore the soil vitality of any area by introducing worm activity and even prepare a

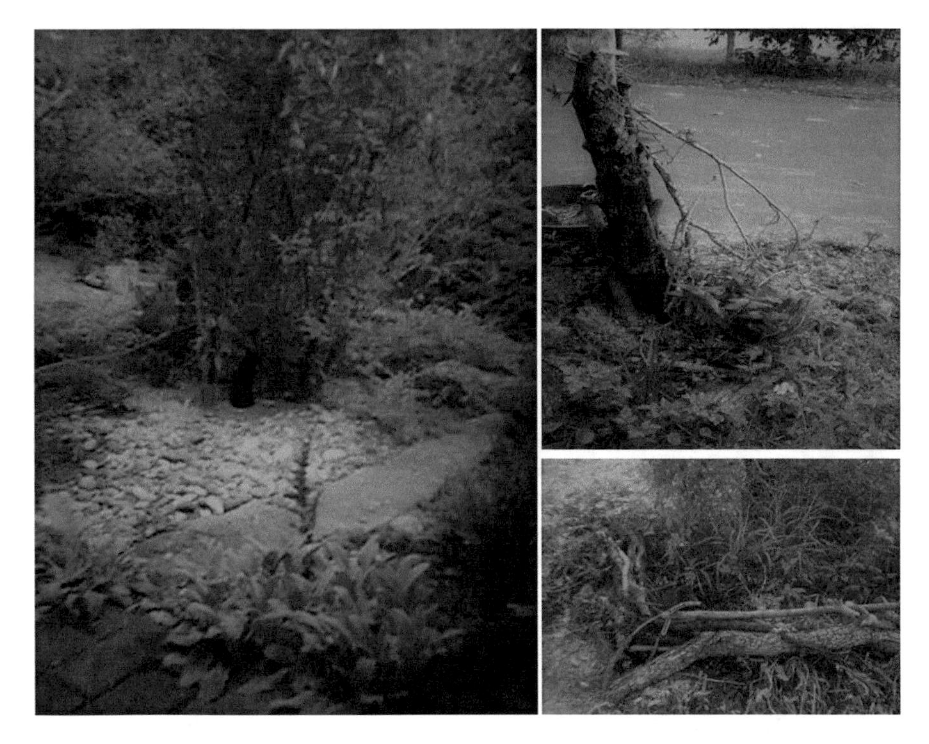

Fig. 13.1 Incorporating landscape features such as stones for natural pathways and oasis, maintaining pockets of natural flora landscapes to attract bees and other useful insects and reusing downed tree limbs for edging conserve resources and promote a strong ecosystem (photo on *left* taken by Beth Ann Fiedler; photos on *right* courtesy of James Barr and Cynthia Sweet-Barr, used by permission)

portion of your backyard for planting fresh herbs and vegetables. Those old pair of jeans can be donated or transformed into the material for a "new" apron (Tamz-Nan Creations) or your favorite t-shirts into a memory quilt (Fig. 13.3). Think before you purchase. Get creative before you toss. Preserve or reintroduce natural flora. Plan outdoor activities including planting fresh produce in your own back yard.

13.6 Summary

This chapter provides an overview of the impact of environmental conditions on public health discussing two primary risk factors, age and socioeconomic status, and the leading environmental causes of death. But more importantly, the chapter brings forth the need for an individual response to global concerns through civic engagement, by changing harmful behavior patterns, and bringing a little nature

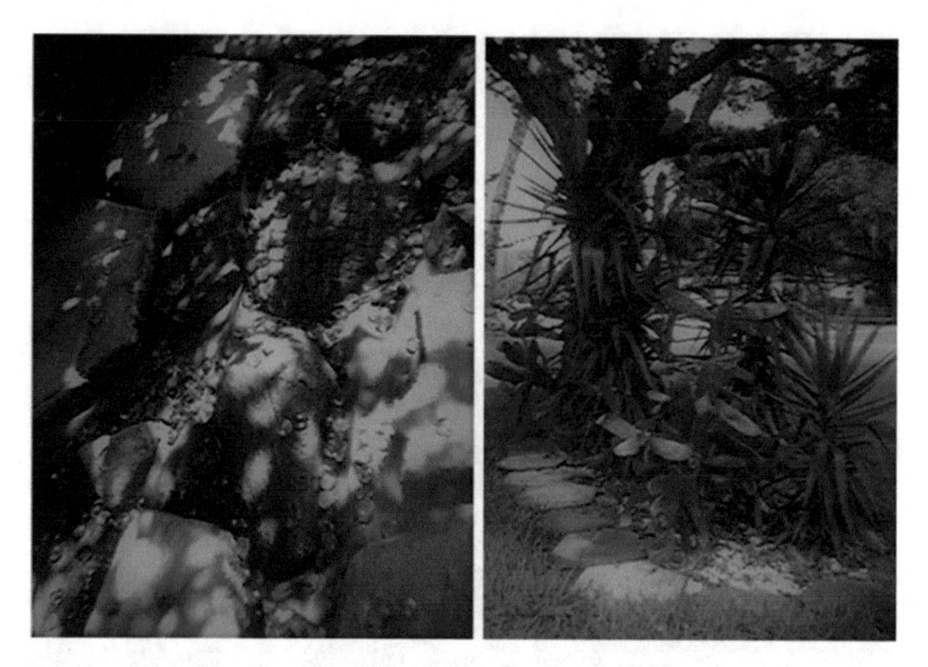

Fig. 13.2 Repurposing broken and intact concrete pavers to create a whimsical rock garden to contain soil for drought-resistant plants is one way to abate weed growth under shrubs, conserve water, keep soil from eroding, and reduce the number of reusable items heading to landfills (photos by Beth Ann Fiedler)

back into the world one person at a time. We show how economic barriers limit the capacity to overcome the negative impact of poverty on public health but also the devastation of ecosystems in developed nations. The introduction of manufacturing facilities in nations with less rigid or absent regulatory systems tarnishing new ecosystems around the globe is not the answer. Global objectives and international collaboration represent an opportunity to address the ills of the past and prevent future harm. But these objectives can only be achieved through active participation in environmental impact assessments as well as the concern for income inequality. Opposing positions were presented on the problem of income inequality and the potential for those with low socioeconomic status to lack government representation as a prelude to decay of the foundation of US government. Others suggest that alternative paradigms could be developed to meet basic needs while protecting the ecosystem. The chapter also considers that those who advocate an ecosystem economy should avoid patterns established in nations who currently demonstrate high levels of sustainability but limit opportunity. Finally, the chapter provides some points of contact to national, state, and local agencies to facilitate civic engagement and encourages personal commitments to what has been previously considered a problem of big business and powerful governments.

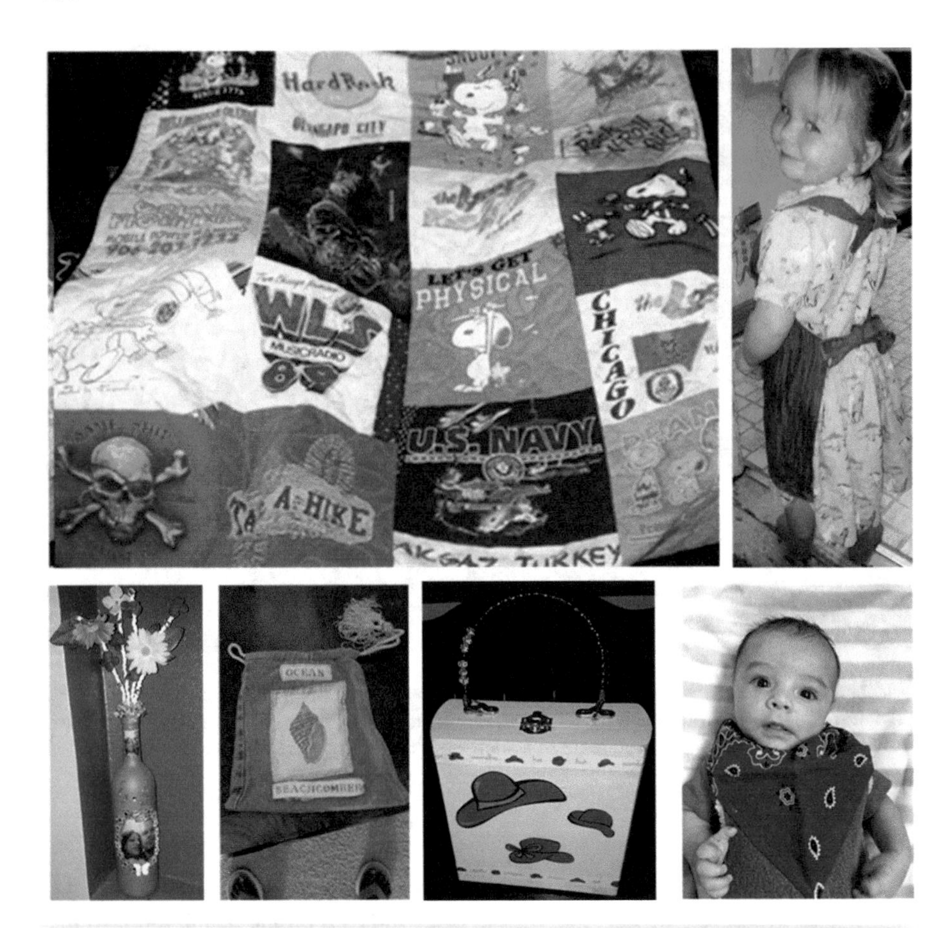

Fig. 13.3 Sandra Pratt transformed Joanie Feledy's favorite t-shirt collection into a custom quilt (clockwise from *top left*) (photo courtesy of Curt Pratt, used by permission); Nancy Stein's granddaughter Tamzin models her upcycled denim kids' apron—complete with front pocket and back bow tie, and Nathan models baby Bandanna bibs from Tamz-Nan creations on Facebook) (photos courtesy of Nancy Stein, used by permission); Margie Lozada demonstrates how a repurposed cigar box and denim pant leg can become a unique purse and beach bag while bottles get new life as a stunning table decoration and special occasion keepsake (photos courtesy of Margie Lozada, used by permission)

Acknowledgments The author would like to thank the World Health Organization (WHO) and the Organization for Economic Development (OECD) for access to their reliable and consistent research. Analysis, interpretation, and conclusions drawn from WHO and OECD source material remain the sole responsibility of the author. Special thanks to Naz Onel for helpful commentary on the final first draft.

Glossary

Benzene Organic compound generated naturally in crude oil, volcanic eruption, and forest fires but used as an additive to produce industrial lubricants, detergents, rubber, plastics, nylon, and pesticides.

Built environment Surrounding features, such as buildings or bridges, that human beings construct.

Capitalism A system of politics and economic development where private versus government ownership of business entities control industry motivated by profit or return on investments.

Climate resilience The process of developing sustainable options in response to environmental stressors intensified by climate change (e.g., limited freshwater supply coupled with drought).

Clinical protocols A treatment regimen for disease management developed in response to evidence-based standards and peer consensus otherwise identified as best practices.

Economic Problem The difficulty in balancing population needs that consume national resources against the reality of limited resources.

Effluents Liquid form of emission waste derived from industrial processing of materials.

Emissions Waste derived from industrial processing of materials into the environment in the form of gas (i.e., carbon emissions) or solids (i.e., lead, particulate matter).

Environmental impact assessment (EIA) Analysis that determines economic, environmental, and political feasibility of projects prior to development to minimize environmental impact.

Feasibility The likelihood of a plan or project to achieve success.

Formaldehyde Strong-smelling gas used in constructing walls and furniture appearing in glue, insulation, and particle board; appear in some personal hygiene products such as soap, toothpaste, and cosmetics labeled are urea, methanol, and others.

Income inequality An unequal distribution of national wealth that sharply divides members of that economy by their status as rich or poor; a measure of the unequal wealth distribution generating a widening gap or indicating a hole in reported individual income where socioeconomic classes are concentrated at the high end for relatively few and low for an increasing number of people.

Infrastructure Infrastructure is the interconnected system of the physical, natural, and social components that societies need to survive and function (NSCE 2017).

Ischemic heart disease The most common of several cardiovascular diseases resulting in damage or disease to the coronary arteries (major vessels supplying the heart with blood, nutrients, and oxygen).

Natural/physical environment Natural features of the geographical surroundings such as mountains, lakes, and plants; natural landscape.

Particulate matter Small, harmful airborne particles (e.g., lead, aerosols) suspended in the atmosphere that impact climate and human health.

Persistent Organic Pollutants (POPs) The capacity of certain chemicals to travel over long distances.

Polychlorinated biphenyls (PCBs) An example of a persistent industrial use organic pollutant that causes environmental harm at locations beyond the area of original use.

Social environment Personal impact of cultural influence, level of institutional development, and physical location influencing the capacity to interact with others.

Social foundation Various interpretations including a list of basic needs found in access to such items as water, nutrition, and healthcare but inclusive of human rights such as fair political representation and equitable governance.

Systolic blood pressure The peak pressure occurring at the end of the cardiac cycle when the ventricles (pumping chambers of the heart) contract, reported as the first number; whereas diastolic in the second and minimum number reported, measures the beginning of the cardiac cycle when the ventricles fill with blood.

Trichloroethylene Clear, flammable industrial solvent toxic to nervous system and normally found in aerosol form used as a degreaser in cleaning products for cars or dry cleaning for clothing.

Volatile organic compounds (VOCs) Organic chemicals normally produced consequently to industrial processing (e.g., solvents) generating emissions harmful to human health.

Vulnerable Can refer to a specific population identified by certain characteristics (i.e., low income, ethnic, female) that place them at greater risk of poor health; populations that are exposed to the conditions of climate change with limitations on their capacity to adapt.

References

Aday L. At risk in America. 2nd ed. San Francisco, CA: Jossey-Bass; 2001.

Agency for Healthcare Administration (AHCA). 2017. About the agency for healthcare administration. http://ahca.myflorida.com/Inside_AHCA/index.shtml. Accessed 16 July 2017.

Al-Delaimy WK. The JPC-SE *position statement on asbestos*: a long-overdue appeal by epidemiologists to ban asbestos worldwide and end related global environmental injustice. Environ Health Perspect. 2013;121:A144–5. https://doi.org/10.1289/ehp.1306892; [online 01 May 2013]

Allard SW. *Places in need:* the changing geography of poverty. New York: Russell Sage Foundation; 2017.

Alvarez MD. 2012. Sustainable food & sustainable economics. http://pages.vassar.edu/sustainability/video-home/. Accessed 2 July 2017.

Anand SV. Global environmental issues. Sci Rep. 2013;2(2):1–9. https://doi.org/10.4172/scientificreports.632.

Association of State and Territorial Health Officials. 2017. Federal government relations. http://www.astho.org/Public-Policy/Federal-GR/. Accessed 16 July 2017.

Barton D. 2011. Corporate governance: capitalism for the long term. Harv Bus Rev. https://hbr.org/2011/03/capitalism-for-the-long-term. Accessed 15 July 2017.

Boden TA, et al. 2014. Total fossil-fuel CO_2 emissions. http://cdiac.ornl.gov/trends/emis/top2014.tot. Accessed 27 June 2017.

Boden TA, et al. 2017. National CO_2 emissions from fossil-fuel burning, cement manufacture, and gas flaring: 1751-2014, Carbon Dioxide Information Analysis Center, Oak Ridge National Laboratory, U.S. Department of Energy. https://doi.org/10.3334/CDIAC/00001_V2017.

Bradford WD. 2000. Global capitalism and sustainable development. Macquarie economics working paper no. 10/2000. https://doi.org/10.2139/ssrn.291749. Accessed 2 July 2017.

Breivik K, et al. Tracking the global generation and exports of e-waste. Do existing estimates add up? Environ Sci Technol. 2014;48:8735–43.

Breivik K, et al. Tracking the global distribution of persistent organic pollutants accounting for e-waste exports to developing regions. Environ Sci Technol. 2016;50:798–805. https://doi.org/10.1021/acs.est.5b04226; Accessed 15 July 2017

Brook RD, et al. Particulate matter air pollution and cardiovascular disease: an update to the scientific statement from the American Heart Association. Circulation. 2010;121:2331–78. https://doi.org/10.1161/CIR.0b013e3181dbece1.

Cassar M. 2005. Climate change and the historic environment. Center for Sustainable Heritage. University College London, London, UK. http://discovery.ucl.ac.uk/2082/1/2082.pdf

Center for International and Environmental Law (CEIL). 2015. A comparison of six environmental impact assessment regimes. http://www.ciel.org/Publications/AComparisonof6EnvReg.pdf. Accessed 29 June 2017.

Central Intelligence Agency (CIA). 2016. The world fact book-Cuba. https://www.cia.gov/library/publications/the-world-factbook/geos/cu.html. Accessed 2 July 2017.

Cervantes J. Ideology, neoliberalism and sustainable development. J Stud Res Hum Geogr. 2013;7(2):25–34.

Clean Air Gardening. 2017. Top houseplants for improving indoor air quality. http://www.cleanairgardening.com/houseplants/. Accessed 29 July 2017.

Cohen AJ, et al. Estimates and 25-year trends of the global burden of disease attributable to ambient air pollution: an analysis of data from the Global Burden of Diseases Study 2015. Lancet. 2017;389:1907–18.

Colao A, et al. Environment and health: not only cancer. Int J Environ Res Public Health. 2016;13(724):2–9. https://doi.org/10.3390/ijerph13070724.

European Union (EU) (2014) Directive 2014/52/EU http://ec.europa.eu/environment/eia/pdf/transposition_checklist.pdf. Accessed 1 July 2017.

Florida Department of Health (DOH). n.d. Licensing and regulation. http://www.floridahealth.gov/licensing-and-regulation/index.html. Accessed 16 July 2017.

Florida Department of Transportation. 2017. FDOT. http://fdot.gov/. Accessed 17 July 2017.

Generation Investment Management LLP. 2012. Sustainable capitalism. https://www.genfound.org/media/1136/advocacy-3-sustainable-capitalism.pdf. Accessed 15 July 2017.

Global Burden of Disease Study (GBD). Mortality and causes of death collaborators. Global, regional, and national life expectancy, all-cause mortality, and cause-specific mortality for 249 causes of death, 1980–2015: a systematic analysis for the Global Burden of Disease Study 2015. Lancet. 2016;388:1459–544.

Global Footprint Network. 2017a. Ecological wealth of nations. http://www.footprintnetwork.org/content/documents/ecological_footprint_nations/. Accessed 5 Sept 2017.

Global Footprint Network. 2017b. Footprint calculator faqs. http://www.footprintnetwork.org/footprint-calculator-faq/. Accessed 5 Sept 2017.

Guan W-J, et al. Industrial pollutant emission and the major smog in China: from debates to action. Lancet Planet Health. 2017;1:e57.

Heacock M, et al. E-waste and harm to vulnerable populations: a growing global problem. Environ Health Perspect. 2016;124(5):550–5. https://doi.org/10.1289/ehp.1509699.

Honda S, et al. 2016. Regional E-waste monitor: East and Southeast Asia, United Nations University ViE—SCYCLE, Bonn, Germany. http://ewastemonitor.info/pdf/Regional-E-Waste-Monitor.pdf. Accessed 15 July 2017.

International Association for Impact Assessment (IAIA). 1999. Principles of environmental impact assessment best practice. https://web.archive.org/web/20120507084339/http://www.iaia.org/publicdocuments/special-publications/Principles%20of%20IA_web.pdf). Accessed 3 June 2017.

Ireland Environmental Protection Agency (IEPA). 2017. Environmental impact assessment. http://www.epa.ie/monitoringassessment/assessment/eia/. Accessed 1 July 2017.

Lambin J-J. Capitalism and sustainable development. Theatr Symp. 2009;2:3–9. https://doi.org/10.4468/2009.2.02lambin.

Lancet Respiratory Medicine. Health inequality: a major driver of respiratory disease. Lancet. 2017;5:235. https://doi.org/10.1016/S2213-2600(17)30092-9.

Leech G. 2015. The elephant in the room: capitalism and sustainable development. Transcend Media Service. https://www.transcend.org/tms/?p=65133. Accessed 2 July 2017.

Lewis T. 2015. The world's most sustainable country: what? Cuba? http://www.dailyimpact.net/2015/02/09/the-worlds-most-sustainable-country-what-cuba/. Accessed 2 July 2017.

Liodokis G. Political economy, capitalism and sustainable development. Sustainability. 2010;2:2601–16. https://doi.org/10.3390/su208260

Lundgren K. 2012. The global impact of e-waste: addressing the challenge. International Labour Office, Programme on Safety and Health at Work and the Environment (SafeWork), Sectoral Activities Department (SECTOR). Geneva: International Labour Office. http://www.ilo.org/wcmsp5/groups/public/@ed_dialogue/@sector/documents/publication/wcms_196105.pdf. Accessed 15 July 2017.

Mirsa T. 2017. Confronting the myths of suburban poverty. https://www.citylab.com/solutions/2017/07/confronting-the-myths-about-suburban-poverty/532680/. Accessed 15 July 2017.

Nachmany M, et al. 2017. Global trends in climate change legislation and litigation: 2017 update. http://www.lse.ac.uk/GranthamInstitute/publication/global-trends-in-climate-change-legislation-and-litigation-2017-update/. Accessed 10 June 2017.

National Council for Science and the Environment (NCSE). 2017. Defining sustainable infrastructure. http://files.constantcontact.com/ce6a496a001/882b1881-aa62-41de-91aa-26ae4b7b5723.pdf. Accessed 19 July 2017.

Official Portal of the State of Florida. 2017 State of Florida agencies. http://www.myflorida.com/directory/. Accessed 16 July 2017.

Organization for Economic Cooperation and Development (OECD). Sustainable development: critical issues. 2001. OECD Publishing, Paris. https://doi.org/10.1787/9789264193185-en. Accessed 7 July 2017.

Organization for Economic Cooperation and Development (OECD). 2008a. OECD key environmental indicators. https://www.oecd.org/env/indicators-modelling-outlooks/37551205.pdf. Accessed 20 May 2017.

Organization for Economic Cooperation and Development (OECD). 2008b. OECD environmental outlook to 2030 (summary), OECD Publishing, Paris. https://doi.org/10.1787/9789264040519-sum-en.

Organization for Economic Cooperation and Development (OECD). 2017a. Governance of land use. http://www.oecd.org/regional/governance-of-land-use.htm. Accessed 5 July 2017.

Organization for Economic Cooperation and Development (OECD). 2017b. Sustainable development: critical issues—free overview of the report. http://www.oecd.org/greengrowth/sustainabledevelopmentcriticalissues-freeoverviewofthereport.htm. Accessed 5 July 2017.

Quinn M. 2006. The power of community: how Cuba survived peak oil. http://www.resilience.org/stories/2006-02-25/power-community-how-cuba-survived-peak-oil/. Accessed 2 July 2017.

Raworth K. A doughnut for the anthropocene: humanity's compass in the 21st century. Lancet Planet Health. 2017a;1:e48–9.

Raworth K. Doughnut economics: seven ways to think like a 21st-century economist. White River Junction, VT: Chelsea Green Publishing; 2017b.

Rector R, Sheffield R. Understanding poverty in the United States: surprising factors about America's poor. The Heritage Foundation, No. 2607. 2011. http://report.heritage.org/bg2607

Regional Office for Europe of the World Health Organization (WHO Europe). 2013. Health and the environment in the WHO European region: creating resilient communities and supportive environments.

Rull V. Sustainability, capitalism and evolution: nature conservation is not a matter of maintaining human development and welfare in a healthy environment. The European Molecular Biology Organization EMBO reports, published online 2011 Jan 14. EMBO Rep. 2011;12(2):103–6. https://doi.org/10.1038/embor.2010.211.

Schweickart D. Selected papers of Beijing forum 2008 is sustainable capitalism possible? Procedia Soc Behav Sci. 2010;41:6739–52.

Simon H, et al. The development and uses of EPA's SPECIATE database. Atmos Pollut Res. 2010;1(4):196–206. https://doi.org/10.5094/APR.2010.026.

Sitaraman G. The crisis of the middle class: why economic inequality threatens our democracy. New York: Alfred A. Knopf; 2017.

Solomon PA. Air pollution and health: bridging the gap from sources to health outcomes. Environ Health Persp. 2011;119(4):A156–7. https://doi.org/10.1289/ehp.1103660volume.

Srinivasan S, et al. Creating healthy communities, healthy homes, healthy people: initiating a research agenda on the built environment and public health. Am J Public Health. 2003;93(9):1446–50.

United Kingdom Department for Communities and Local Government. 2014. Guidance environmental impact assessment. https://www.gov.uk/guidance/environmental-impact-assessment. Accessed 30 June 2017.

United Nations. 2017. Sustainable development goals, Goal 3: Ensure healthy lives and promote well-being for all at all ages. http://www.un.org/sustainabledevelopment/health/. Accessed 5 Sept 2017.

United Nations Environment Programme (UNEP). 2002. UNEP briefs on economics, trade and sustainable development: information and policy tools from the United Nations Environment Programme. http://unep.ch/etu/publications/UNEP_EIA_Manual.pdf. Accessed 29 June 2017.

United Nations Environment Programme, World Conservation Monitoring Centre (UNEP-WCMC). 2015. An introduction to environmental assessment. http://www.ecosystemassessments.net/resources/an-introduction-to-environmental-assessment.pdf. Accessed 1 July 2017.

United Nations Framework Convention on Climate Change (UNFCCC). 2014. Kyoto protocol. https://unfccc.int/kyoto_protocol/items/1678.php. Accessed 16 July 2017.

United States Center for Disease Control and Prevention (CDC). 2017a. Health effects notebook for hazardous air pollutants. https://www.epa.gov/haps/health-effects-notebook-hazardous-air-pollutants. Accessed 3 July 2017.

United States Center for Disease Control and Prevention (CDC). 2017b. Public health preparedness and response national snapshot 2017. https://www.cdc.gov/phpr/whyitmatters/00_docs/2017_PublicHealthPreparednessSnapshot_508.pdf. Accessed 4 July 2017.

United States Center for Disease Control and Prevention (CDC). 2017c. National Center for Environmental Health. https://www.cdc.gov/nceh/. Accessed 16 July 2017.

United States Centers for Disease Control and Prevention (CDC). 2016a. Air pollution and respiratory health. https://www.cdc.gov/nceh/airpollution/default.htm. Accessed 3 July 2017.

United States Centers for Disease Control and Prevention (CDC). 2016b. Environmental health media toolkits. https://www.cdc.gov/nceh/toolkits/index.html. Accessed 16 July 2017.

United States Environmental Protection Agency (EPA). 2012. National ambient air quality standards (NAAQS). https://www.leg.state.mn.us/docs/2015/other/150681/PFEISref_2/USEPA%202012a.pdf. Accessed 4 July 2017.

United States Environmental Protection Agency (EPA). 2017a. Air topics. https://www.epa.gov/environmental-topics/air-topics. Accessed 5 July 2017.

United States Environmental Protection Agency (EPA). 2017b. International cooperation: technical review guidelines for environmental impact assessments in the tourism, energy and mining sectors. https://www.epa.gov/international-cooperation/eia-technical-review-guidelines-energy-sector. Accessed 30 June 2017.
United States Environmental Protection Agency (EPA). 2017c. Environmental impact statement (EIS) database. https://cdxnodengn.epa.gov/cdx-enepa-public/action/eis/search. Accessed 1 July 2017.
United States Environmental Protection Agency (EPA). 2017d. SPECIATE data browser. https://cfpub.epa.gov/speciate/. Accessed 5 July 2017.
United States Global Change Research Program (USGCRP). The impacts of climate change on human health in the United States: a scientific assessment. In: Crimmins A, Balbus J, Gamble JL, Beard CB, Bell JE, Dodgen D, Eisen RJ, Fann N, Hawkins MD, Herring SC, Jantarasami L, Mills DM, Saha S, Sarofim MC, Trtanj J, Ziska L, editors. U.S. Global Change Research Program. Washington, DC; 2016. 312 pp. https://doi.org/10.7930/J0R49NQX
United States Office of Disease Prevention and Health Promotion (ODPHP). 2017. Environmental health. https://www.healthypeople.gov/2020/topics-objectives/topic/environmental-health. Accessed 12 June 2017.
World Bank. 2017a. Number of Under 5 Deaths [Data source: estimates developed by the UN Inter-agency Group for Child Mortality Estimation (UNICEF, WHO, World Bank, UN DESA Population Division) at www.childmortality.org]. https://data.worldbank.org/indicator/SH.DTH.MORT?view=chart. Accessed 5 Sept 2015.
World Bank. 2017b. Cause of death, by non-communicable diseases (% of total) [Data World Health Organization World Health Statistics]. https://data.worldbank.org/indicator/SH.DTH.NCOM.ZS?view=chart. Accessed 5 Sept 2017.
World Bank. 2017c. Cause of death, by communicable diseases and maternal, prenatal and nutrition conditions (% of total) [Data World Health Organization World Health Statistics]. https://dataworldbankorg/indicator/SHDTHCOMMZS?view=chart. Accessed 5 Sept 2017.
World Bank. 2017d. CO_2 emissions (metric tons per capita) [Data Carbon Dioxide Information Analysis Center, Environmental Sciences Division, Oak Ridge National Laboratory, Tennessee, United States]. https://data.worldbank.org/indicator/EN.ATM.CO2E.PC?view=map. Accessed 4 Sept 2017.
World Health Organization (WHO). 2017a. PHE environmental impacts on health. What is the big picture? http://www.who.int/phe/infographics/en/. Accessed 20 May 2017.
World Health Organization (WHO). 2017b. Almost half of all deaths now have a recorded cause, WHO data show. http://www.who.int/mediacentre/news/releases/2017/half-deaths-recorded/en/. Accessed 5 Sept 2017.
World Health Organization (WHO). 2017c. Noncommunicable diseases. http://www.who.int/mediacentre/factsheets/fs355/en/. Accessed 5 Sept 2017.
World Health Organization (WHO). 2017d. Fact sheets: infectious disease. http://www.who.int/topics/infectious_diseases/factsheets/en/. Accessed 5 Sept 2017.
World Health Organization (WHO). 2017e. Protecting children from the environment. Infographic, 1–3. http://www.who.int/phe/infographics/protecting-children-from-the-environment/en/. Accessed 20 May 2017.
World Health Organization (WHO). 2017f. Environment and health in developing countries: future trends and developing issues. The Health and Environment Linkage Initiative. http://www.who.int/heli/risks/ehindevcoun/en/index1.html. Accessed 10 June 2017.
York JW. Does rising income inequality threaten democracy? The Heritage Foundation, No. 3227. 2017. http://report.heritage.org/bg3227

Further Reading

Global Environmental Health. https://www.niehs.nih.gov/research/programs/geh/index.cfm Accessed 12 June 2017.

Greengrants Fund (GGF) of USA. https://www.greengrants.org/. Accessed 12 June 2017.

Global Health Security Agenda (GHSA). https://www.ghsagenda.org/. Accessed 3 Sept 2016.

Gould S, Rudolph L. Challenges and opportunities for advancing work on climate change and public health. Int J Environ Res Public Health. 2015;12:15649–72. https://doi.org/10.3390/ijerph121215010.

National Council for Science and the Environment (NCSE). 2017. The science, business, and education of sustainable infrastructure—building resilience in a changing world. https://vimeo.com/226211680. Accessed 22 July 2017.

Organization for Economic Development and Cooperation (OECD). 2003. OECD indicators: development, measurement and use. https://www.oecd.org/env/indicators-modelling-outlooks/24993546.pdf. Accessed 10 June 2017.

Speake J, Pentaraki M. Living (in) the city centre, neoliberal urbanism, engage Liverpool and citizen engagement with urban change in Liverpool, UK. Hum Geogr. 2017;11(1):41–63.

United Nations Environment Programme (UNEP). 2002. UNEP environmental impact assessment training resource manual. 2nd ed. http://unep.ch/etu/publications/eiaman_2edition_toc.htm. Accessed 1 July 2017.

The United Nations University, RMIT University, and the United Nations Environment Programme (UNEP). n.d. Environmental impact assessment: open educational resource. http://eia.unu.edu/. Accessed 1 July 2017.

United States Environmental Protection Agency. 2011. Final report: estimation of the risks to human health of pm and pm components. https://cfpub.epa.gov/ncer_abstracts/index.cfm/fuseaction/display.abstractDetail/abstract/7781/report/F. Accessed 3 July 2017.

Chapter 14
Streetwise Community Policing to Inform United States National Policy

Vincent N. Van Ness III

Abstract The provisions of the 10th Amendment of the United States Constitution defer policing as a reserved and sovereign power of the States, representing a significant obstacle for community law enforcement. The problem is embedded in the complex nature of local policing strategies enforced in communities in direct public contact but without sovereign status. Cities, where police report to local jurisdictions, are considered non-sovereign. Nevertheless, police must respond to a variety of looming social issues, such as the opioid crisis, immigration, and sex trafficking with limited or no formal guidance. This chapter suggests that sovereign entities (e.g., federal, state) empowered with authority to create law can generate policy by using a "ground up" approach. In this scenario, local police solutions can be used to inform and establish national and state policy to avoid cultural clashes between police authority and citizens that have devastated the fabric of American society. This chapter provides an overview of vexing social problems and the need to develop solutions that provide local law enforcement agencies the protocol to uniformly address violations. The recommendations effectively "uncuff" the hands of police officers by removing the variety of independent actions decided in a split second and replacing them with successful alternatives found to be effective in various localities.

14.1 Introduction

Policing in the United States has entered a new and challenging period, with a combination of changing roles and missions, fiscal constraints, more intense public scrutiny and enhanced service expectations. Cutbacks in other areas of government services have made many police agencies the service provider of last resort in many nontraditional areas such as social service referral, family outreach, mental health screening, and drug abuse control, to name a few.

V. N. Van Ness III (✉)
Orange County (FL) Sheriff's Office (Retired), Lee, MA, USA

B. A. Fiedler (ed.), *Translating National Policy to Improve Environmental Conditions Impacting Public Health Through Community Planning*,
https://doi.org/10.1007/978-3-319-75361-4_14

Despite the fiscal and social challenges of the current policing climate, public needs have borne a period of innovation for many policing entities. When coupled with a developing sense of innovation, interagency collaboration and evidence-based practice, many vexing social problems are being given a fresh look by the police.

This chapter examines local police response to three such vexing social problems in the United States, and how those responses have helped inform national policy toward these issues, and indeed, how such problems are viewed at the national level. The seemingly intractable issues of opioid drug abuse, illegal transnational migration, and human trafficking. Interventions have met with varying degrees of success. While local agency "grassroots" problem-solving has been the key to informing national policy and government response, this chapter suggests that the expedient envelopment of successful policing strategies into national and state policies can provide substantial relief to the individuals struggling with the problems and to overburdened police forces across the nation.

14.2 Population Impact of Policing in America

The likelihood of overstating the impact policing has in the United States would be difficult. Police officers at the local level reach deep into the fabric of American society, and the decisions individual officers make can have profound population impact. Many of the cultural touchstone incidents of the last 25 years have been predicated, at least in part, on policing decisions. The Rodney King incident, the OJ Simpson arrest and prosecution, U.S. riots, and major shifts in how the American public perceive notions of criminal justice, are all informed or shaped by policing decisions. Many of the effects of police decision-making are due to the outsize role that crime and policing play in the news media and popular culture. One of the several factors contributing to this problem is the lack of U.S. national policy in policing—a right granted to States by the sovereignty of federal laws embedded in the 10th Amendment of the U.S. Constitution and delegated to States that, in turn, hold policing rights in their State Constitutions. However, the application of policing is rarely conducted at the national or state level, except in the time of emergencies or other natural disasters, causing a disconnect in local police response.

Unlike many other developed countries, U.S. policing is thought to be a fragmented discipline, owing to the fear of the founding fathers of a strong, monolithic government. Instead of an overarching, nationalized police force, U.S. policing is primarily conducted by small agencies under the control of local governments. At the federal level, the preeminent agency is the Federal Bureau of Investigation (FBI) , however the FBI's investigative mandate is rather narrow in scope, and many of the traditional roles of the police (e.g., preventative patrol, response to emergency situations) fall far outside of the Bureau's bailiwick. There are other federal agencies, such as the Bureau of Alcohol, Tobacco, and Firearms (ATF) or the United States Bureau of Customs and Border Protection (CBP) , but these federal agencies have a very narrow investigative bandwidth. For example, they generally conduct a limited investigative mission, or in the case of CBP, conduct a very specific type of policing, such as border protection. At the state level, police agencies tend to mimic their federal counterparts, conducting strategic, long-term, statewide investigations, or in many cases handling a limited policing mandate, usually statewide traffic safety and crash investigation. While the work state agencies do is important, they are often not thought of as full-service police departments, with a few exceptions, primarily in the northeast U.S.

Primary response to the needs of citizens then normally falls to local law-enforcement agencies: municipal police departments and county sheriff's offices. There are over 17,000 local police agencies in the United States, and their capabilities vary widely, from the 40,000 strong New York City Police Department to many rural agencies where there might be only one serving officer, and a part-time one at that (Reaves 2011). These local agencies are responsive to their parent municipal or county government, and to the issues their residents feel are priorities, and derive their legitimacy from what Crank and Langworthy describe as "sovereigns" (1992, p.342).

Despite efforts to improve information sharing after the tragic events of September 11, 2001, many of these agencies interact with each other on an ad-hoc basis, with a minimum of information and resource sharing, and a maximum of autonomy. This makes coordinated responses to developing issues difficult. Police agencies also have a mixed record of information sharing with their federal partners. While the local-federal relationship often works well in case-specific instances, at the macro level information sharing is complicated by law, policy, and institutional challenges on both the federal and local ends of the information pipeline.

Many of the contemporary issues and problems facing these local agencies are not viewed as traditional local police responsibilities. Opioid crisis response, illegal immigration, and the trafficking of human beings for sexual purposes are often not seen as a police problem, and are many times handled by nonpolice governmental entities, or even nongovernmental organizations (NGOs) . These other entities may have little to no experience dealing with the police, or in some cases may even have an adversarial relationship with the criminal justice system. This makes the role of police agencies responding to these issues even more problematic, beginning with the police response to the national opioid problem.

14.3 Police Response to the Opioid Crisis

The use of opioid pain relief medications in the U.S. more than doubled in the years 1999–2011, and consumption of oxycodone (a synthetic opioid) increased more than 500% during the same period (Kolodny et al. 2015, p.560). Along with the rise in opioid abuse rates, drug overdoses caused by the ingestion of opioid analgesics led to what the Centers for Disease Control and Prevention (CDC) called "the worst drug overdose epidemic in history" (Kolodny et al. 2015, p.560; Paulozzi 2010).

Criminal justice representatives, public health leaders, and government officials determined that opioid addictions were being caused by a combination of over-prescribing the pain killers, the use of pain clinics and "pill mill" operations to distribute the medications, as well as diversion of legal opioid pharmaceuticals to a black-market sales network. Government entities at all levels responded by cracking down on pill mill and pain management operations by implementing enhanced tracking of opioid prescriptions and receiving patients. This policy response led to a reduction in the availability of prescription opioids for abuse, and the addict community turned to an old street drug, heroin, to fill the void (Davis et al. 2015). Heroin abuse rates and overdoses surged at the tail end of the prescription opioid epidemic, with accompanying concerns about the death rate (Fig. 14.1).

14.3.1 Organizational and Policy Adjustment

Traditionally, opioid addiction has been viewed by law-enforcement as a criminal justice issue, requiring arrest and prosecution of drug abusers. Other actors in the criminal justice system have embraced a more expansive view of drug crimes as a public health as well as a criminal justice problem. Corrections agencies have long used incarceration and community supervision plans that include drug offender treatment and monitoring as part of a sentence for drug offenses. More recently, state and local court systems have begun to embrace drug courts as a model for the diversion of lower-level drug offenders. Policing, however, has been slow to embrace treatment and diversion of drug abuse patients, preferring to adhere to the "war on drugs" philosophy.

The epidemic of opioid overdoses forced law-enforcement to confront drug abuse as something other than a criminal justice problem. Police officers are often first on the scene of drug overdose events, arriving prior to fire or emergency medical units. Law-enforcement investigative units often generate investigative casework as part of the response to an overdose. A wrongful death or homicide investigation is often required in the case of a fatal overdose investigation, and many times this has lead to a resource-consuming and frustrating investigative search for the person who supplied the fatal drug dose. This investigative mandate became even more pronounced when it was discovered that many batches of heroin were mixed with other potent drugs, such as the synthetic opioid Fentanyl. Child abuse, neglect, and narcotic sales investigations were often generated from even nonfatal overdose instances, further taxing police department resources. Faced with a mounting burden on resources, police executives began searching for a novel way to counteract the issue of heroin overdose cases.

The key development that facilitated innovative police participation in overdose response was the introduction of naloxone hydrochloride in an inhalant form. Naloxone (marketed under the trade name Narcan, as well as other names) is an opioid antagonist drug that reverses the effect of an opioid overdose when administered in a timely manner. Naloxone had been previously available to healthcare

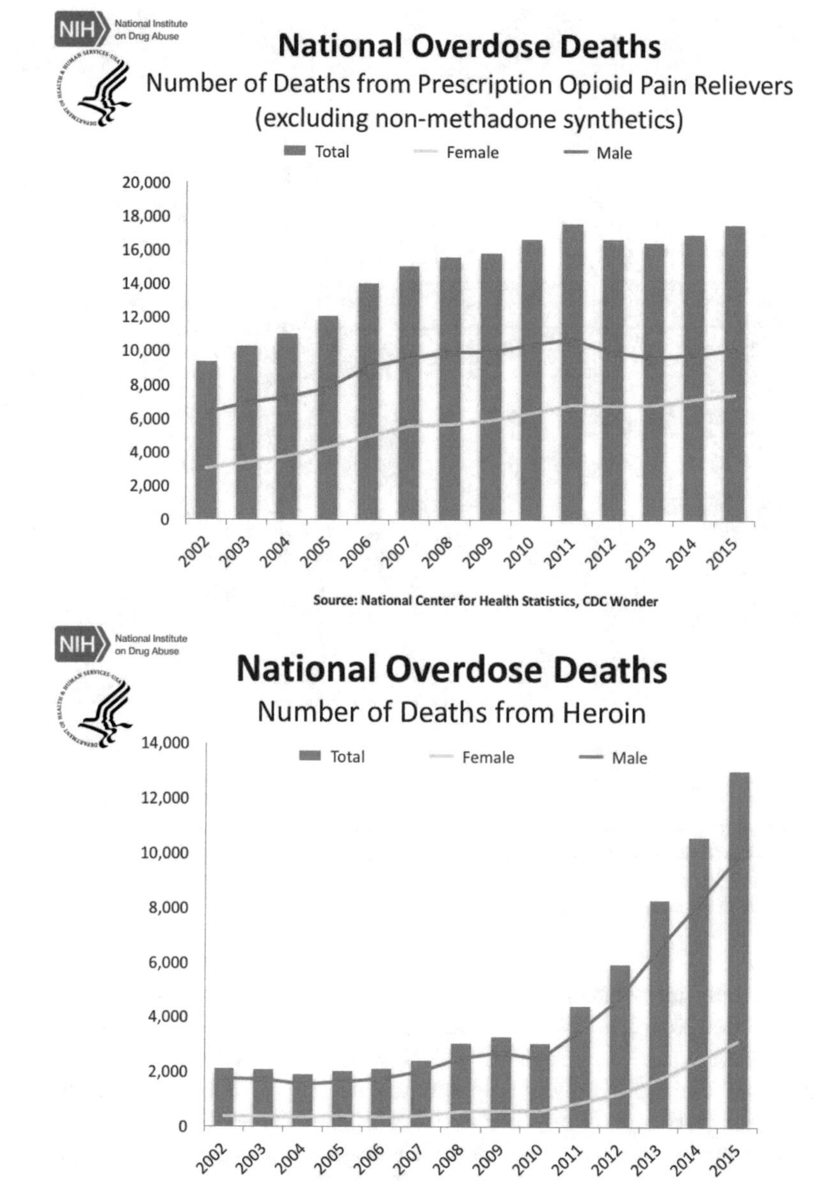

Fig. 14.1 Prescription opioid and heroin overdose death rates, 2001–2014 (National Institute of Health, National Institute on Drug Abuse 2015, used by permission granted under public domain)

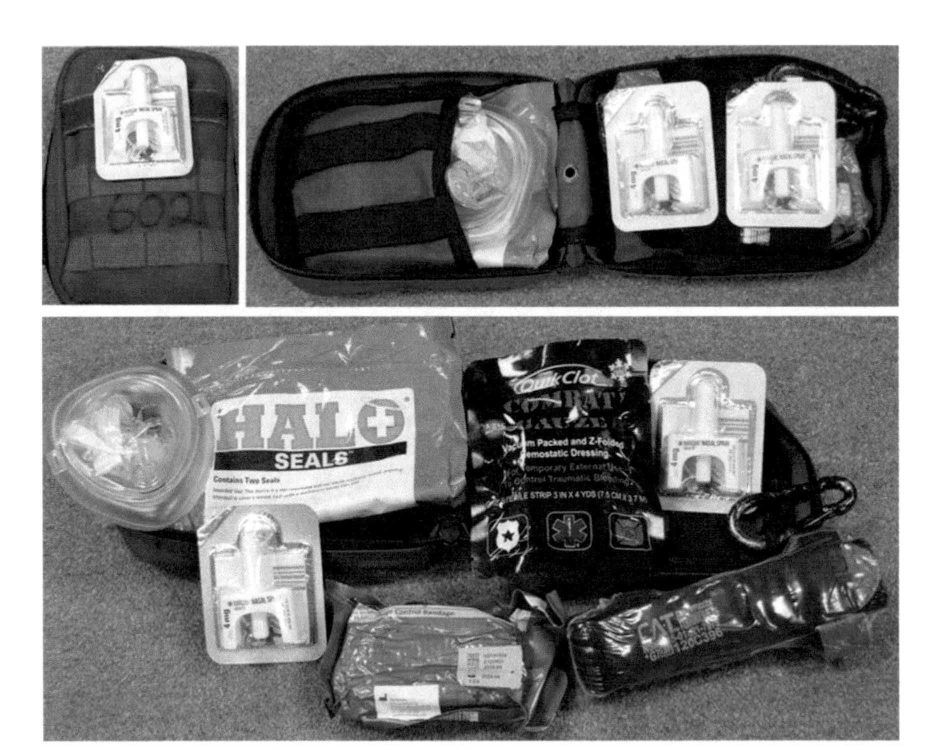

Fig. 14.2 A key development in the fight against opioid overdoses, naloxone hydrochloride inhalers (seen here under the trade name Narcan® nasal spray *top left* and *right*) allows first responders and members of the Crestwood Police Department in Illinois to administer life-saving drugs and other care items (*bottom* from *left clockwise*: CPR breathing mask, Israel bandage for deep wounds, quick clot bandage, first of two Narcan, and tourniquet) from emergency kits called jump bags there that are also carried in squadrons across the United States (photographs courtesy of Detective Sergeant Steven J. Gomboz, used by permission)

providers only in injectable form, which required an advanced level of medical training. Pilot programs involving take-home injectable naloxone among the drug user community had been found to reduce the fatal overdose rate by 30% (Piper et al. 2008). The availability of naloxone in a nasal spray allowed first responders with a basic level of training, such as police officers and EMT's to administer the drug upon arrival on-scene. Each dose of naloxone costs approximately $12, and can be carried in an officer's shirt pocket (Fig. 14.2).

Another key development was the application of good-Samaritan laws in jurisdictions that authorize naloxone administration by first responders (Wermeling 2013). Such laws absolve those administering lifesaving care of civil liability, if the person administering care does so within the limits of their training. Administering naloxone to a patient who is not experiencing an opioid overdose, but is having another type of medical emergency, has no negative effect on the patient.

14.3.2 Population Impact/Community Response

The Quincy, MA Police Department was one of the first police agencies to authorize the administration of naloxone to overdose victims. The department serves a Boston suburb municipality of approximately 92,000 residents. Quincy has two ambulance stations, while patrolling police officers are far more numerous, and are dispatched to every 911 medical call (Davis et al. 2014).

Beginning in 2010, every sworn member of the police department was trained on the administration of naloxone, and every agency police vehicle and the headquarters building was equipped with a dosage kit. Between 2010 and 2013, Quincy police administered naloxone to suspected overdose victims over 200 times. By 2014, the Massachusetts Department of Public Health had begun supplying naloxone inhalant kits to additional fire and police departments (Davis et al. 2014). Other agencies adopted naloxone inhalers to combat heroin overdoses and by the end of 2016 over 1200 US police agencies were carrying naloxone (Childs 2016).

14.3.3 Evidence to Support Life-Saving Application

The Police Executive Research Forum (PERF) is a policy think tank for emerging criminal justice problems. A 2017 PERF survey showed that between 2014 and 2016, PERF member agencies issuing naloxone rose from 4 to 61%. The same survey cited over 3500 naloxone interventions and "overdose reversals" by 164 respondent agencies (PERF 2017a, p.11). Other innovations being explored by PERF member agencies to combat heroin overdoses include:

- Improved information sharing about heroin overdose trends, both among police agencies as well as with other local government entities and public health organizations;
- Direct intervention, in concert with public health officials, with nonfatal heroin overdose patients, within 24 h of an overdose event;
- Support and facilitation of "drop in" centers where addicts can receive counseling, and a range of other addiction support services;
- Increased outreach to inmates in local jails and lockups regarding the prevalence of opioid addiction (PERF 2017a).

Contrastingly, federal officials have played a limited role in responding to the opioid crisis, primarily by the Centers for Disease Control in tracking the overdose epidemic, and through the various US Attorney's Offices, who are responsible for strategic prosecutions of heroin traffickers and large-scale drug sellers. Even here, federal prosecutorial and sentencing guidelines are "not calibrated to solve the heroin crisis" (PERF 2017a, p.73). Instead, federal guidelines require the possession of more than 100 g of heroin before a prosecution can be considered. The average street-level dose of heroin is well under 1 g.

The use of naloxone as part of a suite of drug abuse reduction tools represents a shift in the mindset from enforcers to problem solvers on the part of local police agencies, as well as a policy solution derived from local experience with a public health crisis. Naloxone promises to continue to be a powerful weapon in the fight against overdose deaths and represents a successful innovation on the part of police practitioners.

14.4 Local Police Involvement with National Immigration Policy

Like the opioid overdose issue, the emergent issue of legal and illegal migration, economic displacement, and refugees has forced local law-enforcement agencies to innovate. But unlike drug overdoses, here the policy issues are much more complex, and the track record is mixed. Two primary issues exist when considering local police response to immigration. The first issue is how local police interface with national policy regarding illegal immigration; and the second is how local policing agencies deal with immigrant communities, many of which contain a shadow population of residents highly fearful of police.

14.4.1 Organizational Policy Issues and Immigration Enforcement Policy

Issues arising from local police involvement in immigration enforcement policy emanate from lack of jurisdiction. Control of immigration into the U.S. is a federal responsibility, enabled primarily by the Immigration and Naturalization Act of 1952, as amended. There are several mirroring statutes in the Code of Federal Regulations that make the screening of people entering the United States as well as the handling and deporting of illegally arrived migrants a responsibility of the federal government. Other federal laws deal with the process of obtaining or renouncing of American citizenship, the visa process for foreign nationals, and various diplomatic protocols when interfacing with non-US citizens on American soil. The primary federal player in immigration is the Department of Homeland Security, an umbrella agency containing Customs and Border Protection, the U.S. Border Patrol, and Citizenship and Immigration Services.

Historically, state and local police agencies had very little interaction with immigration authorities except in isolated circumstances, such as discovery that a party to police activity was in the U.S. contrary to federal law. For an example, if a criminal suspect was arrested and the defendant was discovered to be illegally in the U.S., immigration authorities might place a "detainer" on the defendant with the local jail, an administrative order requesting the local jail not to release the individual back into the community until there was a disposition on the individual's immigration status. However, it was just as likely that the local police would never discover that the suspect was out of status and the defendant would be released on bond back into the community.

The events of September 11, 2001 brought about many changes in federal immigration policy, placing a new emphasis on securing the borders and improving accountability for non-US citizens visiting and residing in the U.S. Due to increased immigration enforcement and information sharing with state and local police, immigrants who were out of status were much more likely to be discovered after being arrested on local charges.

Over time, increased detention of illegal immigrants by local police led to a political response from local governments. Local governments began forbidding their police agencies and jails from disclosing to federal authorities the immigration status of arrestees, as well as proscribing street officers from asking probative questions regarding immigration status in street encounters. Finally, some local governments refused to honor federal immigration detainers, labeling themselves "sanctuary cities." Federal agencies have responded to the sanctuary city phenomenon by threatening to withhold grant money from those local entities that refuse to cooperate with federal immigration authorities.

A second consequence of immigration is the establishment of large legal immigrant populations in local communities who fear police contact. These communities often consist of a great number of out-of-status immigrants, who are subject to detention and deportment if discovered by immigration authorities. The illegal immigrant community often exists as a shadow community, involved in an unofficial economy and fearful of any cooperation with government authorities. This shadow community is frequently targeted by the criminal element. Immigrants are frequently paid in cash, and are unwilling to put their earnings in banks or other institutions, and criminals know these ripe targets are unlikely to contact the police should they be a victim of crime.

14.4.2 Impact of Police Involvement in Immigration Issues; a Mixed Blessing

The involvement of local police in immigration, which has been traditionally seen as a federal issue, has had mixed results, and has become mired in both politics and legal entanglements.

A post-9/11 development of local police involvement in immigration laws was the inclusion of local police in the enforcement of immigration law violations.

Violations occur in two primary forms. The first form occurs when an individual enters the U.S. through an unlawful border crossing—either by walking across the border or being smuggled via various modes of transport. This type of violation is in and of itself a violation of the Immigration and Naturalization Act. The second type of violation involves what is widely referred to as a "visa overstay." This scenario involves a non-U.S. person who enters the United States in a legal manner such as a visa approved by the federal government. Visas are generally good for a fixed period, or for a duration of employment, after which time the individual must leave the country or begin proceedings to obtain citizenship or lawful permanent resident status (a so-called green card).

There is no enabling law that explicitly allows for state and local police to detain persons who are "out of status" with regard to federal immigration law. However, some legal scholars argue that no explicit authorization is needed for local police to enforce federal immigration law (Kobach 2005). Several local police agencies, especially in border areas, availed themselves to the concept of using their resources to enforce immigration law with results that were both legally mixed and harmful to their standings in the immigrant community regardless of their legal or illegal status. These agencies were aided by a federal government program that explicitly empowered designated local police officers with immigration enforcement authority, via a Memorandum of Understanding (MOU) (Kobach 2005, p.196).

While some state and local agencies embraced a new role as immigration enforcers, others explicitly rejected the notion of local police in this role (Harris 2006). Police officials opposed to acting as immigration agents argued enforcement of immigration law was not a local police responsibility, and moreover, cut into hard-won gains of trust in minority and immigrant communities. Immigration enforcement, they argued, was in opposition to the tenets of community-oriented policing, which sought to improve communications with members of neighborhoods and social groups. Harris argues, "officers and departments using community policing know that they can only make their communities safe—from criminals, from terrorists, or from any other threat- by working with communities, and decidedly not by instilling the type of fear that working as adjunct immigration agents will create" (2006, p.7).

Additionally, many local police agencies, especially county sheriffs who run the bulk of local jails and lockups in the U.S., began to refuse cooperation with immigration officials by not honoring immigration detainers (Fig. 14.3). This gave rise to the "sanctuary city" movement, where local governments forbade police department involvement with immigration enforcement on any level.

Outreach efforts to immigrant communities has been an example of a police success story. Unlike the contentious issue of local police immigration enforcement, a more positive aspect of police-immigrant relations is the development of outreach efforts to local immigrant communities. As mentioned, immigrant groups often have a difficult relationship with police agencies. Portions of immigrant populations may be in violation of immigration laws, and therefore fearful of the police, and even populations which follow immigration regulations may harbor historical grievances and fears, due to corrupt police practices in their home country. As a result, immigrant communities often suffer a higher crime rate than nonimmigrant populations while under-reporting criminal activity in their neighborhoods to the police.

Local police, recognizing the need for improved relationships with immigrant populations, adapted the tenets of community policing to face the challenges of

DEPARTMENT OF HOMELAND SECURITY
IMMIGRATION DETAINER - NOTICE OF ACTION

Subject ID:
Event #:

File No:
Date:

TO: (Name and Title of Institution - OR Any Subsequent Law Enforcement Agency)

FROM: (Department of Homeland Security Office Address)

MAINTAIN CUSTODY OF ALIEN FOR A PERIOD NOT TO EXCEED 48 HOURS

Name of Alien: ____
Date of Birth: ____ Nationality: ____ Sex: ____

THE U.S. DEPARTMENT OF HOMELAND SECURITY (DHS) HAS TAKEN THE FOLLOWING ACTION RELATED TO THE PERSON IDENTIFIED ABOVE, CURRENTLY IN YOUR CUSTODY:

☐ Determined that there is reason to believe the individual is an alien subject to removal from the United States. The individual (*check all that apply*):

☐ has a prior a felony conviction or has been charged with a felony offense;
☐ has three or more prior misdemeanor convictions;
☐ has a prior misdemeanor conviction or has been charged with a misdemeanor for an offense that involves violence, threats, or assaults; sexual abuse or exploitation; driving under the influence of alcohol or a controlled substance; unlawful flight from the scene of an accident; the unlawful possession or use of a firearm or other deadly weapon, the distribution or trafficking of a controlled substance; or other significant threat to public safety;
☐ has been convicted of illegal entry pursuant to 8 U.S.C. § 1325;
☐ has illegally re-entered the country after a previous removal or return;
☐ has been found by an immigration officer or an immigration judge to have knowingly committed immigration fraud;
☐ otherwise poses a significant risk to national security, border security, or public safety; and/or
☐ other (specify): ____.

☐ Initiated removal proceedings and served a Notice to Appear or other charging document. A copy of the charging document is attached and was served on ____ (date).

☐ Served a warrant of arrest for removal proceedings. A copy of the warrant is attached and was served on ____ (date).

☐ Obtained an order of deportation or removal from the United States for this person.

This action does not limit your discretion to make decisions related to this person's custody classification, work, quarter assignments, or other matters. DHS discourages dismissing criminal charges based on the existence of a detainer.

IT IS REQUESTED THAT YOU:

☐ Maintain custody of the subject for a period **NOT TO EXCEED 48 HOURS**, excluding Saturdays, Sundays, and holidays, beyond the time when the subject would have otherwise been released from your custody to allow DHS to take custody of the subject. This request derives from federal regulation 8 C.F.R. § 287.7. For purposes of this immigration detainer, **you are not authorized to hold the subject beyond these 48 hours.** As early as possible prior to the time you otherwise would release the subject, please notify DHS by calling____ during business hours or____ after hours or in an emergency. If you cannot reach a DHS Official at these numbers, please contact the ICE Law Enforcement Support Center in Burlington, Vermont at: (802) 872-6020.

☐ Provide a copy to the subject of this detainer.

☐ Notify this office of the time of release at least 30 days prior to release or as far in advance as possible.

☐ Notify this office in the event of the inmate's death, hospitalization or transfer to another institution.

☐ Consider this request for a detainer operative only upon the subject's conviction.

☐ Cancel the detainer previously placed by this Office on ____ (date).

(Name and title of Immigration Officer) (Signature of Immigration Officer)

TO BE COMPLETED BY THE LAW ENFORCEMENT AGENCY CURRENTLY HOLDING THE SUBJECT OF THIS NOTICE:
Please provide the information below, sign, and return to DHS using the envelope enclosed for your convenience or by faxing a copy to ____. You should maintain a copy for your own records so you may track the case and not hold the subject beyond the 48-hour period.

Local Booking/Inmate #: ____ Latest criminal charge/conviction: ____ (date) Estimated release: ____ (date)

Last criminal charge/conviction: ____

Notice: Once in our custody, the subject of this detainer may be removed from the United States. If the individual may be the victim of a crime, or if you want this individual to remain in the United States for prosecution or other law enforcement purposes, including acting as a witness, please notify the ICE Law Enforcement Support Center at (802) 872-6020.

(Name and title of Officer) (Signature of Officer)

DHS Form I-247 (12/12) Page 1 of

Fig. 14.3 Department of Homeland Security DHS Form I-247 (12/12) is a detainer used by the federal agency to request temporary detention of a defendant in a local jail or lockup as local law enforcement agencies struggle to arrive at a consensus on how best to respond to DHS detainer requests (U.S. Customs and Immigration Enforcement (2012), used by permission of public domain)

policing in immigrant dense neighborhoods. Innovative police agencies used problem-solving tools developed by community-policing advocates to identify key issues with policing in immigrant communities:

- Language barriers;
- Reluctance of immigrants to engage with police due to historically abusive and corrupt officials in their home countries;
- Inability of immigrants to differentiate between local police and federal immigration officers;
- Differing cultural norms between officers and immigrants;
- Negative experiences with individual officers.

Police officials overcame these issues through many innovative outreach programs. In some instances, this meant deploying dedicated teams of bilingual officers into immigrant communities, with a mandate to cultivate trust, and to become seen as more than enforcers. Other agencies, such as the Palm Beach, FL Sheriff's Office, found that a full-time civilian liaison employee was key to improving relations with the community. They also found that sending a team of relief officers and supplies to Haiti in the aftermath of the 2010 earthquake paid dividends in terms of community mutual respect and trust. Although the forms of outreach vary widely, local agencies have found that investing in relationships with immigrant populations both improves the relationship and increases the effectiveness of crime-fighting efforts (Saint-Fort et al. 2012).

Another development in police outreach toward immigrant communities is the strategic use of the U-Visa which was authorized by Congress in 2002. U-Visas are a discretionary type of immigration law relief, allowing the victim of a serious crime to remain in the U.S. for up to 4 years, without fear of detention or deportation. State and local police agencies play an integral role in the use of the U-Visa, certifying the applicant has been the victim of a qualifying offense, such as domestic or sexual abuse, or the victim of human trafficking. The San Francisco Police Department pioneered the use of the U-Visa in 2003, and as of January 2017 was typically certifying more than 600 U-Visa applications per year, cultivating trust and goodwill among immigrant communities. Other cities such as Tucson, Arizona, Minneapolis, MN, and Dayton, Ohio have adopted U-Visa outreach programs (PERF 2017b).

Much like the grassroots development of naloxone use by police to thwart opioid overdose deaths, the successful use of outreach by law-enforcement organizations to immigrant communities represents a diffusion of innovation across the police community. A few innovator agencies saw the need to apply a proven policing tool (community policing) to a novel problem (policing the immigrant community). Other agencies observed the success of innovator departments and applied the successes and lessons learned from failures to their own efforts.

The success of local police as immigration enforcement officers is less clear. The use of local officers to detain illegal immigrants has yet to prove reliably successful at lowering the crime rate or protecting against terrorist attack. In places where the concept of local police immigration officers has been fully implemented there have been both legal challenges and public relations problems for the participant agencies. An example of this is Maricopa County, Arizona, where the Sheriff's Office was an early advocate for a proactive approach to immigration enforcement by local authorities. Indeed, the passage of Senate Bill 1070 in Arizona in 2010 signaled the preference for a muscular local approach to immigration enforcement. SB1070 was promptly mired in civil litigation, while Maricopa County was ultimately enjoined by a federal court order from enforcing immigration law.

Immigrant populations in the United States, both legal and illegal, suffer from many disadvantages compared to native-born Americans. Lower educational attainment, higher poverty rates, and lower rates of healthcare coverage are some of the unfortunate benchmarks of immigrant communities (Walters 2012). Predation by criminals and an indifferent, sometimes harmful policing environment can only add to the troubles of the immigrant population. However, innovative outreach by local police officials can play a positive role in immigrant assimilation into the U.S.

14.5 Police Responses to the Issue of Human Trafficking

Another contemporary issue facing local police agencies is the crime of human trafficking. Human trafficking is broadly defined as coercion or exploitation of a person for the purpose of labor or sexual industry. Human trafficking need not involve movement of persons across international or trans-state boundaries to qualify, nor does the victim's status as a minor or illegal migrant determine if a person is the victim of trafficking. Here the police response is promising but still developing.

The crime of human trafficking can be subdivided into two categories. Labor exploitation occurs when a victim is enslaved, forced to work, or indentured by the perpetrator to obtain work from the victim. Sexual exploitation involves compelling the victim to engage in sex work: sexual activity, pornography, working in strip clubs or massage parlors, etc. (Logan et al. 2009). The Department of Justice reported between 2008 and 2010 its task forces (primarily made up of local police officers) investigated over 2500 incidents of suspected human trafficking in the United States (Banks et al. 2011, p.1).

14.5.1 Organizational Policy Issues and History of Human Trafficking

More than 8 in 10 cases of human trafficking in the United States involve sex trafficking or the sexual exploitation of trafficking victim (Banks et al. 2011, p.1). Typically, a sex trafficking victim is lured into a coercive relationship with the perpetrator, or in the case of an immigrant victim, perhaps sold into the situation by a smuggler or handler. Human traffickers then systematically deprive the victim of

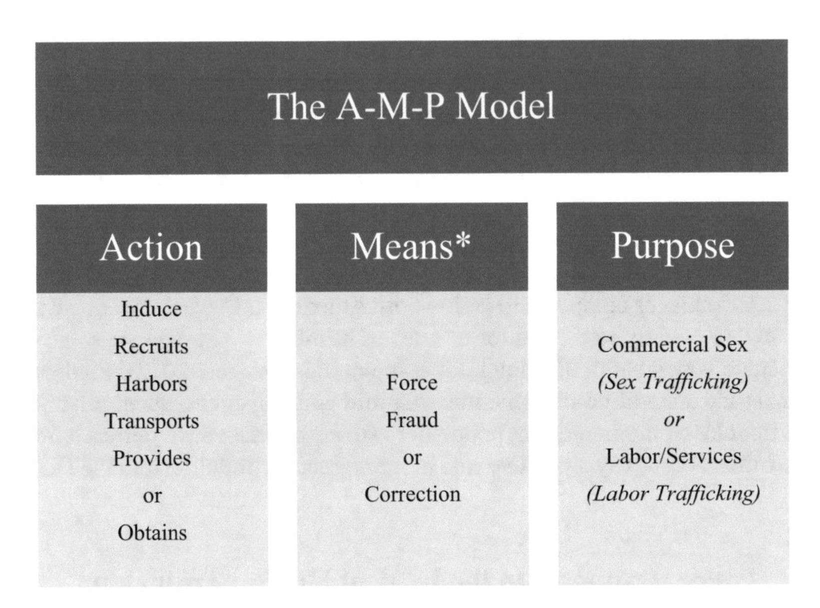

Fig. 14.4 Training resources like the A-M-P model help local Police identify the traits of a human trafficking operation (National Human Trafficking Resource Center 2012, used by permission)

access to money, means of communication such as a cellphone, and even their identification documents. Isolated from family and friends, intimidated and perhaps abused, the victims soon find themselves engaging in illegal sexual activity and unable to escape.

Until recently, human trafficking as a U.S. domestic problem was largely ignored. The federal government passed the Victims of Trafficking and Violence Protection Act in 2000, and between 2000 and 2015 expanded legislation designed to both combat human trafficking and provide support to victims. During the same time span, over 20 states passed legislation to combat human trafficking, primarily the type caused by sexual exploitation.

14.5.2 Police Response to Human Trafficking as a Crime Issue

Historically, state and local law-enforcement has viewed the sex industry and component parts (e.g., prostitution, massage parlors, pornography, and adult-entertainment businesses) as criminal activity to be policed by vice crimes investigators. Local law-enforcement agencies often treated the sex worker as a criminal suspect under this paradigm regardless of whether they were also the victim of human trafficking.

With a rise in awareness of human trafficking as a crime that impacted cities and towns in the United States, many local agencies have begun to see sex workers as more than vice criminals. Front line officer awareness and training (Fig. 14.4) by victim advocacy groups and nongovernmental organizations, such as the Polaris Project, has facilitated a paradigm shift in responding to complaints of vice crime, and has helped police identify previously undetected criminal activity occurring in their jurisdiction. With some important caveats, changes in how police agencies investigated vice crimes have facilitated human trafficking investigations at the local level.

14.5.3 Trafficking Response: A Work in Progress

Despite the increased awareness of human trafficking as a criminal issue, Farrell and Pfeffer (2014) argue there is much room for improvement. In a study of local police response to potential human trafficking cases, the authors found that local police agencies were limited in their response to human trafficking incidents, concentrating primarily on child exploitation cases. Sex trafficking cases involving adult victims, and especially same-sex victims, were investigated at a much lower rate. Human trafficking cases involving coercive labor exploitation practices were essentially invisible to investigators. The study found the following determinants as primarily responsible for the variation in effectiveness of local police agency response to human trafficking:

- A lack of consistent understanding of what human trafficking is among police officials;
- Lack of resources, primarily budget and staffing;
- Variation in community opinions in how important human trafficking was as a local issue;
- A lack of awareness on the part of initial responders as to the signs of a human trafficking operation.

Farrell and Pfeffer (2014) recommend cultivation of relationships between police and community groups who serve at-risk populations, such as legal aid and prostitution survivor help groups. While these groups often have a poor relationship with police agencies, they can assist officers both in identifying potential investigative targets and providing aid and comfort to trafficking victims.

Innovative police practices involving vice crime and enforcement have allowed local law-enforcement to address a previously transparent type of crime that went unaddressed in their communities. While there is work yet to be done, the willingness of police to view an old crime through a new lens is encouraging.

14.6 Recommendations and Conclusion

Opioid overdoses, immigrant populations, and human trafficking are issues that have not traditionally fallen within the purview of local-law enforcement agencies. Local police officers have historically engaged in order maintenance, response to emergencies, and the systematic investigation of traditional criminal activity occurring in their jurisdictions. Nontraditional, persistent social issues have compelled police agencies to engage in innovative responses to these issues, and to learn from each other's successes and failures.

While police agencies have shown their ability to innovate and collaborate, there is wide variation in how well police agencies both adapt to emerging issues, and learn from each other. The spread of innovative police responses aligns well with Rogers' Diffusion of Innovation Theory (1962), which attempts to explain how novel ideas or practices spread through a community. While a thorough treatment of Diffusion of Innovations Theory is beyond the scope of this work, it is important to recognize that police agencies are generally averse to innovation, due to their fear of criticism, sanction, and liability for their actions. Nonetheless some agencies have taken the risk to innovate and the following recommendations would encourage greater innovation among police agencies.

Steal. Local police agencies swim in an ocean filled with other fish—other police agencies, prosecutor's offices, advocacy groups, and NGO's. Many of these groups have implemented their own innovative practices and these innovations could be adapted to other intractable problems the police face. In this case plagiarism is the sincerest form of flattery.

Communicate. Due to the innate fragmentation of policing in the U.S., turf protection, and simple ego, police agencies are often reluctant to share success stories and ideas with one another. Achievements are often not shared with other agencies until after the developing agency basks in the glow of government awards, grant funding, and positive media attention. While police agencies crave approbation and guard their turf, public policy problems know no jurisdictional boundaries. Successful innovation and solving of persistent policy problems requires both good ideas and information sharing. Academia, groups such as PERF, and organizations like the International Associations of Chiefs of Police (IACP) are excellent conduits with which to share ideas.

Listen. Just as innovation often comes from the bottom up among police organizations, innovations often start as an idea that percolates up from the line level *within* a police organization. The solutions mentioned here often started in a department as a result one employee having a good idea. Police organizations would do well to foster an internal culture where thoughtfulness, innovative thinking, and speaking up are rewarded, and not stifled. Given the traditional, paramilitary culture within many police agencies, this is often a difficult task for the police manager.

Innovative thinking will continue to be one of the most powerful weapons in the American policing arsenal. New public policy problems will continue to arise, just as those of terrorism, civil rights, drug abuse, and school shootings did in the past.

A culture of innovation and information sharing will enable local agencies to set the bar and respond to the intractable policy problems of society.

Glossary

A-M-P Model Consists of a framework of actions, means, and purpose for police to identify sex trafficking.

Community policing A philosophy that promotes organizational strategies that support the systematic use of partnerships and problem-solving techniques to proactively address the immediate conditions that give rise to public safety issues such as crime, social disorder, and fear of crime.

Detainer Judicial tool of U.S. immigration authorities; an administrative order compelling the local jail not to release the individual back into the community until there was a disposition on the individual's immigration status.

Human trafficking The illegal movement of people, typically for the purposes of forced labor or commercial sexual exploitation.

Memorandum of understanding (MOU) An agreement between parties to act or respond to a situation or circumstance in a prescribed and uniform manner.

Nongovernmental organizations (NGOs) Nongovernmental organization.

Opioid Highly addictive pain relief medication.

Sex trafficking Sexual exploitation of trafficking victim.

Sovereignty The power of a government or entity to self-regulate.

Visa A **U.S. Visa** is a document, or official endorsement, obtained from a U.S. consul (abroad), that allows its holder to apply for entry to the United States; two primary types are Immigrant Visas and Nonimmigrant Visas.

References

Banks D, Kyckelhahn T, Bureau of Justice Statistics. Characteristics of suspected human trafficking incidents, 2008-2010. https://www.bjs.gov/index.cfm?ty=pbdetail&iid=2372 (2011).

Childs R. US law enforcement who carry naloxone. 2016. http://www.nchrc.org/law-enforcement/us-law-enforcement-who-carry-naloxone/. Accessed 8 Oct 2017.

Crank JP, Langworthy R. An institutional perspective of policing. J Crim Law Criminol. 1992;83(2):338–63.

Davis CS, et al. Expanded access to naloxone among firefighters, police officers, and emergency medical technicians in Massachusetts. Am J Public Health. 2014;104(8):e7–9. https://doi.org/10.2105/AJPH.2014.302062.

Davis CS, et al. Overdose epidemic, prescription monitoring programs, and public health: a review of state laws. Am J Public Health. 2015;105(11):e9–e11.

Farrell A, Pfeffer R. Policing human trafficking: cultural blinders and organizational barriers. Ann Am Acad Pol Soc Sci. 2014;653(1):46–64.

Harris DA. The war on terror, local police, and immigration enforcement: a curious tale of police power in post-9/11 America. Rutgers Law J, 38(1). University of Pittsburgh Legal Studies Research Paper No. 2007-04. https://ssrn.com/abstract=1008927 (2006).

Kobach KW. The quintessential force multiplier: the inherent authority of local police to make immigration arrests. Albany Law Rev. 2005;69:179–235.

Kolodny A, et al. The prescription opioid and heroin crisis: a public health approach to an epidemic of addiction. Annu Rev Publ Health. 2015;36(1):559–74. https://doi.org/10.1146/annurev-publhealth-031914-122957.

Logan TK, et al. Understanding human trafficking in the United States. Trauma Violence Abuse. 2009;10(1):3–30.

National Human Trafficking Resource Center (NHTRXC). The actions means purpose (AMP) model. 2012. https://humantraffickinghotline.org/resources/actions-means-purpose-amp-model. Accessed 3 Oct 2017.

National Institute of Health, National Institute on Drug Abuse. Overdose death rates. [Data sources: National Center for Health Statistic and the Centers for Disease Control and Prevention, CDC Wonder]. 2015. https://www.drugabuse.gov/related-topics/trends-statistics/overdose-death-rates. Accessed 3 Oct 2017.

Paulozzi LJ. 2010. The epidemiology of drug overdoses in the United States. Presented at Promis. Leg. Responses to the Epidemic of Prescr. Drug Overdoses in the U.S., Maimonides Med. Cent. Dep. Psychiatry, Dec. 2, Grand Rounds, Brooklyn.

Piper TM, et al. Evaluation of a naloxone distribution and administration program in New York City. Subst Use Misuse. 2008;43(7):858–70.

Police Executive Research Forum (PERF). The unprecedented opioid epidemic: as overdoses become a leading cause of death, police, sheriffs and health agencies must step up their response. 2017a. http://www.policeforum.org/assets/opioids2017.pdf. Accessed 2 Oct 2017.

Police Executive Research Forum (PERF). U visas and the role of local police in preventing and investigating crimes against immigrants. 2017b. http://www.policeforum.org/assets/docs/Subject_to_Debate/Debate2017/debate_2017_junaug.pdf31(2):1-20. Accessed 2 Oct 2017.

Reaves BA. Census of state and local law enforcement agencies, 2008. [Data source: United States Department of Justice, Bureau of Justice Statistics]. 2011. https://www.bjs.gov/content/pub/pdf/csllea08.pdf. Accessed 2 Oct 2017.

Saint-Fort P et al. Engaging police in immigrant communities. 2012. https://www.vera.org/publications/engaging-police-in-immigrant-communities-promising-practices-from-the-field. Accessed 2 Oct 2017.

United States Customs and Immigration Enforcement. Department of Homeland Security DHS Form I-247. 2012. https://www.ice.gov/doclib/secure-communities/pdf/immigration-detainer-form.pdf. Accessed 17 Oct 2017.

Walters NP. The foreign-born population in the United States: 2010. [Data source: United States Census Bureau (ACS-19)]. 2012. https://www.census.gov/prod/2012pubs/acs-19.pdf. Accessed 2 Oct 2017.

Wermeling D. Survey of naloxone legal status in opioid overdose prevention and treatment. J Opioid Manag. 2013;9(5):369–77.

Further Reading

Gibbs JT. Race and justice: Rodney King and OJ Simpson in a house divided. San Francisco: Jossey-Bass; 1996.

Green TC, et al. Law enforcement attitudes toward overdose prevention and response. Drug Alcohol Depend. 2013;133(2):677–84. https://doi.org/10.1016/j.drugalcdep.2013.08.018.

Nadelmann E, LaSalle L. Two steps forward, one step back: current harm reduction policy and politics in the united states. Harm Reduct J. 2017;14:37. https://doi.org/10.1186/s12954-017-0157-y.

PR Newswire. Narcan nasal spray approved by FDA for opioid withdrawal. 2017. https://www.pharmpro.com/news/2017/01/narcan-nasal-spray-approved-fda-opioid-withdrawal. Accessed 3 Oct 2017.

Rogers EM. Diffusion of innovations. New York: Simon & Schuster; 2010.

Trojanowicz R, Bucqueroux B. Community policing. Cincinnati, OH: A contemporary perspective. Anderson Publishing Co.; 1990.

Index

B. A. Fiedler (ed.), *Translating National Policy to Improve Environmental Conditions Impacting Public Health Through Community Planning*,
https://doi.org/10.1007/978-3-319-75361-4

D

Printed in the United States
By Bookmasters